1999
YEAR BOOK OF
HAND SURGERY®

Statement of Purpose

The YEAR BOOK Service

The YEAR BOOK series was devised in 1901 by practicing health professionals who observed that the literature of medicine and related disciplines had become so voluminous that no one individual could read and place in perspective every potential advance in a major specialty. In the final decade of the 20th century, this recognition is more acutely true than it was in 1901.

More than merely a series of books, YEAR BOOK volumes are the tangible results of a unique service designed to accomplish the following:

- to *survey* a wide range of journals of proven value
- to *select* from those journals papers representing significant advances and statements of important clinical principles
- to provide *abstracts* of those articles that are readable, convenient summaries of their key points
- to provide *commentary* about those articles to place them in perspective.

These publications grow out of a unique process that calls on the talents of outstanding authorities in clinical and fundamental disciplines, trained literature specialists, and professional writers, all supported by the resources of Mosby, the world's preeminent publisher for the health professions.

The Literature Base

Mosby and its editors survey approximately 500 journals published worldwide, covering the full range of the health professions. On an annual basis, the publisher examines usage patterns and polls its expert authorities to add new journals to the literature base and to delete journals that are no longer useful as potential YEAR BOOK sources.

The Literature Survey

The publisher's team of literature specialists, all of whom are trained and experienced health professionals, examines every original, peer-reviewed article in each journal issue. More than 250,000 articles per year are scanned systematically, including title, text, illustrations, tables, and references. Each scan is compared, article by article, to the search strategies that the publisher has developed in consultation with the 270 outside experts who form the pool of YEAR BOOK editors. A given article may be reviewed by any number of editors, from one to a dozen or more, regardless of the discipline for which the paper was originally published. In turn, each editor who receives the article reviews it to determine whether or not the article should be included in the YEAR BOOK. This decision is based on the article's inherent quality, its probable usefulness to readers of that YEAR BOOK, and the editor's goal to represent a balanced picture of a given field in each volume of the YEAR BOOK. In addition, the editor indicates

The 1999 Year Book Series

Year Book of Allergy, Asthma, and Clinical Immunology: Drs. Rosenwasser, Boguniewicz, Borish, Routes, Spahn, and Weber

Year Book of Anesthesiology and Pain Management®: Drs. Tinker, Abram, Chestnut, Roizen, Rothenberg, and Wood

Year Book of Cardiology®: Drs. Schlant, Collins, Gersh, Graham, Kaplan, and Waldo

Year Book of Chiropractic®: Dr. Lawrence

Year Book of Critical Care Medicine®: Drs. Parrillo, Balk, Calvin, Franklin, and Shapiro

Year Book of Dentistry®: Drs. Meskin, Berry, Jeffcoat, Leinfelder, Roser, Summitt, and Zakariasen

Year Book of Dermatology and Dermatologic Surgery™: Drs. Thiers and Lang

Year Book of Diagnostic Radiology®: Drs. Osborn, Dalinka, Groskin, Maynard, Pentecost, Ros, Smirniotopoulos, and Young

Year Book of Emergency Medicine®: Drs. Wagner, Dronen, Davidson, King, Niemann, and Hamilton

Year Book of Endocrinology®: Drs. Bagdade, Braverman, Horton, Kannan, Landsberg, Molitch, Morley, Odell, Poehlman, Rogol, and Fitzpatrick

Year Book of Family Practice®: Drs. Berg, Bowman, Davidson, Dexter, and Scherger

Year Book of Gastroenterology: Drs. Aliperti and Fleshman

Year Book of Hand Surgery®: Drs. Amadio and Hentz

Year Book of Medicine®: Drs. Klahr, Frishman, Malawista, Mandell, Jett, Young, Barkin, and Bagdade

Year Book of Neonatal and Perinatal Medicine®: Drs. Fanaroff, Maisels, and Stevenson

Year Book of Nephrology, Hypertension, and Mineral Metabolism: Drs. Schwab, Bennett, Emmett, Hostetter, and Moe

Year Book of Neurology and Neurosurgery®: Drs. Bradley and Gibbs

Year Book of Nuclear Medicine®: Drs. Gottschalk, Blaufox, Coleman, Strauss, and Zubal

Year Book of Obstetrics, Gynecology, and Women's Health: Drs. Mishell, Herbst, and Kirschbaum

Year Book of Oncology®: Drs. Ozols, Eisenberg, Glatstein, Loehrer, and Urba

Year Book of Ophthalmology®: Drs. Wilson, Augsburger, Cohen, Eagle, Grossman, Laibson, Maguire, Nelson, Penne, Rapuano, Sergott, Spaeth, Tipperman, Ms. Gosfield, and Ms. Salmon

Year Book of Orthopedics®: Drs. Morrey, Beauchamp, Currier, Tolo, Trigg, and Swiontkowski

when to include figures and tables from the article to help the YEAR BOOK reader better understand the information.

Of the quarter million articles scanned each year, only 5% are selected for detailed analysis within the YEAR BOOK series, thereby assuring readers of the high value of every selection.

The Abstract

The publisher's abstracting staff is headed by a seasoned medical professional and includes individuals with training in the life sciences, medicine, and other areas, plus extensive experience in writing for the health professions and related industries. Each selected article is assigned to a specific writer on this abstracting staff. The abstracter, guided in many cases by notations supplied by the expert editor, writes a structured, condensed summary designed so that the reader can rapidly acquire the essential information contained in the article.

The Commentary

The YEAR BOOK editorial boards, sometimes assisted by guest commentators, write comments that place each article in perspective for the reader. This provides the reader with the equivalent of a personal consultation with a leading international authority—an opportunity to better understand the value of the article and to benefit from the authority's thought processes in assessing the article.

Additional Editorial Features

The editorial boards of each YEAR BOOK organize the abstracts and comments to provide a logical and satisfying sequence of information. To enhance the organization, editors also provide introductions to sections or individual chapters, comments linking a number of abstracts, citations to additional literature, and other features.

The published YEAR BOOK contains enhanced bibliographic citations for each selected article, including extended listings of multiple authors and identification of author affiliations. Each YEAR BOOK contains a Table of Contents specific to that year's volume. From year to year, the Table of Contents for a given YEAR BOOK will vary depending on developments within the field.

Every YEAR BOOK contains a list of the journals from which papers have been selected. This list represents a subset of approximately 500 journals surveyed by the publisher and occasionally reflects a particularly pertinent article from a journal that is not surveyed on a routine basis.

Finally, each volume contains a comprehensive subject index and an index to authors of each selected paper.

Year Book of Otolaryngology–Head and Neck Surgery®: Drs. Paparella, Holt, and Otto

Year Book of Pathology and Laboratory Medicine®: Drs. Raab, Cohen, Dabbs, Olson, and Stanley

Year Book of Pediatrics®: Dr. Stockman

Year Book of Plastic, Reconstructive, and Aesthetic Surgery®: Drs. Miller, Bartlett, Garner, McKinney, Ruberg, Salisbury, and Smith

Year Book of Psychiatry and Applied Mental Health®: Drs. Talbott, Ballenger, Frances, Lydiard, Meltzer, Jensen, and Tasman

Year Book of Pulmonary Disease®: Drs. Jett, Castro, Maurer, Peters, Phillips, and Ryu

Year Book of Rheumatology, Arthritis, and Musculoskeletal Disease™: Drs. Panush, Hadler, Hellman, LeRoy, Pisetsky, and Simon

Year Book of Sports Medicine®: Drs. Shephard, Drinkwater, Eichner, Torg, Alexander, and Mr. George

Year Book of Surgery®: Drs. Copeland, Bland, Deitch, Eberlein, Howard, Luce, Seeger, Souba, and Sugarbaker

Year Book of Urology®: Drs. Andriole and Coplen

Year Book of Vascular Surgery®: Dr. Porter

The Year Book of HAND SURGERY®

1999

Editors
Peter C. Amadio, M.D.
Vincent R. Hentz, M.D.

Editors Emeritus
Robert A. Chase, M.D.
James H. Dobyns, M.D.

International Assistant Editors
Guy Foucher, M.D.
Priv.-Doz. Dr. Med. Christian L. Jantea
Caroline LeClercq, M.D.
Alberto Lluch, M.D., Ph.D.
Yasuo Ueba, M.D., D.M.Sc.

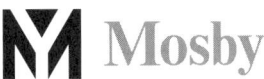

St. Louis Baltimore Boston Carlsbad Naples New York Philadelphia Portland London
Madrid Mexico City Singapore Sydney Tokyo Toronto Wiesbaden

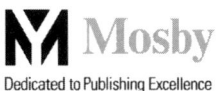
Dedicated to Publishing Excellence

Associate Publisher: Cynthia Baudendistel
Developmental Editor: Jaime Pendill
Manager, Periodical Editing: Kirk Swearingen
Production Editor: Stephanie M. Geels
Project Supervisor, Production: Joy Moore
Production Assistant: Laura Bayless
Manager, Literature Services: Idelle L. Winer
Illustrations and Permissions Coordinator: Chidi C. Ukabam

1999 EDITION
Copyright © 1999 by Mosby, Inc.

All rights reserved. No part of this publication may be reproduced, stored in a retrieval system, or transmitted, in any form or by any means, electronic, mechanical, photocopying, recording, or otherwise, without prior written permission from the publisher.

Permission to photocopy or reproduce solely for internal or personal use is permitted for libraries or other users registered with the Copyright Clearance Center, provided that the base fee of $4.00 per chapter plus $.10 per page is paid directly to the Copyright Clearance Center, 21 Congress Street, Salem, MA 01970. This consent does not extend to other kinds of copying, such as copying for general distribution, for advertising or promotional purposes, for creating new collected works, or for resale.

Printed in the United States of America
Composition by Reed Technology and Information Services, Inc.
Printing/binding by Maple-Vail

Editorial Office:
Mosby, Inc.
11830 Westline Industrial Drive
St. Louis, MO 63146

International Standard Serial Number: 0739–5949
International Standard Book Number: 0–8151–0164–3

Editors

Peter C. Amadio, M.D.
Professor of Orthopedic Surgery, Mayo Medical School; Consultant, Department of Orthopedics and Surgery of the Hand, Mayo Clinic, Rochester, Minnesota

Vincent R. Hentz, M.D.
Professor of Surgery and Chief, Division of Hand Surgery, Stanford University School of Medicine, Stanford, California

Editors Emeritus

Robert A. Chase, M.D.
Emile Holman Professor of Surgery, Emeritus, Stanford University School of Medicine, Stanford, California

James H. Dobyns, M.D.
Emeritus Professor of Orthopedic Surgery, Mayo Foundation, Rochester, Minnesota; Clinical Professor, University of Texas Health Science Center, San Antonio, Texas

International Assistant Editors

Guy Foucher, M.D.
Ancien Chef de Clinique de la Facultí de Strasbourg, Strasbourg, France

Priv.-Doz. Dr. Med. Christian L. Jantea
Associate Professor and Lecturer, Department of Orthopaedics, Heinrich-Heine-University Dusseldorf, Dusseldorf, Germany

Caroline LeClercq, M.D.
Ancien Chef de Clinique des Hospitaux de Paris; Hand Surgeon, Institut de la Main, Paris, France

Alberto Lluch, M.D., Ph.D.
Assistant Professor of Orthopedic Surgery, University of Barcelona, Institut Kaplan for Surgery of the Hand and Upper Extremity, Barcelona, Spain

Yasuo Ueba, M.D., D.M.Sc.
Professor Emeritus, College of Medical Technology, Kyoto University, Kyoto; Chief of Orthopedic Surgery, Shiragikuen Hospital, Tosa City, Kochi, Japan

Contributing Editors

Edward Akelman, M.D.
  Professor and Vice Chairman, Brown University School of Medicine; Chief, Division of Hand, Upper Extremity, and Microvascular Surgery, Rhode Island Hospital, Providence, Rhode Island

Kai-Nan An, Ph.D.
  Professor of Bioengineering; Co-Director, Orthopedic Biomechanics Laboratory, Mayo Clinic, Rochester, Minnesota

Marie A. Badalamente, Ph.D.
  Professor of Orthopedics, State University of New York, Stonybrook, New York

Robert D. Beckenbaugh, M.D.
  Professor of Orthopedic Surgery, Mayo Clinic, Rochester, Minnesota

Keith A. Bengtson, M.D.
  Consultant, Department of Physical Medicine and Rehabilitation, Mayo Clinic, Rochester, Minnesota

Richard A. Berger, M.D., Ph.D.
  Associate Professor of Orthopedic Surgery and Anatomy, Mayo Medical School; Consultant, Departments of Orthopedics, Surgery of the Hand and Anatomy, Mayo Clinic, Rochester, Minnesota

Gabrielle Bergman, M.D.
  Assistant Professor of Radiology, Stanford University School of Medicine, Stanford, California

Thomas H. Berquist, M.D.
  Professor of Diagnostic Radiology, Mayo Clinic, Jacksonville, Florida

William P. Cooney III, M.D.
  Professor of Orthopedic Surgery, Mayo Clinic, Rochester, Minnesota

Jasper R. Daube, M.D.
  Professor of Neurology; Consultant, Department of Neurology, Mayo Clinic, Rochester, Minnesota

Paul C. Dell, M.D.
  Professor and Chief of Hand and Microsurgery, University of Florida, Gainesville, Florida

William D. Engber, M.D.
  Associate Professor of Orthopedic Surgery, University of Wisconsin, Madison, Wisconsin

Roslyn B. Evans, O.T.R./L., C.H.T.
  Director, Indian River Hand Rehabilitation, Inc., Vero Beach, Florida

Joseph M. Failla, M.D.
  Adjunct Assistant Professor of Anatomy, Wayne State University; Chief of Hand Surgery, Department of Orthopaedic Surgery, Henry Ford Hospital, Detroit, Michigan

Stephan J. Finical, M.D.
  Senior Associate Consultant, Mayo Clinic, Rochester, Minnesota

Carolyn Gordon, O.T.R., C.H.T.
  Senior Hand Therapist, UCSF–Stanford Health Services, Palo Alto, California

Michelle A. James, M.D.
Associate Clinical Professor of Orthopaedic Surgery, University of California Davis Medical School; Medical Director of Ambulatory Services, Shriner's Hospital for Children, Sacramento, California

Neil F. Jones, M.D.
Professor, Department of Orthopedic Surgery, Division of Plastic and Reconstructive Surgery, University of California, Los Angeles; Chief of Hand Surgery, UCLA Medical Center, Los Angeles, California

Jesse B. Jupiter, M.D.
Professor of Orthopedic Surgery, Harvard Medical School; Director, Orthopedic Hand Service, Massachusetts General Hospital, Boston, Massachusetts

Morton L. Kasdan, M.D.
Clinical Professor of Surgery, University of Louisville; Clinical Professor, Department of Preventive Medicine and Environmental Health, University of Kentucky, Lexington, Kentucky

Julie A. Katarincic, M.D.
Instructor in Orthopedics, Mayo Clinic, Rochester, Minnesota

L. Andrew Koman, M.D.
Professor and Vice Chair, Department of Orthopaedic Surgery, Wake Forest University School of Medicine; Orthpaedic Surgeon, North Carolina Baptist Hospital, Winston-Salem, North Carolina

Amy L. Ladd, M.D.
Associate Professor, Stanford University Medical Center; Chief, Lucile Saltec Packard Children's Hospital at Stanford, Stanford, California

Prem Lalwani, O.T.R., C.H.T.
Lead Hand Therapist, UCSF–Stanford Health Services, Palo Alto, California

Lewis B. Lane, M.D.
Associate Clinical Professor of Orthopedic Surgery, Albert Einstein College of Medicine; Chief, Hand Surgery, Long Island Jewish Medical Center, New Hyde Park, New York

Donna Lashgari, O.T.R., C.H.T.
UCSF–Stanford Health Services, Palo Alto, California

William C. Lineaweaver, M.D.
Associate Professor, Division of Plastic Surgery and Hand Surgery, Stanford University School of Medicine, Stanford, California

Ronald L. Linscheid, M.D.
Professor Emeritus of Orthopedic Surgery, Mayo Medical School, Rochester, Minnesota

Susan E. Mackinnon, M.D., F.R.C.S.C.
Shoenberg Professor and Chief, Division of Plastic and Reconstructive Surgery, Washington University School of Medicine; Plastic Surgeon in Chief, Barnes-Jewish Hospital, St. Louis, Missouri

Peter A. Nathan, M.D.
Providence St. Vincent Medical Center, Portland, Oregon

John M. Navarro, M.D.
  Clinical Instructor, Fellow in OR Management, Stanford University, Stanford, California
Edward R. North, M.D.
  Washington Hand Surgery, Kirkland, Washington
Shawn W. O'Driscoll, M.D., Ph.D., F.R.C.S.C.
  Associate Professor of Orthopedics, Mayo Medical School; Consultant, Orthopedic Surgery, Mayo Clinic, Rochester, Minnesota
Leonard K. Ruby, M.D.
  Professor of Orthopedic Surgery, Tufts University School of Medicine; Chief, Division of Hand Surgery, New England Medical Center, Boston, Massachusetts
William J. Shaughnessy, M.D.
  Assistant Professor of Orthopedic Surgery; Chair, Division of Pediatric Orthopedics, Mayo Clinic, Rochester, Minnesota
Anthony A. Smith, M.D.
  Associate Professor of Plastic Surgery; Senior Associate Consultant, Section of Hand Surgery, Mayo Clinic, Scottsdale, Arizona
Peter J. Stern, M.D.
  Norman S. and Elizabeth C.A. Hill Professor and Chairman, Department of Orthopaedic Surgery, University of Cincinnati, Cincinnati, Ohio
Robert M. Szabo, M.D., M.P.H.
  Professor of Orthopaedics and Plastic Surgery, University of California, Davis; Chief, Hand and Microvascular Surgery, University of California—Davis Health Systems, Sacramento, California
Steven M. Topper, M.D.
  Assistant Professor; Chief, Hand and Microsurgery Section, Department of Orthopaedics and Rehabilitation, Oregon Health Sciences University, Portland, Oregon
Francisco J. Valero-Cuevas, Ph.D.
  Research Associate and Lecturer, Department of Mechanical Engineering, Biomechanical Engineering Division, Stanford University, Stanford, California
Steven F. Viegas, M.D.
  Professor and Chief, Division of Hand Surgery, Department of Orthopaedic Surgery and Rehabilitation; Professor, Department of Anatomy and Neurosciences and Department of Preventive Medicine and Community Health, University of Texas Medical Branch, Galveston, Texas
Peter B.J. Wu, M.D., M.P.H.
  Assistant Professor, Stanford University School of Medicine, Stanford, California
Felix E. Zajac, Ph.D.
  Director, Rehabilitation R&D Center, VA Palo Alto Health Care System; Professor, Departments of Medical Engineering and Functional Restoration, Stanford University, Stanford, California

Table of Contents

JOURNALS REPRESENTED	xvii
INTRODUCTION	xix
1. Anatomy and Biomechanics	1
2. Diagnosis, Evaluation, and Anesthesia	27
3. Skeletal Trauma and Reconstruction	43
4. Soft-Tissue Trauma and Reconstruction	59
5. Tendon Trauma and Reconstruction	73
6. Nerve Trauma and Reconstruction	87
7. Compression Neuropathy	99
8. Wrist	133
General	133
Carpus	140
Distal Radius	167
Distal Radioulnar Joint	187
9. Neuromuscular Disorders	197
10. Arthritis	207
11. Tumors	227
12. Congenital Problems	239
13. Physical and Occupational Medicine	247
14. Microsurgery	265
15. Vascular and Dystrophic Problems	279
16. Research	287
SUBJECT INDEX	301
AUTHOR INDEX	331

Journals Represented

Mosby and its editors survey approximately 500 journals for its abstract and commentary publications. From these journals, the editors select the articles to be abstracted. Journals represented in this YEAR BOOK are listed below.

Acta Orthopaedica Scandinavica
American Industrial Hygiene Association Journal
American Journal of Industrial Medicine
American Journal of Physical Medicine
Annales de Chirurgie Plastique et Esthetique
Annales de Chirurgie de la Main
Annals of Plastic Surgery
Archives of Orthopaedic and Trauma Surgery
Archives of Physical Medicine and Rehabilitation
Archives of Surgery
Arthritis and Rheumatism
Atlas of the Hand Clinics
Brain
British Journal of Plastic Surgery
British Medical Journal
Canadian Journal of Anaesthesia
Canadian Journal of Plastic Surgery
Canadian Medical Association Journal
Clinical Orthopaedics and Related Research
Clinical Radiology
European Journal of Plastic Surgery
Handchirurgie, Mikrochirurgie, Plastische Chirurgie
Injury
International Orthopaedics
Investigative Radiology
Journal of Biomechanics
Journal of Bone and Joint Surgery (American Volume)
Journal of Bone and Joint Surgery (British Volume)
Journal of Hand Surgery (American)
Journal of Hand Surgery (British)
Journal of Hand Therapy
Journal of Occupational and Environmental Medicine
Journal of Orthopaedic Research
Journal of Pediatric Orthopaedics
Journal of Reconstructive Microsurgery
Journal of Rheumatology
Journal of Surgical Research
Journal of the Japanese Society for Surgery of the Hand
La Main
Medical Problems of Performing Artists
Neurosurgery
Occupational Medicine
Occupational and Environmental Medicine
Orthopedics
Pain
Plastic and Reconstructive Surgery

Radiology
Revista de Ortopedia y Traumatologia
Revista Espanola de Cirugia de la Mano
Scandinavian Journal of Plastic and Reconstructive Hand Surgery

STANDARD ABBREVIATIONS

The following terms are abbreviated in this edition: acquired immunodeficiency syndrome (AIDS), cardiopulmonary resuscitation (CPR), central nervous system (CNS), cerebrospinal fluid (CSF), computed tomography (CT), deoxyribonucleic acid (DNA), electrocardiography (ECG), health maintenance organization (HMO), human immunodeficiency virus (HIV), intensive care unit (ICU), intramuscular (IM), intravenous (IV), magnetic resonance (MR) imaging (MRI), and ribonucleic acid (RNA).

NOTE

The YEAR BOOK OF HAND SURGERY® is a literature survey service providing abstracts of articles published in the professional literature. Every effort is made to assure the accuracy of the information presented in these pages. Neither the editors nor the publisher of the YEAR BOOK OF HAND SURGERY® can be responsible for errors in the original materials. The editors' comments are their own opinions. Mention of specific products within this publication does not constitute endorsement.

To facilitate the use of the YEAR BOOK OF HAND SURGERY® as a reference tool, all illustrations and tables included in this publication are now identified as they appear in the original article. This change is meant to help the reader recognize that any illustration or table appearing in the YEAR BOOK OF HAND SURGERY® may be only one of many in the original article. For this reason, figure and table numbers will often appear to be out of sequence within the YEAR BOOK OF HAND SURGERY®.

Introduction

Fifteen years ago, Jim Dobyns and Bob Chase brought a vision to fruition: the first issue of the YEAR BOOK OF HAND SURGERY appeared. They had the help of a baker's dozen of contributors, all from a single institution. The articles covered a broad spectrum of topics, and by all appearances the product was well-accepted; sales have continued at a steady pace ever since, despite the advent of newer reference sources, the internet probably first among those.

This YEAR BOOK, of course, has not stood still. The content and organization has changed, reflecting new interests. Chapters on burns and infections have disappeared; a chapter on the wrist is now included and has become our largest single section. The YEAR BOOK OF HAND SURGERY continues to offer a major advantage over other bibliographies, in that experts have selected the best articles for inclusion and have added comments, sometimes longer than the abstracts they refer to, to put the work in perspective and to add to the enlightenment of the reader.

The ranks of contributors have grown through the years and now include a stellar international cast of characters. This is fitting because the field of hand surgery now truly includes an international community. Hand surgeons seem to have a peculiar wanderlust; most of us have developed an international array of friends whom we meet in a variety of locations around the world. This globalization has been reflected in hand surgery publications as well; it is not unusual for authors of one country to publish not only in their own national journals but also in those of other lands. This is reflected in our book's contents, which include publications and authors mixed and matched from around the globe. We are grateful especially to our international associate editors, who filter literature from France, Japan, Spain, and Germany. The family of contributing editors has grown to more than 50, from 30 institutions across the United States. We are thankful, too, for the continuity provided by the never-flagging participation of our predecessors, Jim Dobyns and Bob Chase, and of those contributors who have added to the wisdom of every volume of the YEAR BOOK OF HAND SURGERY: Ron Linscheid, Bob Beckenbaugh, and Bill Cooney. Finally, we thank Mosby, Inc., and especially Jaime Pendill, our developmental editor, for unflagging support over the past year.

In the inaugural volume, Jim Dobyns predicted that the YEAR BOOK OF HAND SURGERY would grow and change over time, and indeed it has. We hope that this fifteenth edition meets with your approval.

Peter C. Amadio, M.D.
Vincent R. Hentz, M.D.

1 Anatomy and Biomechanics

Colour Doppler Analysis of Tendon and Muscle Movements
Sugamoto K, Ochi T (Osaka Univ, Japan)
J Hand Surg [Br] 23B:237–239, 1998
1–1

Background.—Though CT and MRI can be used to assess tendon and muscle structure, analysis of movement may be more important. The use of a color Doppler device in the assessment of tendon and muscle movement was reported.

Methods.—A Quantum 2000 Doppler color-flow imager with a 7.5-MHz linear-type probe was employed. Two healthy subjects, 3 patients with tendon ruptures, and 2 patients with muscle and tendon adhesions underwent imaging.

Findings.—In the healthy subjects, only gliding tendons and muscles were seen as color images. In patients with tendon rupture, the point of rupture could be identified. In some cases of finger tendon ruptures, the presence of the rupture could be seen. The whole area of the muscle could be visualized as a color image on flexion and extension of the finger in patients with partial ruptures of muscle bellies. Partial muscle rupture could not be detected. Adhesion sites in patients with tendon and muscle adhesions could be identified easily on color Doppler images.

Conclusions.—Active and passive movement of tendons and muscles can be visualized successfully using color Doppler US. The preliminary findings in this study suggest that color Doppler may be very useful in assessing tendon and muscle movement.

▶ It would not be surprising to me if some day color Doppler were used not only to assess tendon integrity after injury but also in cases of synovial proliferation, such as trigger finger and carpal tunnel syndrome. Such data may allow noninvasive study of tendon adhesions, friction, and the effects, if any, of repetitive activity on tendon or synovial biology.

P.C. Amadio, M.D.

The Blood Supply of the Lumbrical Muscles

Zbrodowski A, Mariéthoz E, Bednarkiewicz M, et al (Univ Med Ctr, Geneva)
J Hand Surg [Br] 23B:384–388, 1998   1–2

Purpose.—The lumbrical muscles play a key role in the hand's normal functions, including fine coordinated finger movements, flexion and stabilization of the metacarpophalangeal joint, and extension of the interphalangeal joint. However, there is little information about the blood supply to these muscles. An anatomic study was performed to demonstrate the blood supply of the lumbrical muscles.

Methods.—Studies were performed in 100 cadaver upper extremities. Some specimens were injected with latex and others with gelatin, both injections mixed with Indian ink. Dissections were then performed to demonstrate the arterial network and sources of blood supply for the lumbrical muscles.

Results.—Each of the lumbrical muscles was found to have 4 distinct sources of blood supply: the superficial palmar arch, the common palmar digital artery, the deep palmar arch, and the dorsal digital artery. These vessels anastomosed with each other, resulting in smaller branches that penetrated the muscle intrafascicular space. The blood vessels supplying the flexor digitorum profundus tendon did not anastomose with those supplying the lumbrical muscles. The details of blood supply to the lumbrical muscles varied significantly among muscles, among individuals, and between sides in the same individual.

Conclusions.—The blood supply to each lumbrical muscle is segmental, with the proximal third supplied by branches from the superficial palmar arch, the middle third directly from the common digital artery, and the distal third by branches from the dorsal metacarpal arteries. The arteries of the hand may be viewed as a system, with each supplying a specific territory.

▶ The segmental nature of lumbrical blood supply suggests that lumbrical flaps, occasionally used in revision carpal tunnel surgery, may not be reliable because anastomoses among the various segmental distributions may not be robust.

P.C. Amadio, M.D.

Anatomy of the Adductor Pollicis Muscle: A Basis for Release Procedures for Adduction Contractures of the Thumb

Witthaut J, LeClercq C (Clinique Jouvenet, Paris)
J Hand Surg [Br] 23B:380–383, 1998   1–3

Background.—Adduction contracture of the thumb is a common and disabling problem in which the adductor pollicis muscle plays a major role. The authors' experience suggests that in surgical release to correct this deformity, poor results may occur if the origins of the adductor pollicis are not addressed. This anatomic study described the origins of the adductor pollicis muscle.

Methods and Results.—Dissections were performed in 20 cadaver hands. In most cases, the classical double muscle belly of the adductor pollicis was not immediately apparent. In these cases, fibers distal to the deep palmar arch were regarded as the "transverse head" and proximal fibers as the "oblique head." The transverse head always originated in the long metacarpal, but often had additional origins in the distal head of the index metacarpal. The connection between these 2 origins was a fibrous arch that fused with the second interosseous space fascia. The oblique head had origins in the shaft and base of the index and long metacarpals and in the trapezoid and capitate bones. In addition, most specimens showed origins in the ring metacarpal. Fibers originating in the bones of the distal carpal row usually originated in the palmar carpometacarpal ligaments, rather than in the bones.

Conclusions.—The origins of the adductor pollicis muscle are more extensive than generally thought. These findings have important implications for surgical release of the adductor pollicis origins. Complete release of the oblique head must include the soft tissue origins in the fascia of the second interosseous space, as well as osseous origins from the distal third of the index metacarpal. For complete release of the oblique head, fibers from the bases of the ring, long, and index metacarpals, as well as from the capitate and trapezoid, must be divided.

▶ This useful article directs our attention to the extensive origins of the adductor pollicis. When this muscle must be released, exposure needs to reach the ring metacarpal and carpus.

P.C. Amadio, M.D.

An Anatomical Study of the Palmar Ligamentous Structures of the Carpal Canal
Tanabe T, Okutsu I (Japanese Red Cross Med Ctr, Tokyo)
J Hand Surg [Br] 22B:754–757, 1997
1–4

Background.—Treatment for carpal tunnel syndrome has a goal of releasing the palmar structures that are causing compression of the median nerve. This study examined the location and size of palmar structures in the carpal tunnel, to assess the effects of their release on carpal canal pressures.

Methods.—Twelve hands from 12 embalmed cadavers and 8 hands from 4 fresh cadavers were dissected. Age ranged from 48 to 98 years (mean, 76 years). The roof of the carpal canal was opened and the length, breadth, and thickness of the flexor retinaculum and the transverse fibers were measured. In the fresh cadaveric hands, the skin and subcutaneous adipose tissue was removed from the wrist and palm. Then the flexor retinaculum was released (with the same approach as taken during endo-

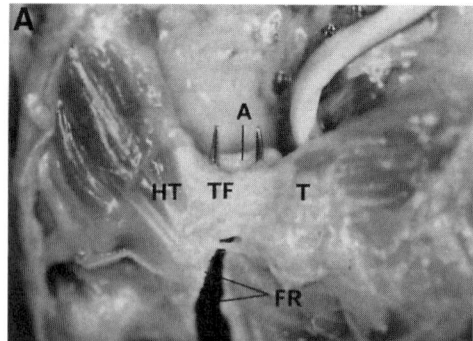
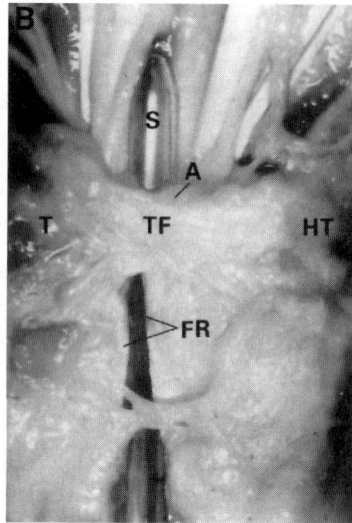

FIGURE 1.—The transverse fibers (*TF*). **A,** hand no. 13. **B,** hand no. 16. The TF is between the thenar and hypothenar fascia. It is separated from the flexor retinaculum (*FR*) by adipose tissue. *Abbreviations*: T, Thenar fascia; HT, hypothenar fascia; A, adipose tissue; FR, resected ends of the flexor retinaculum; S, sheath of the Universal Subcutaneous Endoscope system. (Courtesy of Tanabe T, Okutsu I: An anatomical study of the palmar ligamentous structures of the carpal canal. *J Hand Surg [Br]* 22B:754–757, 1997.)

scopic surgery) and the minimum distance between its severed ends was measured. The transverse fibers were then released, and the minimum distance between the severed ends of the flexor retinaculum was remeasured. Measurements were performed with a caliper (length and breadth) or a micrometer (thickness).

Findings.—All hands showed transverse fibers between the thenar and hypothenar fascia, running transversely in a layer of fat separate from the flexor retinaculum. The transverse fibers were superficial and distal to the flexor retinaculum (Fig 1). For the embalmed and fresh cadaveric hands, the mean measurements for the flexor retinaculum, respectively, were length, 26.3 ± 1.5 and 27.1 ± 1.6 mm; breadth, 19.7 ± 0.7 and 19.9 ± 0.8 mm; and thickness, 2.5 ± 0.2 and 2.5 ± 0.1 mm. For the transverse fibers, the mean measurements, respectively, were: length, 9.0 ± 0.6 and 9.1 ± 0.7 mm; and thickness, 0.7 ± 0.1 and 0.8 ± 0.1 mm. The breadth between the attachment of the thenar and hypothenar fascia averaged 13.3 ± 0.6 and 13.4 ± 0.7 mm, respectively. When the flexor retinaculum was released in the fresh cadaveric hands, the mean distance between its severed ends was 1.3 ± 0.2 mm. However, when both the flexor retinaculum and transverse fibers were released, the distance increased to 6.6 ± 0.2 mm.

Conclusions.—There was a 5-fold increase in the distance between the severed ends of the flexor retinaculum when the transverse fibers were severed as well. Thus for complete release of the carpal canal, both the flexor retinaculum and the transverse fibers should be sectioned.

▶ This paper clearly demonstrated a potential reason for increasing the tissues released with limited incisions or closed carpal tunnel techniques. Specifically, the authors have advocated release of the distal transverse fibers not directly contiguous with the transverse carpal ligament to allow maximum spread of the ligament during surgical intervention. It is presumed that this spread will have a significant effect on decreasing the pressure within the carpal canal, and in separate works (report to the International Federation of Societies for Surgery of the Hand in Helsinki, Finland, in 1995), these authors have also shown differences in carpal tunnel pressures with release of these fibers. Some developers of endoscopic technique (Agee and Chow) have advocated a release of the transverse carpal ligament only, believing that release of the distal fascial fibers and/or the overlying palmar fascia and transverse palmaris muscles will eliminate the benefits of transverse carpal ligament release endoscopically (presumed decreased morbidity). In my experience, release of these additional structures (distal fiber, transverse fibers of Okutsu-Tanabe, and palmar fascia) has not resulted in significantly increased morbidity. It provides for an additional level of assurance of adequate ligament separation and should be considered as an alternative to the more limited releases, although clinically both techniques (ligament only and ligament plus palmar fascia of distal fibers) may be adequate in decompressing the median nerve in the majority of clinical cases.

R.D. Beckenbaugh, M.D.

Anatomical Classification of Sites of Compression of the Palmar Cutaneous Branch of the Median Nerve
Al-Qattan MM (King Saud Univ, Riyadh, Saudi Arabia)
J Hand Surg [Br] 22B:48–49, 1997   1–5

Background.—The anatomical course of the palmar cutaneous nerve was studied in 10 cadavers and classified into 6 zones at which compression may occur.

Methods.—Ten right upper cadaverous limbs were dissected. The anatomical course of the palmar cutaneous nerve was traced and classified into 6 zones. The literature on entrapment neuropathy of this nerve was reviewed and the zone of compression identified.

Results and Discussion..—The palmar cutaneous nerve branch arose from the radial side of the median nerve in all 10 cadavers. It remained bound to the main body of the median nerve for 1.5–10 cm and then separated and emerged from under the radial margin of the flexor digitorum superficialis tendon. It ran deep to the antebrachial fascia in close proximity to the ulnar margin of the flexor carpi radialis tendon. As the nerve became increasingly superficial, it entered its unique tunnel, which

TABLE 1.—Anatomical Classification of the Sites of Compression of the Palmar Cutaneous Branch of the Median Nerve

Site of compression	Cause of compression	References
A: Where the nerve is bound to the body of median nerve	Masses or anomalous tendons compressing the radial aspect of the median nerve in the distal forearm	
B: Site of emergence from the radial margin of the FDS	FDS muscle fascia	Shuntzu et al. 1998
C: Ulnar margin of the flexor carpi radialis and its sheath	Flexor carpi radialis tendinits, ganglia	Buckmiller and Rickard, 1987; Gessini et al. 1983; Naff et al. 1993
D: Within the palmar cutaneous nerve tunnel	Ganglia, atypical palmaris longus muscle	Al-Qattan and Robertson 1993a; Stellbrink, 1972 Duncan et al. 1995
E: In relation to the distal part of palmaris longus tendon	The nerve piercing the distal part of palmaris longus tendon	
F: The subcutaneous course before innervating the skin	Fibrous and scar tissue entrapment following carpal tunnel release	Mackinnon and Dellon, 1988

(Courtesy of Al-Qattan MM: Anatomical classification of sites of compression of the palmar cutaneous branch of the median nerve. *J Hand Surg [Br]* 22B:48–49, 1997.)

varied in both length and location. After exiting the tunnel, the nerve was closely related to the distal part of the palmaris longus (PL) tendon. The palmar cutaneous branch never pierced the PL tendon. The nerve ran subcutaneously and divided into radial and ulnar branches before supplying the skin of the thenar area and palmar triangle. The course of the palmar cutaneous nerve was divided into 6 zones where compression could occur (Table 1). The palmar cutaneous nerve fascicle is in the palmar-radial quadrant of the median nerve and could be compressed before its separation from the main branch. The fascia of the flexor digitorum superficialis tendon could entrap the nerve. The palmar cutaneous nerve runs in close proximity to the flexor carpi radialis sheath and ganglia could entrap the nerve. Compression of the nerve tunnel is also possible. When the nerve does pierce the PL tendon, compression is possible. Scar tissue from carpal tunnel release may cause entrapment of the palmar cutaneous nerve along its subcutaneous course. The definition of the anatomical course of the palmar cutaneous nerve and the location of possible sites of entrapment should be useful to the surgeon dealing with compression of the palmar cutaneous branch of the median nerve.

▶ In addition to their own study of 10 upper limbs, these authors summarize for us the literature on the anatomy and possible compression sites for this important, albeit, tiny sensory nerve branch. Some may consider the separation of areas of compression into 6 zones as overkill, but it is helpful to the surgeon faced with this troublesome and not uncommon problem of median nerve palmar cutaneous neuropathy.

R.A. Chase, M.D.

Distribution of Human Pacinian Corpuscles in the Hand: A Cadaver Study
Stark B, Carlstedt T, Hallin RG, et al (Karolinska Hosp, Stockholm; Karolinska Inst, Stockholm)
J Hand Surg [Br] 23B:370–372, 1998

Background.—Distributed throughout the body, Pacinian corpuscles (PCs) are the largest encapsulated sensory receptors for the perception of skin stimuli or vibration. In this cadaver study, the distribution of these sensory receptors in the hands is analyzed, particularly in relationship to nerves and vessels.

Methods.—Ten fresh hands were dissected from 6 female cadavers (mean age, 83 years) and 4 male cadavers (mean age, 71.5 years). In 4 cases the left hand was analyzed, and in 6 cases the right hand was

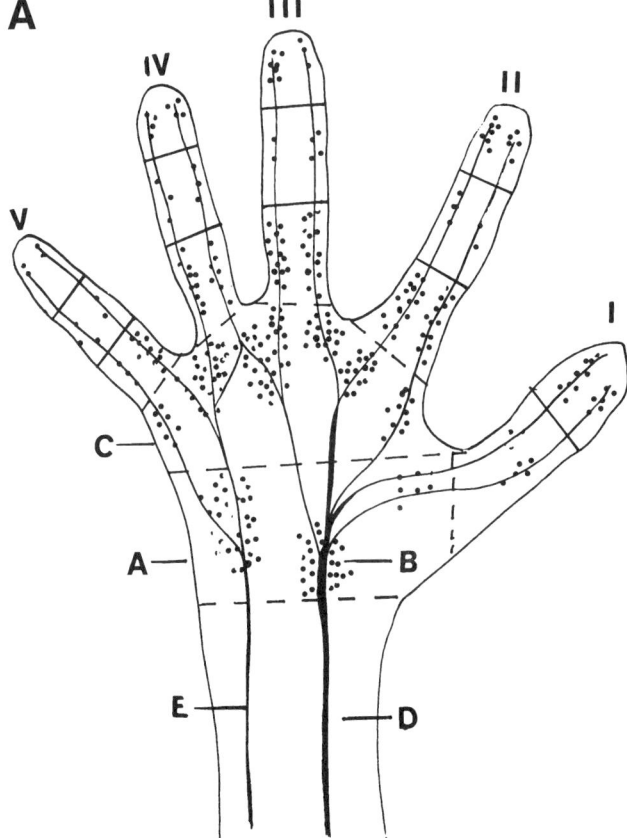

FIGURE 1, A.—Distribution of Pacinian corpuscles in the right hand of an 89-year-old female cadaver. *A*, hypothenar; *B*, thenar; *C*, metacarpus; *D*, median nerve; *E*, ulnar nerve. (Courtesy of Stark B, Carlstedt T, Hallin RG, et al: Distribution of human Pacinian corpuscles in the hand: A cadaver study. *J Hand Surg [Br]* 23B:370–372, 1998.)

analyzed. Only subcutaneous PCs were investigated; deeper receptors or those close to superficial flexor tendons or joints were not included. PCs were recorded from the thenar, hypothenar, and the 3 phalanges of each digit. The sizes of the PCs from the metacarpophalangeal (MCP) region and the distal phalanx of the index finger were also measured.

Findings.—PCs clustered around subcutaneous tissue close to nerves and vessels (Fig 1, A). They were found in greatest numbers in the MCP and proximal phalangeal regions, where they existed in close contact with nerve structures. PCs were found primarily in the fingers (from 44% to 60% of the total amount of PCs), secondarily, in the MP regions (23% to 48%), and lastly in the thenar and hypothenar regions (8% to 18%). The thumb, index, long, ring, and little fingers had mean PC counts of 38, 63, 63, 60, and 41, respectively. The thenar and hypothenar areas had mean PC counts of 16 and 18, respectively. Compared with PCs in the middle phalange (mean, 23), there were twice as many PCs in the distal phalange (mean, 48) and almost 4 times as many PCs in the proximal phalange (mean, 84). The PCs in the distal palmar skin of the index finger were much smaller than those in the MCP region (mean surface area, 0.77 vs. 3.5 mm^2). PC long axes varied from 0.6 to 3.5 mm, and the transverse diameter perpendicular to the long axis varied from 0.30 to 4.84 mm. Overall, the mean number of PCs in the hand was 300 (range, 192–375).

Conclusions.—There was great variation in the number of PCs in these 10 cadaver hands. However, their distribution seemed to be rather constant, with most PCs clustering close to nerves and vessels in the MP area and proximal phalanges of the index, long, and ring fingers. Furthermore, larger PCs were found in the MCP region of the index finger than were found in the distal palmar skin of the index finger. However, whether a relationship exists between size and function is not known.

▶ For those with an esoteric bent, this interesting article gives us a better view of the mechanoreceptors in the human hand.

P.C. Amadio, M.D.

The Detailed Anatomy of the Palmar Cutaneous Nerves and Its Clinical Implications
Matloub HS, Yan J-G, Mink van der Molen AB, et al (Med College of Wisconsin, Milwaukee)
J Hand Surg [Br] 23B:373–379, 1998   1–7

Background.—After carpal tunnel surgery, patients often experience scar tenderness and "pillar pain." Some clinicians suggest that these sensations result from damage to the palmar cutaneous branch of the median nerve (PCBm) or the palmar cutaneous branch of the ulnar nerve (PCBu). The distributions of the PCBm and PCBu in cadaver hands were analyzed to determine the most appropriate nerve-sparing open or semi-open approach to carpal tunnel surgery.

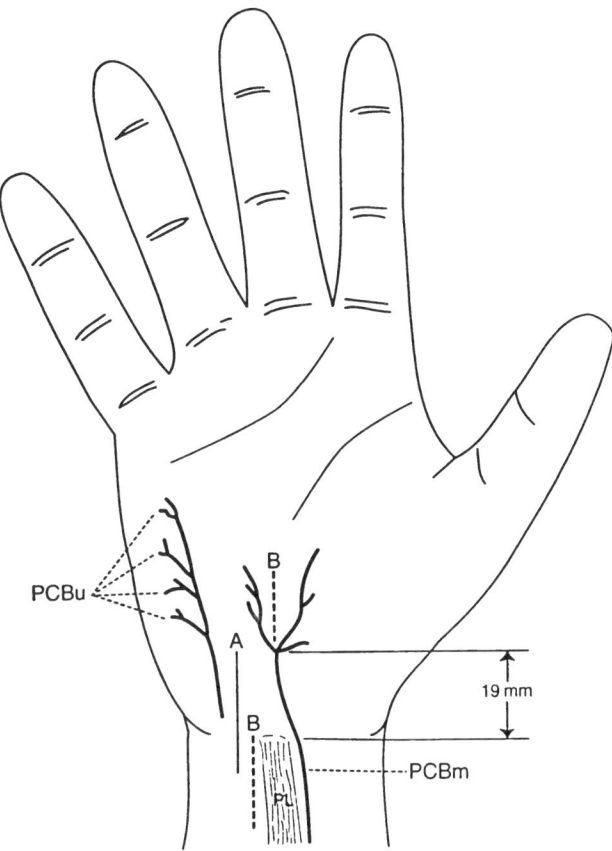

FIGURE 8.—This figure shows 2 possible approaches to the carpal tunnel, designed to minimize the chance of injury of the palmar cutaneous nerves. *Line A* indicates a single short incision parallel and 10 to 15 mm ulnar to the thenar crease. The length of this incision should be a maximum of 15 mm from the distal wrist crease to the distal end of the incision. If needed, it can be extended proximally. *Lines B1* and *B2* indicate a 2-portal approach to the carpal tunnel. *Line B1* shows the proximal incision in the distal forearm along the ulnar margin of the palmaris longus (PL) tendon. *Line B2* shows the short 2-cm long incision in the palm. This incision starts proximally in line with the trunk of the palmar cutaneous branch of the median nerve (PCBm)(3 mm ulnar to the thenar crease) and at least 2 cm distal of the distal wrist crease. The incision extends distally perpendicular to the distal wrist crease for 1.5 to 2 cm. *Abbreviation: PCBu,* Palmar cutaneous branch of the ulnar nerve. (Courtesy of Matloub HS, Yan J-G, Mink van der Molen AB, et al: The detailed anatomy of the palmar cutaneous nerves and its clinical implications. *J Hand Surg [Br]* 23B:373–379, 1998.)

Methods.—The specimens were 40 fresh-frozen cadaver forearms and hands. Specimens were dissected under the microscope to determine the distributions of the PCBm, PCBu, and their branches. The nerves and their branches were traced onto a film, then the skin was replaced and the film was transferred to the skin, so that the innervation was apparent on the skin. Then, 3 standard incisions for open carpal tunnel release were marked on each hand, and the nerves and branches that would be cut off by a particular incision were counted.

Findings.—The PCBm always originated from the radial side of the median nerve, about 4.4 cm proximal to the distal crease of the wrist. It typically passed through the sheath of the flexor carpi radialis (36 cases), and it typically (35 cases) gave off 1 or 2 secondary branches that supplied the scaphoid before it entered a tunnel between the superficial and deeper layers of the flexor retinaculum (37 cases). At the end of the tunnel, the PCBm typically passed over the palmaris longus tendon (37 cases). With respect to the PCBu, in no specimen could a typical single trunk of this nerve be identified; instead, there were several palmar cutaneous branches originating from the ulnar digital nerve to the little finger. The branches pierced the deep fascia and continued to the ulnar side of the palm, where they innervated the skin. A midline incision between the long and ring fingers injured the PCBm in each case; an incision in line with the midline of the ring finger injured the PCBm in 10 cases (25%); and an incision in line with the ulnar side of the ring finger injured the PCBm in fewer than 10% of cases. However, this latter incision carried a 72% risk for injuring branches of the PCBu.

Conclusions.—All 3 standard incisions studied are quite likely to damage branches of the PCBm or PCBu. However, the risk of injury can be minimized in 2 ways (Fig 8). First, a short (no more than 15 mm) longitudinal incision can be made in the heel of the hand, parallel to the thenar crease and 10–15 mm ulnad. Alternatively, 2 minimal incisions can be used, with the first from the center of the palm to the bifurcation of the trunk of the PCBm (perpendicular to the distal crease of the wrist) and the second on the ulnar side of the palmaris longus tendon (proximal to the distal crease of the wrist). Furthermore, when harvesting the flexor carpi radialis tendon for transfer, the sheath should be opened on the radial side to avoid the PCBm. Similarly, when harvesting the palmaris longus tendon, it should be cut proximal to the distal crease of the wrist.

▶ This excellent and provocative study raises once again the question of whether pillar pain is really neuroma pain from injured branches of palmar cutaneous nerves. The authors assume, one hopes incorrectly, that open carpal tunnel releases are performed by cutting down directly along the skin incision all the way down to the flexor retinaculum, without looking for cutaneous nerves. It would seem appropriate to dissect along one's chosen incision, to be sure no small nerve branches are in the way. Usually, at least in my experience using an incision along the ring metacarpal, these can be safely retracted away. Nonetheless, these authors have a valid point, and their suggested safer incisions seem reasonable.

P.C. Amadio, M.D.

Anatomy of the Posterior Interosseous Nerve in Relation to Fixation of the Radial Head
Tornetta P III, Hochwald NL, Bono C, et al (Kings County Hosp, Brooklyn, NY)
Clin Orthop 345:215–218, 1997   1–8

Background.—Although nonoperative management of radial head and neck fractures is accepted, operative management appears to give better results. If internal fixation is employed, the head must be fixed to the shaft, but extension of the approach distal to the annular ligament may put the posterior interosseous nerve at risk. The risk of blind subperiosteal dissection distal to the annular ligament for the placement of a plate across the radial neck was examined in cadaver specimens.

Methods.—The investigations involved 50 fresh cadaver arms. A standard posterolateral approach to the radial head was used in each arm. The forearm was pronated to identify the most anterior aspect of the safe zone, and then supinated to identify the most posterior aspect of the safe zone for plate placement. No specific attempts were made to locate the posterior interosseous nerve. A small key elevator stripped an area large enough for placement of a 4-cm minifragment plate on the radius. The forearm was supinated, and a longitudinal anterolateral incision was made from above the elbow to the midforearm. The radial nerve was dissected under loupe magnification, and all branches were followed distal to the plate. The distance from the radiocapitellar joint to the branch point of the nerve, to the extensor carpi radialis longus, to the posterior interosseous nerve, and from the posterior interosseous nerve to the closing point of the plate with the arm in neutral were measured. Structural damage to the posterior interosseous nerve was assessed.

Results.—The takeoff of the muscular branch to the extensor carpi radialis longus was approximately 7.1 mm proximal to the radiocapitellar joint. The posterior interosseous nerve originated approximately 1.2 mm from the radiocapitellar joint. In 31 arms, the takeoff was proximal, and in 19 it was distal to the joint. The posterior interosseous nerve was intramuscular in 49 of 50 arms and lay on the radius in 1 arm. There was no damage to the posterior interosseous nerve or branches. The plate did not trap any nerve branches. The distance from the posterior interosseous nerve to the plate was about 5 mm. In 2 cases, the nerve passed over the distal end of the plate within the supinator, approximately 3.5 cm and 4 cm distal to the radial neck.

Conclusions.—This investigation of 50 cadaver arms indicates that the posterior interosseous nerve is not at risk of structural injury during distal subperiosteal dissection along the radius. Plating the radial neck by distal extension of the posterolateral approach with subperiosteal dissection is safe. Tension on the nerve should always be avoided because it could lead to physiologic injury.

▶ This study documents the surgical anatomy of the posterior interosseous nerve with reference to the placement of a minifragment plate on the radial head and neck for radial neck (plus or minus head) fractures.

This is worthwhile information for the surgeon, as the threat of posterior interosseous nerve injury looms as a dark cloud of concern in the minds of most surgeons operating in this area. In the literature, lack of familiarity with the details of this anatomy is much more responsible for this concern than the prevalence of nerve injury. Internal fixation of radial neck fractures or radial head and neck fractures with a plate requires exposure close to the posterior interosseous nerve. This leaves surgeons with only 2 options to choose from: (1) familiarization with the detailed anatomy and avoidance of the nerve and (2) compromise on exposure to stay well away from the nerve. It makes sense to choose no. 1.

S.W. O'Driscoll, M.D., Ph.D., F.R.C.S.C.

Venous Drainage of the Radial Forearm and Anterior Tibial Reverse Flow Flaps: Anatomical and Radiographic Perfusion Studies
Nakajima H, Imanishi N, Aiso S, et al (Keio Univ, Tokyo)
Br J Plast Surg 50:389–401, 1997   1–9

Introduction.—A cadaver study was conducted to investigate the anatomy of the venous system in the pedicles of the radial forearm and anterior tibial reverse flow flaps. A radiographic perfusion study examined their drainage pathways in the veins of 2 radial forearm and 2 anterior tibial pedicles.

Methods.—Six fresh cadavers that had a lead oxide/gelatin mixture infused into the veins were used in the anatomic study. The radial arteries and the associated deep veins, the anterior tibial arteries and their associated deep veins, and the deep peroneal nerve were dissected and the specimens examined with a soft x-ray system. In the perfusion study, the flow of Microfil was recorded radiographically over time by a soft x-ray system.

Results.—The anatomic study demonstrated that the venous system consists mainly of 3 types of veins: venae comitantes, communicating veins between the venae comitantes, and vasa vasorum. Some of the communicating veins formed a venous network by branching and anastomosing with each other. Valves were identified in all 3 types of veins. In the small, fine veins, valves were seen at the sites where those veins which ran along the radial artery anastomosed with the venae comitantes and the cutaneous and muscle perforator veins. In the venous system, including the vasa vasorum, all routes of reverse flow passed directly through veins. The radiographic perfusion study revealed valve incompetence, which did not occur in all valves. It was also apparent that a difference in valve resistance against reverse flow pressure existed. Microfil flow indicated that veins with relatively weak valve resistance became the drainage pathway.

Discussion.—Three types of veins form the venous systems in the pedicles in the radial forearm and anterior tibial reverse flow flaps. Small veins anastomosed with the communicating veins and perforator veins as well as with the venae comitantes, and all anastomoses examined had valves. Thus, venous blood must pass retrogradely through at least 1 valve to enter the microvenous connections from the venae comitantes. The perfusion study revealed that reverse flow primarily occurs as direct flow through valves with weak resistance. Differences in valve resistance may result from differences in the anatomy of the valve sinuses. Findings explain the clinical observation that survival is worse for the anterior tibial reverse flow flap than for the radial forearm reverse flow flap.

▶ This is a very elegant anatomic study to explain the venous outflow of a reverse radial forearm flap. The authors demonstrated interconnecting flow between the venae comitantes themselves, the communicating veins between the venae comitantes, and the vasa vasorum on the surface of the radial artery. Valves were found in all 3 components of this venous network and, therefore, retrograde flow can only occur due to valve incompetence or variable valve resistance. This is probably only of academic interest, since the reverse radial forearm flap is a very reliable flap for coverage of soft-tissue defects of the hand and wrist.

N.F. Jones, M.D.

How Muscle Architecture and Moment Arms Affect Wrist Flexion–extension Moments
Gonzalez RV, Buchanan TS, Delp SL (Northwestern Univ, Chicago; Le Tourneau Univ, Longview, Tex; Univ of Delaware, Newark)
J Biomech 30:705–712, 1997   1–10

Introduction.—In initial attempts to characterize the normal function of wrist muscles, the authors found the peak moment generated by the wrist flexors exceeds that generated by the extensors, the maximum flexion moment showed greater variation by wrist flexion angle than the maximum extension moment, and flexion moment peaked with the wrist in flexed position. However, these data do not provide information on how the muscle architecture and moment arms affect the moment-generating characteristics of the wrist muscles. These questions were addressed using a 3-dimensional computer graphics model.

Methods.—The model estimated the moment arms, maximum isometric forces, and maximum isometric flexion-extension moments generated by 15 wrist muscles across a range of wrist flexion angles. The findings were used in an attempt to explain the previously reported moment findings in normal wrists.

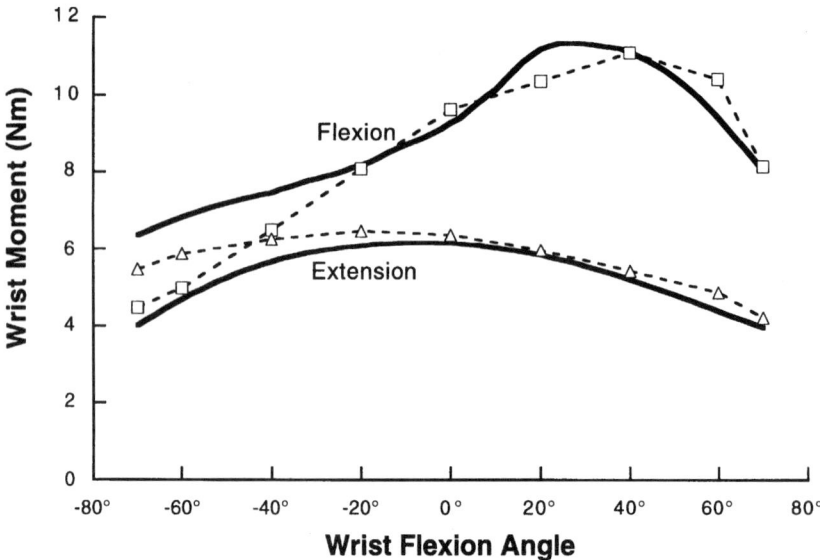

FIGURE 7.—Maximum isometric flexion and extension moments vs. wrist joint angle. The squares and triangles represent the mean of 10 subjects (Delp, et al., 1996). The solid curves represent the maximum isometric moments calculated with the model. Flexion angles are positive, extension angles are negative. The mean flexion moment peaked at approximately 40 degrees; the extension moment peaked at −20 degrees, and varied less with wrist flexion angle. (Reprinted from Gonzalez RV, Buchanan TS, Delp SL: How muscle architecture and moment arms affect wrist flexion–extension moments. *J Biomech* 30:705–712. Copyright 1997, with kind permission from Elsevier Science Ltd, The Boulevard, Langford Lane, Kidlington OX5 1GB UK.)

Results.—The reason peak wrist flexion moment is greater than peak extension moment was the greater summed physiologic cross-sectional area of the flexors (Fig 7). Greater variation of the moment arms of the major wrist flexors with flexion angle accounted for the larger variation of flexion moment with flexion angle. The interaction between flexor moment arms and their force-length behaviors was shown to determine the location of the peak flexion moment (Fig 8).

Conclusions.—The findings of this wrist model suggest variations in wrist maximum isometric moments with flexion angle are determined by variation of the moment arms with flexion angle, and by the operating lengths of muscle fibers. The dedicated wrist flexors apparently account for a relatively small part of total flexion moment-generating potential. The digital muscles may play a major role in the production of wrist moments during maximum voluntary contractions. The authors hope their model will lead to the development of a detailed wrist model to clarify wrist function in health and disease and to plan surgical treatments.

▶ The net moment that an anatomical joint can produce is the combined effect of the tendon moment arm, strength, and relative length of all muscles that cross it. The majority of muscles crossing the wrist are not dedicated wrist muscles, but rather extrinsic finger and thumb muscles.

A: FCU

B: All Flexors

Wrist Flexion Angle

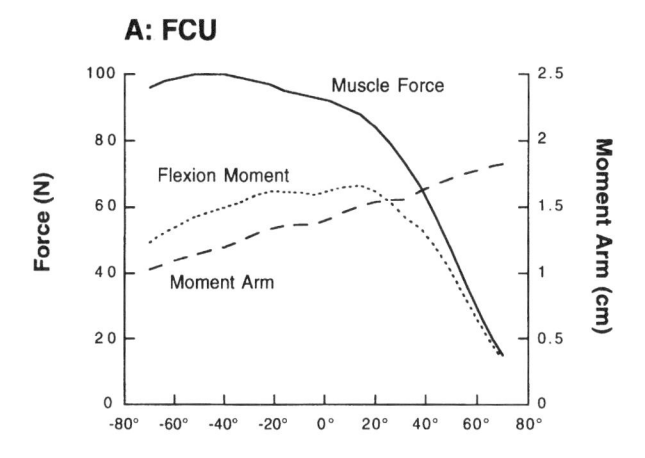

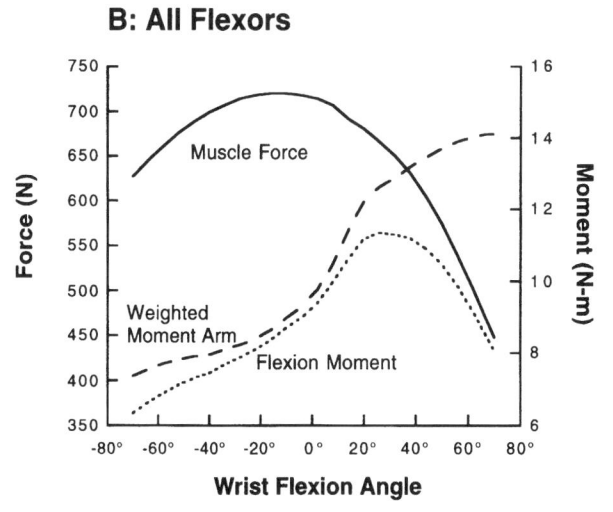

FIGURE 8.—Maximum isometric force, moment arm, and flexion moment vs. flexion angle. In A, the solid curve is the maximum isometric force generated by the flexor carpi ulnaris, FCU, the dashed curve is moment arm, and dotted curve in flexion moment (the peak moment is 1.3 Nm). In B, the solid curve represents the sum of the forces generated by all of the flexors, the dashed curve is the sum of the MA-F^m_o products for all the flexors, and is labeled "weighted moment arm." Flexion angles are positive, extension angles are negative. Note that the positions of the peak moments result from the interplay of moment arm–angle and force–angle relations. (Reprinted from Gonzalez RV, Buchanan TS, Delp SL: How muscle architecture and moment arms affect wrist flexion–extension moments. *J Biomech* 30:705–712. Copyright 1997, with kind permission from Elsevier Science Ltd, The Boulevard, Langford Lane, Kidlington OX5 1GB UK.)

Understanding the role of extrinsic hand muscle on wrist function is important to the understanding of wrist instability and deformity. This paper uses analytical models based on experimental data to reach the following clinically useful conclusions: (1) net wrist joint moment varies irregularly with wrist flexion angle and peaks at around 40 degrees of flexion, (2) changes in muscle fiber length and moment arm with wrist flexion–extension play an important role in the irregularity of flexion moment, (3) finger extrinsic flexors are responsible for a large proportion of net wrist flexion moment. Thus, producing adequate wrist moments and preventing wrist deformity depends as much on dedicated wrist muscles as extrinsic hand muscles.

F.J. Valero-Cuevas, Ph.D.

Effect of Radial Shortening on Muscle Length and Moment Arms of the Wrist Flexors and Extensors
Tang JB, Ryu J, Kish V, et al (West Virginia Univ, Morgantown)
J Orthop Res 15:324–330, 1997
1–11

Background.—In patients with fractures of the distal radius, radial shortening is apparently associated with poor results. Although many studies have examined the treatment of distal radius fractures, few have looked at the biomechanical effects of these fractures. Radial shortening could lead to changes in muscle length and moment arm of the principal wrist flexors and extensors afterwards, possibly resulting in altered loading of the carpal joints. A cadaver study was performed to investigate the effects of shortening of the distal radius on muscle length and moment arm of the wrist flexors and extensors.

Methods.—The investigators performed ostectomy on 8 cadaver upper limbs to simulate the effects of distal radial fractures. By adjusting an external rotation device, the researchers shortened the distal radius progressively by 2.5, 5, 7.5, and 10 mm. With the wrists in neutral position, flexion, extension, and radial and ulnar deviation, rotatory potentiometers were used to measure changes in resting muscle length, including the flexor carpi radialis and ulnaris, extensor carpi radialis longus and brevis, and extensor carpi ulnaris. Simultaneous measurements of tendon excursion and wrist angulation were made as the wrists were moved through passive flexion–extension and radioulnar deviation. This information was used to calculate tendon moment arms.

Results.—Radial shortening significantly altered muscle length or moment arm of the principal wrist flexors and extensors. All of these muscles, except the extensor carpi ulnaris, showed significantly decreased muscle length. During flexion–extension or radioulnar deviation, the moment arm of the extensor carpi ulnaris tendon was significantly decreased. Radioulnar deviation was associated with significant reductions in the moment arms of the extensor carpi radialis brevis and flexor carpi ulnaris tendons. The observed alterations appeared with radial shortening as little as 2.5 mm. At increased shortening lengths, increased biomechanical changes were observed.

Conclusions.—Shortening of the distal radius decreases the muscle length and moment arms of the principal wrist flexors and extensors. Normal radial length is an important factor in wrist kinetics. The results underscore the need to restore normal radial length completely in wrists with distal radial fracture.

▶ This manuscript presents quantitative evidence of the effect of radial shortening on the length and moment arms of wrist muscles, which may explain the poor function of the wrist following distal. It is a well-designed study with a large number of specimens and an experimental paradigm that allowed the isolation of radius length as the independent factor studied. Surgeons repairing radial fractures should take particular care to return the radius to its original length to minimize the disruption of post–operative wrist and hand function.

F.J. Valero-Cuevas, Ph.D.

Transverse Carpal Ligament: Its Effect on Flexor Tendon Excursion, Morphologic Changes of the Carpal Canal, and on Pinch and Grip Strength After Open Carpal Tunnel Release
Netscher D, Mosharrafa A, Lee M, et al (Baylor College of Medicine, Houston; Dept of Veterans Affairs Med Ctr, Houston)
Plast Reconstr Surg 100:636–642, 1997   1–12

Objective.—Some patients continue to have pain and weakness after carpal tunnel release, possibly because of volar migration of the median nerve. Whether transverse carpal ligament division affects flexor tendon excursion and tendon "bowstringing" and whether any adverse effect on tendon excursion might lead to grip and pinch strength weakness was investigated in a cadaver study and in inpatients undergoing transverse carpal ligament reconstruction.

Methods.—The flexor tendons were identified in 8 fresh cadaver arms. Wrists were moved from 30 degrees of extension through 60 degrees of flexion. Carpal tunnel tendon excursion was measured for each finger and at each wrist position before and after transverse carpal ligament repair (Fig 1). Open carpal tunnel release was performed in 45 patients with carpal tunnel syndrome. Fifteen patients had no ligament reconstruction, 15 had a segment of the transverse carpal ligament sutured tension-free to a segment of the palmar aponeurosis, and 15 had transverse carpal ligament repair with the transposition flap. Magnetic resonance imaging was performed preoperatively and at 3 months postoperatively.

Results.—The finger tip failed to contact the palm by an average of 1.8 cm in the flap repair group, 2.15 cm in the aponeurotic group, and 3.41 cm in the no ligament reconstruction group. Whereas grip and pinch strength increased postoperatively in all groups, carpal tunnel cross-sectional area and pinch and grip strength increased significantly only in the flap repair group. Volar displacement of the median nerve was reduced in the flap group.

Conclusion.—Reconstruction of the transverse carpal ligament after carpal tunnel release reduces volar displacement of the median nerve.

▶ After carpal tunnel release, there is a group of patients who fail to recover grip strength, regardless of the approach, whether endoscopic or open. In this study, the authors have shown us that reconstruction of the transverse carpal ligament with a transposition flap after carpal tunnel release results in decreased flexor tendon bowstringing and a more rapid recovery of grip and pinch strength, when compared with no reconstruction or a palmar aponeurosis reconstruction. In fact, all of the authors' patients, regardless of method, regained their strength postoperatively.

However, this is not true in the clinical setting when a vast number of procedures are performed. Sometimes the cause of the persistent pain and weakness is obvious, such as associated thumb carpometacarpal arthritis or underlying wrist arthritis. At other times, the cause is baffling. In such cases, if excessive palmar bowstringing of flexor tendons were demonstrated, would secondary reconstruction with a transposition flap result in restoration of strength?

E.R. North, M.D.

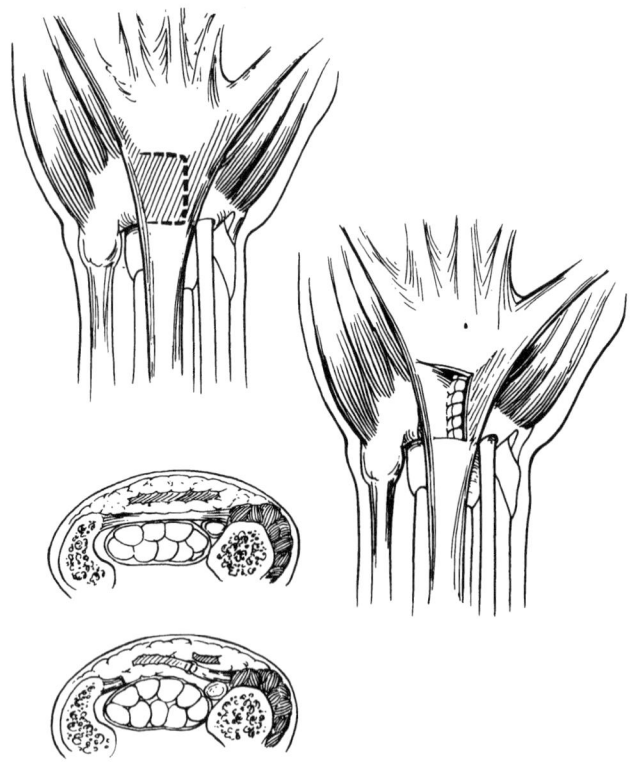

(Continued)

FIGURE 1 (cont.)

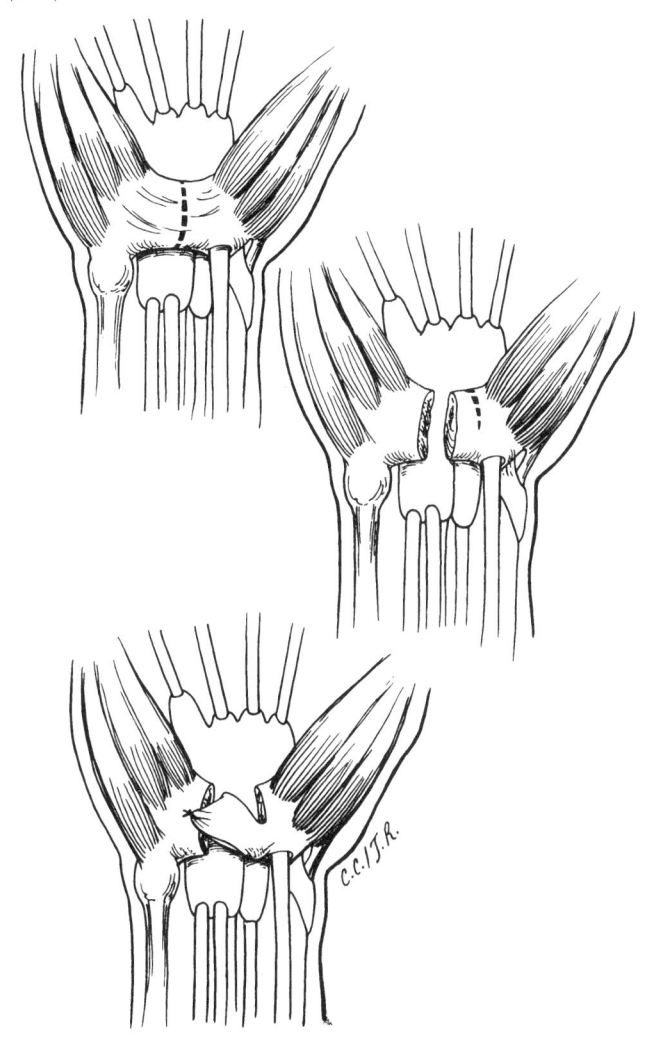

FIGURE 1.—Transverse carpal ligament repair with aponeurotic flap (*left*) and transposition flap (*right*). (Courtesy of Netscher D, Mosharrafa A, Lee M, et al: Transverse carpal ligament: Its effect on flexor tendon excursion, morphologic changes of the carpal canal, and on pinch and grip strength after open carpal tunnel release. *Plast Reconstr Surg* 100:636–642, 1997.)

The Effect of Use of a Wrist Orthosis During Functional Activities on Surface Electromyography of the Wrist Extensors in Normal Subjects

Jansen CWS, Olson SL, Hasson SM (Univ of Texas, Galveston; Texas Woman's Univ, Houston; Univ of Connecticut, Storrs)
J Hand Ther 10:283–289, 1997   1–13

Objective.—Whether use of wrist orthoses by patients with lateral epicondylitis to decrease muscle activity of the wrist extensors during functional activities actually provides protection has not been studied. The difference between muscle activity as measured by electromyography and actual tension in vivo on the tendon of the extensor carpi radialis brevis was measured using 3 types of wrist extensor orthoses under 3 conditions—dorsal, volar, and semicircular—and compared with measurements with no orthosis.

Methods.—Thirteen healthy volunteers (2 men), aged 22–42 years, performed 3 lifting tasks and 2 maximum gripping tasks, repeated on 3 consecutive days, wearing 3 different wrist extensor orthoses or no orthoses. Surface electromyography, the root mean square recorded over the wrist extensor, and maximum voluntary grip strength were measured during the activities. Differences in root mean square while subjects were wearing wrist orthoses were compared with wearing no orthosis.

Results.—Only the semicircular orthotic design significantly decreased the electrical activity of the wrist extensors. Maximum voluntary grip strength was significantly decreased by all 3 orthoses. The root mean square measured during grip strength testing did not change significantly.

Conclusion.—The semicircular wrist orthosis reduced electrical activity less than expected and reduced electrical activity during lifting activities only.

▶ In this study, 13 normal young adults were given protective orthoses positioned in wrist extension to determine which of 3 fabricated styles best reduced the muscular activity of the extensor carpi radialis brevis. Surface electromyographic recordings were used to determine muscle activity in a test of 5 functional activities known to aggravate lateral epicondylitis. It was hypothesized that less muscle activity would translate to less tension on the tendon of the extensor carpi radialis brevis and would most assist clients with lateral epicondylitis to rest the muscle during functional activities. Splinting of the wrist in extension is one of the currently accepted treatments for this problem, but its efficacy has not been adequately tested.

In this well-designed and carefully conducted test, this type of treatment was found to be not nearly as effective as widely accepted. A 6% reduction of tension during lifting was noted with the semicircular wrist orthosis, comparable with a similar study using a counterforce brace on the proximal forearm, but is it questionable whether this is enough to provide long-term advantage. Because this excellent study questioned an accepted treatment method and found it wanting, it should become a challenge to other therapists to repeat this study on a larger scale, with clients demonstrating lateral epicondylitis and with a larger population, including more male subjects. Hopefully, a study on the population of clients with lateral epicondylitis who work at computer keyboards would be included.

D. Lashgari, O.T.R., C.H.T.

Radioulnar Load-sharing in the Forearm: A Study in Cadavera
Markolf KL, Lamey D, Yang S, et al (Univ of California, Los Angeles)
J Bone Joint Surg Am 80A:879–888, 1998   1–14

Objective.—Operations to change the relative lengths of the radius and ulna, or to remove portions of either bone, are commonly performed for disabling conditions of the wrist, forearm, or elbow. Though these procedures are clinically successful, there is little information on their biomechanical bases. There is debate over the load-bearing mechanism of the forearm. An experimental study was performed to measure load-sharing between the radius and ulna at the wrist and elbow.

Methods.—Miniature load-cells were placed into the distal end of the ulna and the proximal end of the radius in 10 cadaver forearms. A constant axial load of 134 N was then applied through the metacarpals, and the forces transmitted through the radius and ulna were measured as the forearm was moved from 60 degrees of supination to 60 degrees of pronation. The data were used to calculate radioulnar load-sharing at the wrist and elbow, as well as force transferred from the radius to the ulna via the interosseous membrane.

Results.—With the elbow in valgus, load was transmitted through the forearm mainly via direct axial loading of the radius. Angle of elbow flexion did not affect loading measurements. With the forearm in neutral, mean force in the distal ulna was 3% of the total load applied to the wrist, and force in the proximal ulna was 12%. Thus, tension in the interosseous membrane was negligible. With the elbow in varus, force was transferred from the radius to the ulna via the interosseous membrane. With the forearm in neutral, mean force in the distal ulna was 3% of the total load applied to the wrist, and force in the proximal ulna was 93%. Forearm supination led to decreased transmission of force through the interosseous membrane. With the elbow in valgus, incremental shortening of the distal radius resulted in increased force in the distal end of the ulna and in decreased force in the radial head. Each increment of radial shortening was followed by continued low forces through the interosseous membrane.

Conclusions.—Many different factors affect the transmission of force from the wrist to the elbow via the radius and ulna. Elbow alignment has a major impact on the mechanism of force transmission through the forearm. With the elbow in valgus, the interosseous membrane does not play an important role in force transmission. However, with the elbow in varus, as in dynamic gripping activities, tension would develop in this membrane. Shortening of the distal radius by as little as 2 mm significantly alters radioulnar load-sharing at the wrist and elbow. With the elbow in valgus alignment, about 4 mm of radial shortening is needed to balance radioulnar loading at the wrist.

▶ This is a very timely and important article which certainly amplifies the results of previous studies defining the relative loads of the proximal radius and ulna, and which confirms the results of those studies focusing on varus and valgus stress. The loss of the mechanical integrity of the interosseous membrane in an Essex-Lopresti injury would certainly be expected to alter the load-sharing construct of the forearm, an alteration which would readily explain the pathomechanics scene in such injuries. The potential influence of a malunion of a distal radius fracture is implied by the significant radioulnar load-sharing at the wrist and the elbow changing when the distal end of the radius was shortened by as little as 2 mm. It is becoming increasingly apparent that some means of reliably reconstituting the effect of the central band in the interosseous membrane, in order to approximate normal physiologic radioulnar load-sharing, will be a critical element in the treatment of patients with interosseous membrane disruption.

R.A. Berger, M.D., Ph.D.

Menisci and Synovial Folds of the Metacarpophalangeal Joint of the Thumb [German]
Putz RV, Sowa G (Aus der Anatomischen Anstalt München)
Handchir Mikrochir Plast Chir 29:316–320, 1997   1–15

Introduction.—Information on the normal anatomy of the thumb metacarpophalangeal (MP) joint is needed to recognize anatomical conditions during thumb joint arthroscopy. The normal findings of the synovial folds and menisci of the thumb MP joint were examined.

Methods and Findings.—The investigators examined the inner surface of 25 thumb MP joints, including the various folds protruding into the joint cavity at the level of the joint cleft (Fig 1). Examination of the ulnar and radial sides revealed compact, wedge-shaped folds. These folds were made up of collagenous fibers, which connected to the fibrous layer of the joint capsule. The fibrous tissue was arranged in a circular fashion and covered by a thin layer of cartilaginous cells. By contrast, the palmar and dorsal aspects of the joint cleft showed typical synovial folds, made up of loose connective tissue with small lobules of fat.

Conclusions.—The normal findings of the thumb MP joint were analyzed. The folds found on the ulnar and radial sides of the joint appear structurally and functionally similar to the menisci of the knee joint. The synovial folds at the palmar and dorsal circumference do not appear to serve any specific mechanical role. Rather, consistent with the requirements of joint mobility, these folds may serve as a malleable spacer.

▶ Arthroscopy of the MP joint of the thumb is becoming more and more popular.

Chapter 1–Anatomy and Biomechanics / 23

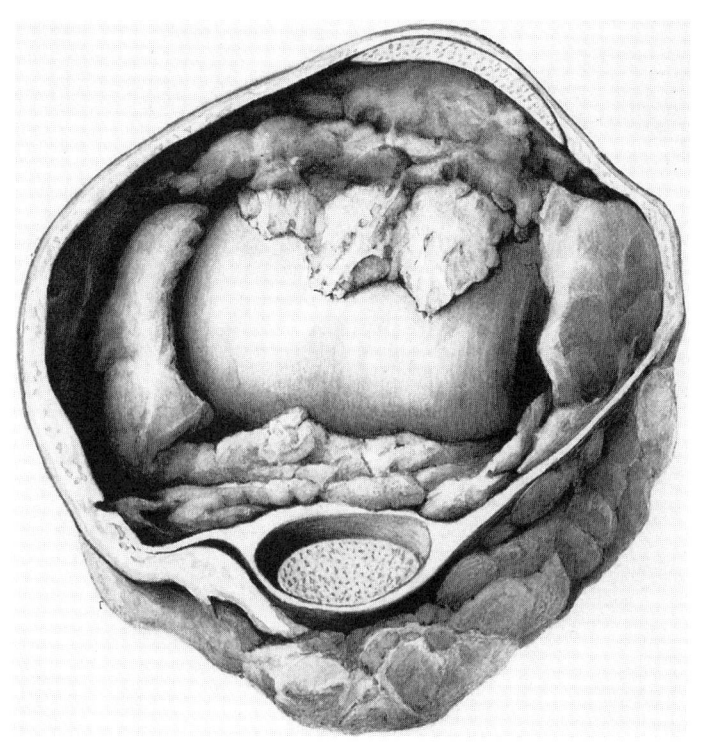

FIGURE 1.—Einblik in ein rechtes Daumengrundgelenk von distal nach Entfernung der Basis der Grundphalanx (Zeichnung nach einem anatomischen Präparat). (Courtesy of Putz RV, Sowa G: Menisci and synovial folds of the metacarpophalangeal joint of the thumb [German]. *Handchir Mikrochir Plast Chir* 29:316–320, 1997.)

In this paper, the normal variation of synovial plicas and menisci, such as tissue configuration within the joint, is described.

This basic anatomical knowledge is necessary so that normal anatomical situations are not confused with pathologic conditions of the MP joint of the thumb during arthroscopy.

In addition, this paper demonstrates nicely that the incongruity of the bony elements within the joint is rectified by soft tissue; thus, a biomechanical task for this tissue configuration can be anticipated.

This paper enhances the anatomical knowledge necessary for successful hand surgery procedures at the MP joint level.

Priv.-Doz. Dr. Med. C.L. Jantea

Suggested Reading

Dvir Z: The measurement of isokinetic finger flexion strength. *Clin Biomechanics* 12:473–481, 1998.

▶ The author cleverly adopted the KinCom 125 Dynamometer for the measurement of concentric and eccentric contraction of hand muscle in grip function. The KinCom Dynamometer was commonly used for the strength evaluation of larger joints where the resolutions for force and angular measurements were different for those of smaller joints. However, the typical curve of the tension–velocity relationship of the muscle physiology was demonstrated. Dynamic hand grip function involved the movement of multiple joints. Ideally, more precise documentation and definition of the angular velocities of individual joints of the hand should be considered. From those data, the muscle contraction speed based on the tendon excursion could then be accurately determined. In addition, the posture of wrist joint had been found to be important for hand grip strength as well. These points should be considered in future studies. The clinical application of such isokinetic strength evaluation of hand is yet to be determined.

K-N. An, M.D.

Grossman JAI, Yen L, Rapaport D: The dorsal cutaneous branch of the ulnar nerve: An anatomic clarification with six case reports. *Ann Chir Main* 17:154–158, 1998.
▶ Injury to the dorsal branch of the ulnar nerve is not rare and may become increasingly common as more percutaneous procedures are done about the wrist. A wise surgeon will use blunt dissection and tissue protectors to minimize the risk of nerve injury when inserting Kirschner wires and endoscopic equipment in this area.

P.C. Amadio, M.D.

Lee JCH: Anatomical basis of the vascularized pronator quadratus pedicled bone graft. *J Hand Surg [Br]* 22B:644–646, 1997.
▶ Sadly, the authors—despite trials—could not give incontrovertible evidence that the anterior interosseous artery alone could nourish a radial bone graft carried on a pronator quadratus pedicle. Nonetheless, the demonstration of a constant anterior interosseous arterial branch found in the pedicle does support the notion that such grafts, done properly, are truly vascularized. I hope the authors persist in attempts to demonstrate flow into the already elevated bone graft by interosseous cannulation.

R.A. Chase, M.D.

Lieber RL, Ljung BO, Fridén J: Sarcomere length in wrist extensor muscles. Changes may provide insights into the etiology of chronic lateral epicondylitis. *Acta Orthop Scand* 68:249–254, 1997.
▶ Using an intraoperative laser diffraction technique to study extensor carpi radialis brevis (ECRB) sarcomere length in 13 patients with tennis elbow undergoing ECRB lengthening, the authors show that ECRB sarcomeres increase in length twice and decrease in length twice over the range of elbow flexion, presumably due to the moment arm of the ECRB at the elbow changing from flexion to extension. The ECRB is estimated to operate on the descending region of the force–length relation. Based on the force–velocity relation for muscles undergoing lengthening (and shortening), the authors also estimate that muscle force changes dramatically during elbow flexion. They suggest that these intense eccentric contractions, which are known to cause muscle damage and inflam-

mation, may be the etiology behind tennis elbow. Further studies are needed on healthy subjects and more patients to assess their assertion.

F.E. Zajac, Ph.D.

Russell GV, Stern PJ: The phylogeny of the wrist. *Am J Orthop* 27:494–498, 1998.
▶ It is unfortunate that this review article does not lend itself to abstracting in the YEAR BOOK format. The commentary and illustrations are excellent; the authors guide us phylogenetically through wrist development, from the dinosaurs through other primates to man. I highly recommend this work to all readers with an interest in comparative anatomy.

P.C. Amadio, M.D.

Valero-Cuevas FJ, Small CF: Load dependence in carpal kinematics during wrist flexion *in vivo*. *Clin Biomechanics* 12:154–159, 1997.
▶ A simple mechanical linkage was designed and built to study in vivo wrist flexion–extension kinematics under load. Ten healthy subjects flexed their wrists under 3 different loads. The center of rotation was found to depend on the load. This technique of testing wrist kinematics may be a sensitive technique to detect wrist pathology. Further studies on patients will be needed, however.

F.E. Zajac, Ph.D.

Voche P, Merle M: Our experience with the anterior interosseous artery. *La Main* 2:219–224, 1997.
▶ The anatomy of the terminal branches of the anterior interosseous artery (AIOA) was clarified by Martin in 1989.[1] There are 2 dorsal branches, proximal and distal, and the latter anastomoses distally with the dorsal carpal vessels, initiating the principle of reverse flow Y-V extension of a pedicle flap (which they fully described in a latter article[2]). Hu et al. described an AIO reverse flow flap based on the proximal artery (with ligation of the AIOA just proximal to the branching of this proximal branch), vascularized through the dorsal carpal network, with a large arc of rotation, down to the fingernails.[3] The authors seem to have been satisfied with this flap, although they had one case of complete loss of the flap, and they state that there is generally an edema of the flap for 3–4 days, which necessitated the use of leeches in 1 case.

Voche and Merle, from Nancy (France), have extensive personal experience in the field of vascularized flaps in the upper limb, as attested by the number and the variety of papers from their team in the recent literature. Among others, their team has reported on the use of the pronator quadratus free flap, based on the volar terminal branch of the AIOA. One is therefore sensitive to their disarray after the third consecutive failure with this flap. There have been examples in the past of new techniques that were reliable in the authors' hands only. Further reports on this flap are needed.

Finally, Voche and Merle recommend the use of only the distal (terminal) dorsal branch of the AIOA for island flaps whether to direct or to reverse flow. This branch has an average diameter of 0.8 mm and its dissection is easier. It is less versatile, however, covering defects only down to the metacarpal heads.

C. LeClercq, M.D.

References

1. Martin D, Rivet D, Boileau R, et al: The posterior radial epiphysis free flap: A new donor site. *Br J Plast Surg* 42:499–506, 1989.
2. Martin D, Legaillard P, Bakhach J, et al: Reverse flow YV pedicle extension: A method of doubling the arc of rotation of a flap under certain conditions [French]. *Ann Chir Plast Esthet* 39:403–414, 1994.
3. Hu W, Martin D, Foucher G, et al: Anterior interosseus flap [French]. *Ann Chir Plast Esthet* 39:290–300, 1994.

2 Diagnosis, Evaluation, and Anesthesia

Validity of Observer-based Aggregate Scoring Systems as Descriptors of Elbow Pain, Function, and Disability
Turchin DC, Beaton DE, Richards RR (Scarborough, Ont; Inst for Work and Health, Toronto; St Michael's Hosp, Toronto)
J Bone Joint Surg Am 80-A:154–162, 1998   2–1

Purpose.—Currently used elbow scoring systems rely on observer assessments of clinical and functional criteria. After these criteria are scored separately and aggregated, the aggregate score is ranked as poor to excellent. The various systems use different outcome criteria, weight the criteria differently, and assign different values to each category ranking. To evaluate the validity of differing elbow scoring systems, 5 systems were used to assess the same group of patients.

Methods.—The study sample comprised 69 patients with elbow problems who sought care at referral clinics. The 5 systems assessed were the Mayo elbow-performance index and the scoring systems described by Broberg and Morrey, Ewald et al., The Hospital for Special Surgery, and Pritchard. Various instruments were used to evaluate the validity of the scoring systems, including visual analogue scales for pain and function, physician and patient ratings of the severity of elbow impairments, and 2 patient-completed functional questionnaires. The raw aggregate scores of the various systems were compared, and the level of agreement among categorical rankings was assessed.

Results.—Comparison of raw scores showed good correlation among the various systems. However, comparison of categorical rankings revealed only slight to moderate correlation. The most discriminating systems on validity testing were that of Ewald et al. and the Mayo elbow-performance index, followed by the systems of The Hospital for Special Surgery and of Broberg and Morrey, and, finally, the system of Pritchard. Correlation with the functional score on the visual analogue scale was only moderate for the 5 scoring systems but moderate to good for the patient-completed functional questionnaires.

Conclusions.—The 5 elbow scoring systems evaluated disagree substantially when used to evaluate the same group of patients. The findings suggest that the results of these systems should be expressed as raw scores rather than as categorical rankings. Patient-completed functional questionnaires give a better picture of perceived functional loss than the elbow scoring systems do. The findings show that it is not valid to compare the results of studies that use different scoring systems. The best approach to evaluating the outcomes of treatment for elbow problems is a patient-derived functional assessment, a clinical examination, and a pain assessment.

▶ Fortunately, the evaluation of clinical outcomes is evolving in a scientific fashion in orthopedics. This excellent study by the Toronto group, which has significant experience in this area of clinical outcomes assessment, brings to our attention a number of facts of which we should be aware.

First, the categorization of patients into excellent, good, fair, or poor outcomes according to a numerical score that has been averaged over a group of categories is not a scientifically reliable method for evaluating or comparing patients. However, the application of a raw score is useful, provided the outcomes tool is used consistently from one patient to the next. The different scores evaluated in this study have their own merits, which is not surprising when one considers that they were derived for different purposes. Self-assessment by the patient correlated best with functional impairment, which has already been shown in other areas involving outcomes assessments.

As orthopedic surgeons, we tend to be unaware of the extent to which the science of questionnaires and outcomes tools has been developed in other fields. These tools have been used for several decades in marketing, industry, and commerce. In other areas of medicine, outcomes assessment tools have been well investigated, tested, and validated. The process of development of a proper outcomes tool must be followed and, inasmuch as these various scales were not derived by employing such techniques, it should not be surprising that they may not be as valid as we would like. This highlights the emphasis on further clinical research in the development of an appropriate scale for measuring outcome after elbow surgery.

S.W. O'Driscoll, M.D., Ph.D., F.R.C.S.C.

Operative Fluoroscopy in Hand and Upper Limb Surgery: One Hundred Cases
Bain GI, Hunt J, Mehta JA (Modbury Public Hosp, South Australia)
J Hand Surg [Br] 22B:656–658, 1997   2–2

Introduction.—Foot and ankle surgery using the C-arm of the new generation of fluoroscopy units has been reported, but its use in hand and upper limb surgery has not been described. The clinical experience with portable operative fluoroscopy in hand and upper limb surgery in 58 trauma and 42 elective procedures was reported.

Methods.—All 100 patients were treated by one surgeon using a 3-inch Fluoroscan unit. The unit is smaller than conventional fluoroscopy machines and has an adjustable boom that allows the mini C-arm to be placed in any position. An onboard computer automatically adjusts voltage and amperage to produce high-quality images with minimal radiation.

Results.—The most common use of fluoroscopy was closed reduction and percutaneous K-wire fixation of distal radial fractures. Other trauma applications included 8 cases of closed reduction of fractures; 25 cases of percutaneous reduction of fractures; 12 cases of arthroscopic-assisted reduction of fractures; 8 cases of application of proximal interphalangeal joint Compass Hinge; 2 cases of humeral closed intramedullary nailing; and 3 cases of foreign bodies. Elective procedures included 7 cases of limited and full wrist fusion; 2 cases of carpometacarpal joint fusion; 4 cases involving examination of joint stability; 3 cases of arthroscopic "ectomy" procedures; 3 cases of diagnostic joint injection; 3 cases of localization of bone tumor; and 20 cases of removal of implants.

Conclusions.—The portable fluoroscopy unit has diagnostic and therapeutic capabilities that are useful in hand and upper limb surgery. The portability of this unit eliminates the need to transport patients to radiology.

▶ The incorporation of image enhancement technology has resulted in the development of small fluoroscopy units that provide relatively good resolution with very minimal radiation exposure. Two units dominate the market in the United States. This article from our Australian colleagues documents the effectiveness of such devices both in the clinic and the operating room for a variety of indications including guiding fracture reduction, diagnostic injections, joint stability, etc. In my hospital, the radiation safety experts recommend lead gloves to avoid hand exposure but don't require us to wear lead aprons if we are more that 12 inches from the beam. I can't imagine doing without these devices today. Our radiology colleagues are not particularly happy, however, because their use results in reduced fees.

V.R. Hentz, M.D.

The Role of Neurophysiological Investigation in Traumatic Brachial Plexus Lesions in Adults and Children
Smith SJM (Natl Hosp, London)
J Hand Surg [Br] 21B:145–147, 1996   2–3

Background.—Neurophysiologic studies are important for establishing the type, severity, and localization of injuries to the brachial plexus and provide valuable information about the degree of recovery after surgery.

Nerve Injury.—Electrophysiologic testing can distinguish among the 3 types of nerve injuries: neurapraxic lesions, axonotmesis, and neurotmesis.

Localization.—Lesion levels and sites can be delineated with a combination of sensory action potentials, somatosensory evoked potentials, and electromyography (EMG).

Neurophysiologic Evaluation in Adults.—Surgical repair, if necessary, is usually performed within a few days of the injury. Neurophysiologic studies can be performed intraoperatively to confirm whether a nerve or root lesion is in continuity and postoperatively to determine the degree of reinnervation. Collateral reinnervation is usually apparent at 3–6 months if less than 60% to 70% of axons are damaged. Regular neurophysiologic assessments during recovery can be used to track improvement and establish the need for surgery if improvement is less than anticipated.

Neurophysiologic Investigation of Obstetric Brachial Plexopathy.—Preoperative neurophysiologic evaluation in 30 patients was valuable in determining the type of lesion and predicting outcome after surgery. Neurophysiologic testing in infants as young as 4 months of age revealed a neurapraxic lesion in 5 infants with normal nerve action potentials and motor unit activity on EMG denoting conduction block. With conservative management, all had full functional recovery at 12 months. Because none of these infants had evidence of biceps recovery at 3 months, all would otherwise have been candidates for surgery. Neurolysis was performed in 13 infants with good neural recruitment on EMG and evidence of collateral reinnervation. Functional outcome in these infants was very good at 12 months. Indications for surgery depend on the size of the nerve action potentials.

Conclusion.—Neurophysiologic evaluation can reveal the size and location of the lesion in obstetric brachial plexopathy, indicate whether surgery is necessary, and distinguish a neurapraxic lesion from more serious lesions. Infants with neurapraxic lesions make excellent recoveries when managed conservatively.

▶ This is a review article with some useful information, from the perspective of the neurophysiologist, regarding the predictive usefulness of EMG and nerve conduction data in adult and obstetric brachial plexus injuries. My experience has not been as rewarding. For example, I have not found EMG helpful in decision making for infants with plexus injuries. It takes only a few regenerating fibers to generate a familiar report: "muscles show evidence of denervation-reinnervation."

Because a number of research and clinical studies have shown no good correlation between the numbers of axons that regenerate across an injury or repair site and ultimate function, one must be circumspect regarding the information that neurophysiologic studies provide. Perhaps there are differences in technique from clinic to clinic that permit more meaningful information.

V.R. Hentz, M.D.

Arthrography Is Superior to Magnetic Resonance Imaging for Diagnosing Injuries of the Triangular Fibrocartilage

Shionoya K, Nakamura R, Imaeda T, et al (Nagoya Univ, Japan; Toyota Mem Hosp, Japan)
J Hand Surg [Br] 23B:402–405, 1998

Background.—In patients with ulnar wrist pain, triangular fibrocartilage (TFC) injury must be part of the differential diagnosis. Imaging modalities used to evaluate TFC injury include wrist arthrography, MRI, and arthroscopy, which is the gold standard. The effectiveness of arthrography and MRI in comparison to arthroscopy for diagnosing TFC injury in patients with ulnar wrist pain were compared.

Methods.—The subjects were 102 patients with wrist pain (80 men and 22 women, mean age, 32 years) who initially underwent physical and radiographic examination. Trauma was the cause in 56 patients, and included 35 cases of nonunion of a scaphoid fracture, 3 cases of an ulnar styloid fracture, 2 cases of a distal radial fracture, and 16 cases in which the radiographs were unremarkable. The wrist pain was spontaneous in the remaining 46 patients; 27 had Kienböck's disease, and 19 had pain but no bone or joint abnormality. All patients underwent single-injection radiocarpal arthrography (contrast leakage from the radiocarpal joint to the distal radioulnar joint was taken as TFC perforation), MRI (only the coronal plane images were examined), and arthroscopy (which was the standard of reference).

Findings.—Arthroscopy identified a full-thickness TFC tear in 41 (40.2%) patients, arthrography identified 35 (34.3%) tears, and MRI identified 47 (46.1%) tears. Compared with arthroscopy, the sensitivity of arthrography was 85%, specificity was 100%, and accuracy was 92%. In 6 patients, arthrography failed to identify TFC injury. Four of these patients had a perforated TFC, and fibrous tissue had regenerated at the perforation site. This situation created a "one-way flap valve" and explained the false-negative results in these 4 patients. In the other 2 patients, large amounts of the contrast medium leaked into the midcarpal joint, which obscured flow into the distal radioulnar joint. Compared with arthroscopy, MRI had a sensitivity of 73%, a specificity of 72%, and an accuracy of 73%. Of 17 patients with false-positive findings, TFC wear or elongation was evident in 7 with arthroscopy but no perforations were observed in the other 10 patients, the surface of the TFC was intact. Of the 11 patients with false-negative findings, arthroscopy found a slit tear in 6, a small perforation in 3, and round tears in 2.

Conclusions.—Single-injection radiocarpal arthrography was more sensitive, specific, and accurate than MRI in the detection of full-thickness TFC tears. Shortcomings of arthrography include difficulties in distinguishing degenerative tears, traumatic tears, and pin-hole perforations. An additional shortcoming of MRI is that its limited spatial resolution makes interpreting images a challenge.

▶ Arthroscopy was the gold standard for this study, and in my practice, arthroscopy has more or less replaced both arthrography and MRI for the evaluation of intra-articular pathology of the wrist.

P.C. Amadio, M.D.

Combining the Clinical Signs Improves Diagnosis of Scaphoid Fractures: A Prospective Study With Follow-up
Parvizi J, Wayman J, Kelly P, et al (Newcastle Gen Hosp, Newcastle upon Tyne, England; Univ of Newcastle upon Tyne, England)
J Hand Surg [Br] 23B:324–327, 1998   2–5

Background.—Scaphoid fractures are a diagnostic dilemma. Although most are diagnosed from radiographs, false positives do occur, and the false negative rate may be as high as 16%. Clinical examination, although a cornerstone of diagnosis, is also fallible. The classic clinical signs of scaphoid fracture were assessed to determine if their combination significantly improved the diagnosis.

Methods.—The subjects were 215 patients (52% male, median age, 28 years) coming to the emergency department within 24 hours after an acute wrist injury that suggested scaphoid fracture. The physical examination included evaluation of tenderness at the anatomical snuff box (ASB), tenderness at the scaphoid tubercle (ST), tenderness with longitudinal compression (LC), and the range of thumb movement (TM). Results were compared with findings in the uninjured hand. Then standard-view radiographs of the scaphoid were taken. All wrists were splinted until patients could be evaluated at the fracture clinic (within 48 hours). Radiographs were repeated at 2 and 6 weeks if clinical or radiologic signs suggested a scaphoid fracture. Based on clinical and radiologic findings, the patients were split into 3 groups. Group 1 comprised patients who had a scaphoid fracture evident on radiographs. Group 2 comprised patients who had a normal radiograph, but whose clinical examination suggested fracture, and group 3 consisted of patients who had pain, but no clinical or radiographic evidence of scaphoid fracture.

Findings.—Initially, there were 48 patients in group 1, 141 in group 2, and 26 in group 3. At the 2-week radiographic evaluation, another 3 fractures were evident, and at 6 weeks another 5 fractures were found (Table 1). Overall, then, approximately 25% of the patients (56 of 215) had a scaphoid fracture. At the initial evaluation, all of these patients had ASB and ST tenderness and tenderness on LC (i.e., sensitivity 100%), and 37 patients had impaired TM (sensitivity 69%). Corresponding specificities at the initial evaluation were 19% (ASB), 30% (AST), 48% (LC), and 66% (TM). Nonetheless, the false-positive rates at initial evaluation were also high, 84% (ASB), 71% (ST), 58% (LC), and 50% (TM). However, if

TABLE 1.—Subgroups of Patients Based on Clinical and Radiologic Findings

	At presentation	At 2 weeks	At 6 weeks
Fracture diagnosed by imaging (Group 1)	48	51	56
Normal imaging (Group 2)	141	138	133*
Normal imaging: clinically non-tender (Group 3)	26	0	0

Note: The figures for group 1 represent the cumulative numbers of patients who were diagnosed as having scaphoid fractures at the different stages of the study. The imaging at presentation and 2 weeks was by plain radiographs and at 6 weeks by radioisotope bone scan (n = 5). Group 3 patients were assumed to have soft tissue injury and had 1 radiograph examination only. The decrease in group 2 throughout the study corresponds to the increase in group 1. Patients in group 1 by the end of the study are termed "fractures." Patients in groups 2 and 3 at the end of the study are the "nonfractures."
*Within this number are included 18 patients who failed to attend for 6-week review.
(Courtesy of Parvizi J, Wayman J, Kelly P, et al: Combining the clinical signs improves diagnosis of scaphoid fractures: A prospective study with follow-up. J Hand Surg [Br] 23B:324–327, 1998.)

ASB, ST, and LC tenderness were all positive at the initial evaluation, then specificity improved to 74%, and sensitivity remained at 100%.

Conclusions.—The initial radiograph examination missed 8 scaphoid fractures (14%). Similarly, all 4 of the individual clinical signs assessed had high false-positive rates. However, ASB, ST, and LC tenderness in combination is a good clue to scaphoid fracture. However, some patients who had negative clinical signs at the initial examination had positive signs at the 2-week check-up, and vice-versa. Thus, these conclusions can be applied only to the initial assessment.

▶ Using a diagnostic gold standard of repeated radiographs and bone scans, the authors of this article teach us 2 things. First, that clinical examination can raise a suspicion of scaphoid fracture and is good at identifying suspect cases. The examination criteria selected picked up all fractures; unfortunately they also falsely identified twice as many unfractured scaphoids. These tests should be used only for screening, and even then many tests perhaps deemed "unnecessary" in retrospect by third parties will have been ordered. The second thing we learn is that when there is no pain on palpation of the scaphoid, either in the ASB, by LC, or at the tubercle, the likelihood of fracture is extremely low (zero, in this series) and in such cases, radiographs or other imaging can be safely forgone (assuming, of course, that examination does not raise suspicion of other injuries!).

P.C. Amadio, M.D.

Gamekeeper Thumb: Comparison of MR Arthrography With Conventional Arthrography and MR Imaging in Cadavers
Ahn JM, Sartoris DJ, Kang HS, et al (Veterans Affairs Med Ctr, San Diego, Calif; Seoul Natl Univ Hosp, Korea)
Radiology 206:737–744, 1998   2–6

Purpose.—The term "gamekeeper thumb" now refers to any chronic or acute injury to the ulnar collateral ligament (UCL) of the first metacarpophalangeal (MCP) joint. The UCL damage occurs because of violent abduction of the thumb; unless the injury is recognized and treated, it can lead to permanent instability or degenerative disease of the MCP joint. Various imaging techniques have been evaluated for use in detecting these injuries, including arthrography, ultrasound, and MRI. The MR arthrography and conventional arthrography findings of gamekeeper thumb were compared.

Methods.—Eighteen cadaver thumbs, 12 with and 6 without experimental abduction stress were studied. All thumbs were imaged by conventional arthrography, standard MRI, and MR arthrography. The MRI studies were performed with both 0.2-T extremity-only and 1.5-T magnets. The images were read in blinded fashion and the results compared with the pathologic findings. Conventional MRI scans and MR arthrograms were paired and compared on a 3-point scale.

Results.—Abduction stress caused tearing of 14 UCLs—57% of the tears were nondisplaced and 43% displaced. Accuracy in detecting the presence of a tear was 83% for conventional arthrography, 89% for low-field-strength MRI, 90% for high-field-strength MRI, 94% for low-field-strength MR arthrography, and 100% for high-field strength MR arthrography. Accuracy in recognizing ligamentous displacement was 61% for conventional arthrography, 89% for low-field-strength MRI, 90% for high-field-strength MRI, 94% for low-field-strength MR arthrography, and 100% for high-field-strength MR arthrography. Magnetic resonance arthrography was rated superior to standard MRI on low-field-strength scans in 72% of cases and on high-field-strength scans in 90%.

Conclusions.—Magnetic resonance arthrography appears to be the most sensitive technique for the diagnosis of gamekeeper thumb. Compared with standard arthrography and standard MRI scanning, MR arthrography is more accurate in recognizing tearing of the UCL of the first MCP joint, as well as displacement of the torn ligament.

▶ There is a general consensus that the UCL should be explored and repaired surgically when, after an injury, a complete disruption of the UCL of the thumb MCP joint is suspected and no avulsion fracture is present. The reason for this consensus is that if the ligament avulsion is off the base of the proximal phalanx and the ligament has folded back upon itself proximally, as described by Stenner, immobilization alone, without surgical repair, will be unsuccessful. Surgical exploration is a reasonable approach because there has not been an imaging study that can reliably identify UCL injuries that are of the Stenner type.

The authors have tried to address this deficit by comparing MR arthrography with conventional arthrography and MR imaging in a cadaver population in which a hyperabduction force has been inflicted with the thumb MCP joint in flexion. Whenever consideration is given to using such specialized imaging studies, the cost, as well as the availability of necessary coil size, an up-to-date MRI and software, as well as technical expertise in using MR arthrographic techniques, are often questioned. However, the reliability and specificity of the MR arthrography that the authors report, at the very least, would suggest additional consideration should be given to this technique, and should encourage the authors to assess MR arthrography in the clinical setting of patients with thumb MCP joint UCL injuries. It is always valuable to be able to identify which patients can benefit from surgery and which can improve with nonsurgical treatment.

S.F. Viegas, M.D.

The "Tic-Tac-Toe" Classification System for Mutilating Injuries of the Hand
Weinzweig J, Weinzweig N (Brown Univ, Providence, RI; Univ of Illinois, Chicago)
Plast Reconstr Surg 100:1200–1211, 1997

Objective.—The mutilated hand has lost prehension, and without surgical reconstruction will be virtually functionless. A classification system is necessary to describe injuries accurately and reproducibly. The "Tic-Tac-Toe" classification system incorporates the degree and precise location of soft tissue and/or bony destruction and the vascular integrity, in addition to the predominantly involved part of the hand.

Methods.—Injuries are categorized into type I, dorsal mutilation; type II, palmar mutilation; type III, ulnar mutilation; type IV, radial mutilation; type V, transverse amputations; type VI, degloving injuries; and type VII, combination injuries. Injury subtypes include soft tissue loss (A); bony loss (B); and combined tissue loss (C). Vascular integrity, recorded as a subscript, is classified as 0, vascularization intact or 1, devascularization.

Conclusions.—The "Tic-Tac-Toe" classification system divides the hand into 9 zones and permits a description of injuries by location.

▶ The authors present a classification system for mutilating injuries of the hand. The system seeks to integrate description of injury orientation (radial, ulnar, dorsal, volar), mechanism (degloving), soft tissue and skeletal involvement, and vascularity with a 9-zone regional anatomical classification grid for localization.

Examples of complex hand injuries presented by the authors do fit their classification scheme. Ultimately, the classification could produce data allowing comparison of different kinds of injuries and treatment variables within a specific injury classification.

The authors neglect to provide a way of including nerve injuries in their classification. This deficit will need to be addressed if this scheme is applied to outcome studies where nerve function can be a critical factor.

Reviewing this paper is a good exercise for a hand surgeon and provokes thought on how we record our findings and results in these difficult injuries. The value of the scheme will ultimately be established by whether it provides a useful framework for collecting and analyzing data from these complex cases.

W.C. Lineaweaver, M.D.

Normal Digit Tip Values for the Weinstein Enhanced Sensory Test
Schulz LA, Bohannon RW, Morgan WJ (Univ of Massachusetts, Worcester; Univ of Connecticut, Storrs)
J Hand Ther 11:200–205, 1998   2–8

Background.—A variety of tools have been developed to objectively measure specific nerve function. The Weinstein Enhanced Sensory Test (WEST), a noninvasive evaluation of threshold of light touch, was designed to test cutaneous sensibility. It is performed with a calibrated monofilament esthesiometer. Normal values for the WEST are established and whether certain factors can affect normal WEST values is determined.

Methods.—One hundred twenty persons with no clinical evidence of peripheral neuropathy or subjective changes in digit tip sensation were tested. In addition, the subjects completed a questionnaire and underwent neurometric median nerve testing and a brief clinical assessment.

Findings.—Age significantly affected WEST values. An interaction effect was noted between age and gender. The WEST values for individual digits in an individual were strongly correlated, as were WEST and electroneurometer values. Normal values were 0.035 g for men and women aged 55 years or younger, 0.15 g for women older than 55 years, and 0.385 g for men older than 55 years.

Conclusions.—The WEST seems to be useful for assessing digit tip sensibility. It can be applied quickly and easily in a clinical setting using the rapid threshold procedure. Age- and sex-specific normal values must be considered when interpreting the test results.

▶ For those who prefer monofilament testing for sensibility measurement, these normal values should be a help. The WEST test seems reliable. Other reports should address its validity, sensitivity, and responsiveness for various clinical uses.

P.C. Amadio, M.D.

Recovery of Sensory and Motor Function After Nerve Repair: A Rationale for Evaluation
Rosén B (Lund Univ, Malmö, Sweden)
J Hand Ther 9:315–327, 1996

Background.—Recovery of hand function relies on 4 key factors: (1) the structural and functional status of peripheral sensory and motor components; (2) tactile gnosis; (3) integrated sensory and motor functions; and (4) the degree of hyperesthesia and cold intolerance. A battery of tests that measures these 4 factors was sought.

Methods and Findings.—Twenty-five patients, aged 10–53 years, were assessed 2–5 years after median or ulnar nerve repair at the distal forearm level. The results of clinical tests for reinnervation were uncorrelated with results from neurophysiologic assessment. Together, grip strength and cold intolerance accounted for a significant 51% of the variance in capability for activities of daily living (ADL). Tactile gnosis was weakly associated with ADL capability and strongly with age.

Conclusions.—Reinnervation (structural and functional status) after median and ulnar nerve repair should be assessed by Semmes-Weinstein monofilaments and manual muscle-testing. Tactile gnosis should be assessed by 2-point discrimination (static and moving) tests and by shape indentification tests. Integrated sensory and motor functions are best measured by Sollerman's grip test and by Jamar's dynamometer grip-strength test. Assessment of hyperesthesia and cold intolerance in ADL can be done by a self-administered questionnaire with patient answers ranked on a 4-point scale from 1 (no effect) to 4 (hinders function).

▶ Sophisticated tests of nerve function may quantify neurophysiology, but they do little to predict clinical function. Age has been shown to be the strongest predictor, as anyone who has done a nerve repair in an infant will attest. Simple measures such as grip, minikit Semmes-Weinstein monofilament testing, shape identification, static 2PD, and a simple pain scale seem sufficient to capture the main parameters. The article contains useful detail on each of the 25 patients studied. I recommend a close reading to all those interested in nerve repair and rehabilitation.

P.C. Amadio, M.D.

Lack of Difference in Sensibility Between the Dominant and Non-Dominant Hands as Tested With Semmes–Weinstein Monofilaments
Van Turnhout AAWM, Hage JJ, De Groot PJM, et al (Vrije Universiteit, Amsterdam)
J Hand Surg [Br] 22B:768–771, 1997

Objective.—Previous studies have shown differences in sensibility between dominant and nondominant index fingers in a minority of individuals. Whether a difference in sensibility is also present in the palmar side of the hand was investigated using the Semmes-Weinstein monofilament test.

Methods.—Testing was performed by 1 investigator using 8 different monofilaments on 22 areas on the palmar aspects of both hands in 50 normal volunteers (21 men), aged 21–60 years. Sensibilities between dominant and nondominant hands were compared.

Results.—Six volunteers (1 man) were left-handed. The sensibility of dominant and nondominant hands was similar in 51% of volunteers, superior in the nondominant hands in 34%, and superior in the dominant hands in 15%.

Conclusion.—There is no difference in distribution of difference in sensibility between dominant and nondominant hands in over half of subjects. Sensibility is superior in the nondominant hand in approximately one third of subjects and in the dominant hand in about 15%.

▶ A previous study showed equal or better sensibility in the pulp of the nondominant vs. the dominant index finger. These authors tested multiple sites in 50 healthy volunteers and found no difference between these palmar sites in 51%, better sensibility in all the nondominant sites in 34%, and better sensibility in the dominant hand in 15%.

V.R. Hentz, M.D.

Pharmacoeconomics of Intravenous Regional Anaesthesia vs General Anaesthesia for Outpatient Hand Surgery
Chilvers CR, Kinahan A, Vaghadia H, et al (Univ of British Columbia, Vancouver)
Can J Anaesth 44:1152–1156, 1997   2–11

Background.—Regional anesthesia seems to have many advantages over general anesthesia (GA) for outpatient surgery. However, there are few available comparisons of regional and general anesthesia for ambulatory surgery, and many of the advantages of regional anesthesia have not been verified. The efficacy and costs of IV regional anesthesia (IVRA) and GA for outpatient hand surgery were compared.

Methods.—One hundred twenty-one patients given IVRA were compared with 64 patients given GA. The 2 groups were well matched for weight, sex, and American Society of Anesthesiologists class. However, patients given IVRA were older and had a lower frequency of 2 types of surgery. Efficacy was determined by time to anesthesia, recovery, and discharge; percentage of patients with unsatisfactory anesthesia; and complications.

Findings.—Median direct variable costs were $24.60 and $48.66 for the IVRA and GA groups, respectively. Anesthesia was unsatisfactory in 11% of the patients given IVRA and in none given GA. Patients receiving IVRA recovered faster, with a median time to discharge of 70 and 118 minutes in the IVRA and GA groups, respectively. Five percent of the patients given

GA had vomiting that necessitated treatment. In addition, 5% had dizziness that delayed discharge. Neither of these complications occurred in the IVRA group.

Conclusions.—Compared with GA, IVRA was less effective in satisfactory anesthesia, equally effective in time to administer anesthesia, and more effective in speeding recovery and minimizing complications after surgery. The cost of IVRA was only half that of GA.

▶ Chilvers, et al., perform a cost-effective analysis comparing 2 anesthetic techniques, IVRA and GA, for outpatient hand surgery during 1 year.

The significance of this article is that the authors considered the importance of cost accounting in defining cost. The cost of anesthesia and the cost of recovery were accurately reflected in this study. By Chilvers' report, IVRA creates value. While total cost was reduced, with IVRA the outcomes did not change. One not-so-obvious limitation of the authors' accounting technique was the neglect of variable to total cost ratio. Total cost is made up of fixed costs (overhead, the operating room, control desk, equipment) and variable costs (disposables, drugs, endotracheal tubes, needles). Marcario et al. identified the variable to total cost of many departments within a teaching hospital and the impact of using this ratio to determine cost.[1] The importance of knowing which parts of total costs are fixed and which are variable is that only reductions in variable costs will result in total cost reduction. Examples of variable-cost reductions are pharmacy wastage minimization, reducing recovery time, and using less expensive supplies and pharmaceuticals.

The importance of cost-effective analysis is comparing outcomes. Although this was a retrospective study and the authors could not ascertain patient satisfaction directly, the authors conjectured that patient satisfaction with IVRA could be related to anesthesia success. Previous studies demonstrated 96% patient satisfaction with 84% anesthesia success rate.[2] It is difficult to argue that a similar patient satisfaction would not result with the IVRA success rate of 89%.

In a cost-conscious environment, it is important that physicians be able to evaluate the financial costs and medical benefits from their medical decisions that may conflict with an overall attempt to minimize costs. It is clear that supply costs alone do not provide justification to use 1 anesthesia technique over the other. However, when drug cost and recovery profiles are also measured, then changes in clinical practice should be considered.

J.M. Navarro, M.D.

References

1. Marcario A, Vitez T, Dunn B, et al: What does perioperative care really cost? Analysis of hospital costs and charges for inpatient surgical care. *Anesthesiology* 83:1138–1144, 1995.
2. Brown AR, Weiss R, Greenberg C, et al: Interscalene block for shoulder arthroscopy: Comparison with general anesthesia. *Arthroscopy* 9:295–300, 1993.

A Prospective Trial to Compare Three Anaesthetic Techniques Used for the Reduction of Fractures of the Distal Radius
Funk L (Bolton Royal Infirmary, England)
Injury 28:209–212, 1997

Background.—The reduction of distal radius fractures is usually performed under general anesthesia. This procedure is time consuming for both patients and staff. Hematoma blocks, with or without sedation, are used for fracture reduction by some hospital departments. A hematoma block, with or without sedation, was compared with general anesthesia for the reduction of distal radius fractures.

Methods.—A prospective study was performed in 58 patients seen during a 5-month period with distal radius fractures requiring manipulation. The study group consisted of 6 men and 52 women, aged 16–91 years of age. Of these 58 patients, 21 received a general anesthetic, 19 had a hematoma block, and 19 had a hematoma block with sedation (midazolam). Data were collected on patient pain (using a visual analogue scale), total waiting time for manipulation, length of procedure, radiographic reduction quality, and total cost.

Results.—No pain was experienced during manipulation in the general anesthesia group. Patients receiving hematoma blocks experienced some pain. The level of pain was higher in those who did not receive a sedative. After manipulation, the general anesthetic group experienced a return of initial pain. This pain was significantly reduced in the other 2 groups. Radiographically assessed reduction was good in all groups. There was a significantly longer waiting period before general anesthesia than for a hematoma block. The procedure time was also significantly longer in the general anesthetic group. Recovery time was longer with a general anesthetic. The cost of the general anesthetic was significantly higher than that for the hematoma block.

Conclusions.—This study compared the use of a hematoma block, with or without sedation, to general anesthesia in the reduction of fractures of the distal radius. A hematoma block with sedation was less expensive, was more efficient, and achieved excellent results with minimal patient pain.

▶ Fifty-eight patients with distal radial fractures underwent closed reduction using either a hematoma block, a hematoma block with sedation, or general anesthesia. The authors concluded that an adequate reduction can be achieved by any of the 3 types of anesthesia; however, the general anesthetic was obviously more expensive. The severity of the fracture configuration will often dictate the type of anesthesia. More severe comminution may require a general anesthetic to allow the surgeon to perform additional instrumentation such as percutaneous pinning or external fixation. In the same inclusion period for these 58 patients, an unknown number of patients were certainly not candidates for hematoma blocks but were not designated within the study.

P.C. Dell, M.D.

Suggested Reading

Brahme SK, Hodler J, Braun RM, et al: Dynamic MR imaging of carpal tunnel syndrome. *Skeletal Radiol* 26:482–487, 1997.
▶ In an attempt to increase the diagnostic utility of MRI in patients with dynamic carpal tunnel syndrome (causes symptoms only after repetitive motions of the wrist), MR of the wrist was performed both before and immediately after performance of standardized wrist exercises. MR changes previously described to indicate carpal tunnel syndrome were scored. It was shown that interval changes of these parameters had a high specificity but low sensitivity for diagnosing the dynamic type of carpal tunnel syndromes. Therefore, this exam may be of use in a subset of patients undergoing wrist MR.

G. Bergman, M.D.

Gillenson SP, Parets N, Bear-Lehman J, et al: The effect of wrist position on testing light touch sensation using the Semmes-Weinstein pressure aesthesiometer: A preliminary study. *J Hand Ther* 11:27–31, 1998.
▶ In normal subjects, Semmes-Weinstein filament sensibility is not altered if the wrist is held in extremes of flexion or extension. Loss of pressure sensibility at extremes of wrist position is likely to be a sign of nerve pathology.

P.C. Amadio, M.D.

McCabe SJ, Breidenbach WC, Herrand HA: The once-twice test for evaluation of the completely anesthetic digit. *Can J Plast Surg* 6:21–22, 1998.
▶ Here's a clever trick. Clinical assessment of sensibility requires patient cooperation, but how do you know if the patient is shamming? In patients who appear to have anesthesia without evident cause, after testing 2-point determination, the patient is asked whether the examiner has touched the affected digit once or twice in succession. This ability relies on proprioception, not cutaneous sensibility, and is almost always preserved unless the entire limb is affected, as in a complete brachial plexus injury or after replantation. If the patient reports that he or she is unable to distinguish 1 touch from 2, with the 2 touches administered a half-second or so apart, the test is considered positive and evidence of a nonphysiological response. The once–twice test seems worth a try, at least once or twice!

P.C. Amadio, M.D.

Tsujino A, Macnicol MF: Finger flexion sign for ulnar neuropathy. *J Hand Surg [Br]* 23B:240–241, 1998.
▶ It is not that difficult to diagnose early ulnar intrinsic motor palsy by a variety of known tests, but it is still appalling how seldom nerve function is adequately tested. Perhaps tests that involve visible malpositioning of digits, such as the Froment weak thumb pinch test or the authors' "finger flexion to augment weak adduction between the long and ring fingers" test, have a more dramatic impact and may therefore be more easily remembered AND DONE!

J.H. Dobyns, M.D.

Zanetti M, Hodler J, Gilula LA: Assessment of dorsal or ventral intercalated segmental instability configurations of the wrist: Reliability of sagittal MR images. *Radiology* 206:339–345, 1998.

▶ This study compared MR and x-ray images of the wrist in 10 normal volunteers. The MR images tended to depict the proximal row in more extension than did the x-rays, suggesting a DISI pattern (lunate extension) in 4 subjects with the wrist in neutral deviation and in 8 of the 10 with the wrist ulnarly deviated. Caution is necessary when interpreting carpal alignment from MR images.

P.C. Amadio, M.D.

3 Skeletal Trauma and Reconstruction

A Treatment Approach for Isolated Unicondylar Fractures of the Proximal Phalanx
Ramos LE, Becker GA, Grossman JAI (Miami Children's Hosp, Fla; Cabrini Med Ctr, New York)
Ann Chir Main 16:305–309, 1997   3–1

Background.—In patients with unicondylar fractures of the head of the proximal phalanx, surgical treatment usually gives poor results. The authors have developed a new rigid fixation protocol including a lag screw technique and continuous passive motion (CPM). Results in 5 patients are reported.

Technique.—The fractures were approached through a dorsal flap using loupe magnification. Entry to the joint was gained between the central extensor tendon and lateral band, with special care to avoid detaching the collateral ligament. The fracture fragment was reduced, stabilized with a Kirschner wire, and rigidly fixed using the lag screw technique. On the second or third day after surgery, a dorsal extension was applied with the proximal interphalangeal joint secured at approximately 15 degrees. CPM exercise, every other hour while the patient was awake, was started at this time. The frequency of use decreased to 1 hour on and 2 hours off at 4 weeks; CPM use was stopped at 6 weeks. The patients also performed active, isolated motion of the distal interphalangeal joint, with the metacarpophalangeal joint in 5–10 degrees of flexion, 10 times per hour. Patients with residual, symptomatic flexion contractures received a night extension splint or serial casting. For the first 6 months after surgery, the position of the digit was controlled with splints and Coban wrap.

Results.—The authors used this technique in 5 consecutive patients over a 4-year period. Active motion of the proximal interphalangeal joint averaged 87 degrees, with 2 patients having residual flexion contractures of 10–20 degrees. Total active motion averaged 241 degrees. No patient required additional surgery or reported subjective disability.

Conclusions.—This rigid fixation technique for the treatment of isolated unicondylar fractures of the proximal phalanx, followed by early CPM, provides excellent results. Control of postoperative pain and swelling through meticulous dissection and oral anti-inflammatory medications is an important part of the technique. As in other forms of hand therapy, excellent results are more likely to be achieved in patients who are compliant with therapy.

▶ The authors have reported excellent results in 5 of 5 cases of isolated unicondylar fractures treated with rigid fixation and immediate motion, with a combined use of CPM and controlled active motion. The 5 consecutive cases were all young men (aged 16–25) who were motivated to follow this demanding protocol. Four of the 5 were athletes.

The protocol calls for CPM use initiated 42–72 hours postoperatively and applied for 1 hour every other waking hour. A dorsal digital splint prevents proximal interphalangeal (PIP) extension beyond 15 degrees for the first 4 postoperative weeks. Active distal interphalangeal motion is performed 10 times every hour (presumably the PIP joint is manually stabilized to the dorsal splint for protection while flexor digitorum profundus gliding is effected). The patient applies active tension to the extensor system by actively extending the PIP joint to the limits of the dorsal digital splint, while positioning the metacarpophalangeal joint at 5–10 degrees of flexion (the most advantageous position for transmitting force to the zone 3 and 4 extensor digitorum communis).[1]

Although the excellent results support this postoperative management protocol, the use of CPM in a cost-containment health climate may not be practical or necessary. The authors acknowledge the problem of cost. Continuous passive motion machines rent at an average of $50.00 per day; 6 weeks of CPM could add another $2,100 or more to a case. Also, it is my clinical experience that it is difficult to get a precise fit for the ulnar fingers on most CPM models. The authors do not tell us which fingers were involved in these 5 cases. I would be concerned about accurate application by the patient, inappropriately applied external forces, and the application of appropriate forces to maintain the desired soft-tissue extensibility.

A compliant patient referred early (24–48 hours postoperatively) to a competent hand therapist for controlled active and passive motion, edema control, and precision splinting can probably obtain similar results. Hastings and Carrol[2] report an average of 12–91 degrees of PIP motion in 13 unicondylar fractures of the PIP joint treated with Kirschner wire (8), and screw (5) fixation and active range of motion started an average of 20 days postoperatively. Patient age ranged from 12 to 65; 3 fractures were to the small digit. While the patients' average PIP motion was 8 degrees less than that obtained by Ramos et al., initiating immediate controlled motion and precision digital splinting at the maximal allowed position of PIP extension, as tolerated by the fracture, would likely equalize these outcomes. Extensor tendon gliding, especially with a dorsal incision, should be the focus of hand rehabilitation in these cases.

R.B. Evans, O.T.R./L., C.H.T.

References

1. Evans RB, Thompson DE: An analysis of factors that support early active short arc motion of the repaired central slip. *J Hand Ther* 15:187–201, 1992.
2. Hastings H, Carrol C: Treatment of closed articular fractures of the metacarpophalangeal and proximal interphalangeal joints. *Hand Clin* 3:503–527, 1988.

Use of a Multiplanar Distracter for the Correction of a Proximal Interphalangeal Joint Contracture
Kasabian A, McCarthy J, Karp N (New York Univ)
Ann Plast Surg 40:378–381, 1998   3–2

Introduction.—Contractures of the proximal interphalangeal (PIP) joint may develop in patients with hand injuries or Dupuytren's contracture. Surgical release may be required in cases that do not respond to splinting or serial casting. During surgery, neurovascular overstretch may occur, causing digital nerve injury or vascular compromise. One approach to preventing this form of neurovascular injury may be gradual distraction of the contracted joint. This principle was applied using a multiplanar distracter developed for 3-dimensional distraction of the mandible.

Case Report.—Man, 22, sustained amputations of the second and third digits. Only the third digit was replantable, and this was done at the level of the proximal phalanx. The patient was later seen with a 95-degree flexion contracture of the PIP joint. After failure of splinting and casting, surgical release of the PIP joint was planned. However, the finger became ischemic after very minor manipulations of the joint. A multiplanar distracter, capable of altering the relationship between 2 planes, was applied to the finger. The patient was instructed to increase the angle of the distracter each day by approximately 5 degrees by means of a simple screw on the device. The distracter caused no neurovascular compromise. The finger had reached approximately 20 degrees of flexion by 2 weeks; the distracter was left in place for an additional 4 weeks. About 10 degrees of extension was lost after removal of the distracter, but the results have remained stable for 6 months.

Conclusion.—A multiplanar distracter was successfully used to correct a PIP joint contracture. This technique provides a useful new approach to the treatment of PIP joint contractures that fail conventional therapy, without risking neurovascular injury.

▶ Distraction across joints has great potential, as indicated in this case study of a patient with a severe (95-degree) PIP joint flexion contracture. By slow distraction (1 mm/day), joint realignment and soft-tissue stretch can be achieved. Recurrence of deformity, however, is a risk. In this study, although the technique was quite successful, the authors did not tell us how they aligned the fixator pivot joint with respect to the joint center of rotation. Secondly, it was not clear how the fixator was "multiplanar." Distraction appears to occur in only the flexion-extension plane. More experience with this device (the Hotchkiss Compass PIP Hinge Distracter) and similar devices is needed.

W.P. Cooney III, M.D.

The Treatment of Fractures of the Ring and Little Metacarpal Necks: A Prospective Randomized Study of Three Different Types of Treatment
Hansen PB, Hansen TB (Odense Univ Hosp, Denmark)
J Hand Surg [Br] 23B:245–247, 1998   3–3

Background.—Though reducing fractures of the metacarpal neck is fairly easy, retaining the reduction is difficult without using the flexed proximal interphalangeal joint splinting method, which is associated with

TABLE 1.—Summary of the Results

	Plaster-of-Paris	Functional brace	Elastic bandage	P-value
Pain during 4 weeks treatment on VAS scale 0–10 (range)	1.5 (0–4)	1.8 (0–5)	2.7 (0–6)	<0.05
Median restriction (range) of MCPJ movement at 4 weeks	20° (−10 to 60)	0° (−5 to 20)	10° (−30 to 50)	<0.05
Median fracture tenderness (range)	1.1 (1–3)	1.0 (1–2)	1.2 (1–2)	NS
Median restriction (range) of MCPJ movement at 3 months	0° (−10 to 35)	0° (0 to 20)	10° (0 to 45)	<0.05
Patient satisfaction at 3 months				
–Fully satisfied	14 (54%)	15 (60%)	13 (46%)	
–Satisfied	10 (38%)	9 (36%)	14 (50%)	NS
–Dissatisfied	2 (8%)	1 (4%)	1 (1%)	

(Courtesy of Hansen PB, Hansen TB: The treatment of fractures of the ring and little metacarpal necks: A prospective randomized study of three different types of treatment. *J Hand Surg [Br]* 23B:245–247, 1998.)

a high incidence of joint contracture and skin necrosis. Palmar angulation rarely results in problems after fracture healing. Currently, clinicians tend to treat fractures with functional braces or elastic bandages and early mobilization. Three types of treatment for fractures of the ring and little metacarpal necks were compared.

Methods.—One hundred five patients with such fractures were randomly assigned to treatment with either dorso-ulnar plaster of Paris from the proximal interphalangeal joint to the elbow, functional brace around the wrist, or elastic bandage. Eighty-five patients were included in the final analysis. Assessments were performed at 4 weeks and at 3 months.

Findings.—Patient satisfaction did not differ among the groups. Patients treated with the functional brace had as little pain as those treated with plaster of Paris, and less pain than those treated with elastic bandage. In addition, patients with the functional brace mobilized as quickly as patients with elastic bandage, and more quickly than those with plaster of Paris (Table 1).

Conclusions.—The functional brace is recommended for the treatment of fractures of the ring and little metacarpal necks. Although all 3 methods are satisfactory for the treatment of such fractures, the functional brace enabled the fastest rehabilitation.

▶ Ring and small-finger metacarpal neck fractures are extremely common in young men. The authors compared 3 nonsurgical treatment methods: an elastic bandage, an ulnar gutter splint, and a cast brace. Patients with angulation of more that 60 degrees, deviation in the coronal plane, or malrotation were excluded. Also, no reduction was performed in any of the patients. The authors favor the functional brace, because at 4 weeks it gave better pain relief than the elastic bandage did, and there was no restriction in range of motion at the metacarpophalangeal joint. However, patient satisfaction at 3 months was the same in all 3 groups. I would argue that even though the short-term differences reached statistical significance, they were small (see Table 1) and did not affect the final outcome. For these rather inconsequential injuries, patient comfort rather than immobilization method should be our primary goal. Finally, overtreatment with internal fixation should be avoided, because it may lead to major complications.

P.J. Stern, M.D.

Avulsion Fracture of the Metacarpophalangeal Joint of the Finger
Sakuma M, Nakamura R, Inoue G, et al (Nagoya Univ, Japan)
J Hand Surg [Br] 22B:667–671, 1997   3–4

Objective.—Little has been written about the management of avulsion fractures of the metacarpophalangeal (MP) joints of the fingers. Treatment of 6 patients with internal fixation of the fragment or pull-out suture of the collateral ligament was discussed. The approach to management based on X-ray and operative findings was reported.

Methods.—All injuries involved abduction stress with slight flexion of the MP joint characterized by persistent pain and swelling. All patients had an avulsed fragment. Time to surgery ranged from 5 to 31 days, and patients were followed for 4–6 months. Although the joint capsule appeared normal at surgery, larger-than-expected triangular or rectangular fragments involving the chondral surface or round fragments avulsed from the metacarpal attachment were apparent on opening of the joint. Triangular and rectangular fragments were repaired with wire and screw. Round fragments were repaired with wire fixation or pull-out suture.

Results.—At follow-up, all patients were pain free, with no swelling or instability or alteration in preinjury activity levels. All but 1 patient regained full range of motion. There were no complications.

> *Case 3.*—Man, 22, injured his right ring finger catching a ground ball. A radiograph revealed a rectangular fragment avulsed from the metacarpal. A fracture of the radial collateral ligament was found at exploration. The fragment was reduced and fixed with a Herbert screw. Exercise was begun on day 2 and union was achieved at 2 months. The range of flexion was 0 to 85 degrees, with no pain at 4 months.
>
> *Case 4.*—Man, 18, injured his index finger on a machine. Still in pain at 4 weeks, he was found at surgery to have a fragment located at the origin of the collateral ligament of the metacarpal head; it was repaired with a pull-out suture. After 2 weeks' immobilization, the MP joint flexed to 30 degrees. At 4 months, the patient had full range of motion without pain.

Conclusion.—Injuries with interposed fragments or large avulsion fragments should be treated surgically. Fractures with round fragments can be treated conservatively.

▶ The authors present a series of 6 cases and create a radiographic classification system based on these cases. From the classification system, they propose treatment guidelines. The concept is admirable. It should stimulate the surgeon faced with one of these injuries to consider carefully whether the avulsed fragment is intra-articular or extra-articular and whether to perform surgery or treat the injury nonoperatively.

One weakness is that there are only 6 patients in the study, too few from which to draw such generalized conclusions. A second weakness is that the shape of the fragment may change as the position of the hand and the orientation of the x-ray beam changes.

The authors aptly point out that the management of this injury is controversial. This is caused, in part, by the difficulty of replacing and internally fixing a small avulsion fragment (especially from the base of the proximal phalanx) in the third, fourth, or fifth webspaces, and, in part, because many patients have good results after conservative treatment, despite a small amount of collateral ligament instability. Readers are urged to treat with surgery those injuries with interposed bone fragments or large articular avulsion fragments and to consider conservative treatment for the remainder.

L.B. Lane, M.D.

Distal Forearm Fractures in Children: The Role of Radiographs During Follow Up
Green JS, Williams SC, Finlay D, et al (Leicester Royal Infirmary, England; Glenfield Gen Hosp, Leicester, England)
Injury 29:309–312, 1998   3–5

Purpose.—Fractures of the distal forearm are common in children, especially the distal-most one third. These patients often receive radiographic as well as clinical follow-up to evaluate fracture healing and to screen for reangulation. However, the value of postmanipulation films remains unproven; radiation exposure is a concern in these young patients. This study assessed the clinical use of repeat radiographs of the wrist after initial treatment of children with forearm fractures.

Methods.—The retrospective study included the clinical and radiographic findings of 325 patients under 16 years old who had distal forearm fractures. Degrees of angulation were measured in all follow-up radiographs. The investigators compared the results of treatment in patients with initial angulation of less than 10 degrees with the results in patients with angulation of greater than 10 degrees. The effects of fracture type and degree of reduction were evaluated as well.

Results.—When initial angulation was less than 10 degrees, there was no evidence of reangulation during follow-up. Twenty-six percent of fractures had initial angulation of 10 degrees or greater. The rate of reangulation was about 25%, regardless of whether the fracture was manipulated under anesthesia. Late manipulation was required in only 11 of 85 cases with initial angulation of 10 degrees or greater.

Conclusions.—In the treatment of forearm fractures in children, fractures with initial angulation of less than 10 degrees can be regarded as stable, requiring only an initial diagnostic radiograph. Closer follow-up is warranted for complete fractures, displaced fractures, and fractures of both the radius and ulna. Five to 10 degrees of residual angulation after manipulation under anesthesia does not appear to increase the rate of secondary reangulation.

▶ This collaborative article from departments of radiology and orthopedics in England asks how many radiographs are necessary after forearm fractures in children. The authors' answer suggests that a larger number of radiographs are taken than are actually necessary. Although I agree with many of the authors' suggestions, in practice it is more difficult to implement changes with reangulation rates of between 23% and 34% for angulated greenstick fractures, displaced fractures, and complete fractures. It is hard not to follow these injuries up with repeat radiographs. I do agree that incomplete fractures with less than 10 degrees of initial angulation rarely require follow-up radiographs.

Perhaps the most significant disagreement I have with this article involves the short follow-up (an average of 25 days). The most significant management issue in many of these fractures is when to remove the cast and allow the child to return to activities that involve weight-bearing on the upper extremity. I rely upon radiographs to make these decisions. To do otherwise requires longer immobilization or arbitrarily long limitations of activities. Although the authors do suggest strongly that fewer radiographs be taken, this article demonstrates no adverse consequences in those children who had more radiographs than recommended.

W.J. Shaughnessy, M.D.

Surgical Treatment of Isolated Forearm Non-Union With Segmental Bone Loss
Moroni A, Rollo G, Guzzardella M, et al (Bologna Univ, Italy)
Injury 28:497–504, 1997
3–6

Purpose.—Isolated nonunions of the bones of the forearm cause serious functional impairments. A number of different surgical procedures have been proposed to correct the shape, length, and continuity of these bones. A new technique—including intercalary bone grafting and internal fixation—was evaluated for the treatment of isolated radial and ulnar nonunions.

Methods.—The 14-year experience included 24 patients with isolated nonunions of the radius and ulna with segment bone loss. There were 20 men and 4 women (average age, 30 years). The radius was affected in 9 patients and the ulna in 15. Twenty cases were considered secondary to inadequate surgical treatment for forearm fracture. All nonunions were managed with removal of all necrotic bone, insertion of an autogenous intercalary bone graft, and stable internal fixation with a plate and cortical bone allograft fixed opposite to the plate (Fig 4). Follow-up averaged 40 months.

Results.—After removal of necrotic bone, the defects averaged 3.6 cm in length. A fibular autograft was most often used for the intercalary graft; a tibial allograft was used for the cortical graft in all cases. Radiographic union was achieved in all patients in a mean of 14 weeks. Three patients had postoperative infections. This complication responded to surgical debridement in 2 cases but led to treatment failure in the third. Healing time was 12.5 weeks for ulnar nonunions vs. 16.4 weeks for radial nonunions. Ten patients had excellent functional results, 6 had satisfactory results, and 7 had unsatisfactory results.

Conclusion.—This bone grafting and internal fixation technique offers good results in difficult-to-treat isolated forearm nonunions with segmental bone loss. Given the seriousness of these nonunions, the functional

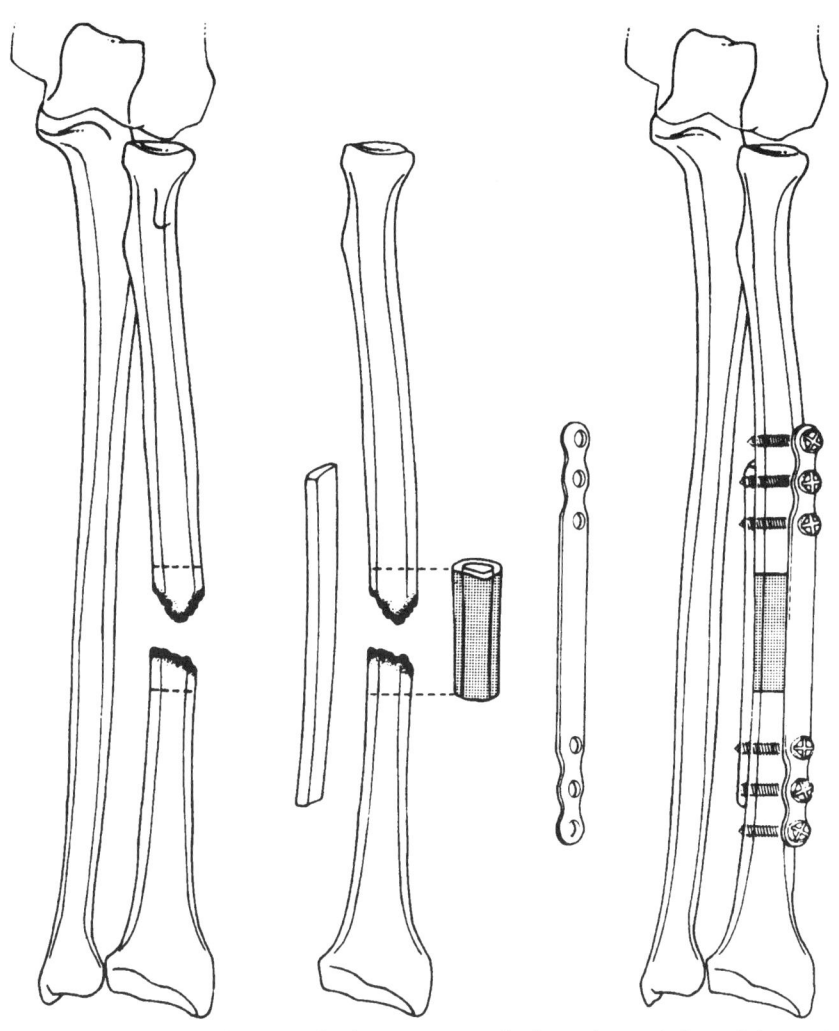

FIGURE 4.—Diagrams show surgical technique consisting of widespread removal of necrotic bone and bridging of the bone defect with an intercalary bone graft of the same size as the final bone defect (intercalary graft). Rigid fixation is obtained by a compression plate and a cortical bone graft on the opposite side joined together with the same screws. (Reprinted from *Injury* courtesy of Moroni A, Rollo G, Guzzardella M, et al: Surgical treatment of isolated forearm non-union with segmental bone loss. *Injury* 28:497–504. Copyright 1997, with permission from Elsevier Science.)

results are good; loss of forearm rotation is the main impairment. Infection is a serious complication, which can lead to treatment failure.

▶ Since the classic papers of Nicoll et al. regarding the reconstruction of diaphyseal, ununited forearm fractures, a number of techniques have been advanced to deal with more complex reconstructive problems. These have extended from noninvasive techniques such as electric stimulation to sophisticated techniques involving the replacement of missing bone with vascularized bone graft or regeneration of diaphyseal defects by the method of Ilizarov. At times the problem is a 3-dimensional one involving a loss of the soft tissue as well as bone. Nevertheless, one is occasionally faced with a rather substantial bony loss in which the conventional techniques of compression plate fixation may not, by themselves, prove to predictably be the conventional technique of compression plate fixation with autogenous bone graft. It is for this reason that the techniques advanced by Moroni et al. in this paper are worthy of the readers' attention, if only to keep "in the bank" as an alternative technique when faced with a unique but formidable bony defect.

Careful scrutiny of this study would suggest, however, that the authors' procedure is potentially fraught with difficulty, particularly in the face of associated prior infection and/or soft deficit. Also, it requires a substantial amount of soft-tissue exposure, which could jeopardize the blood supply required for bony union, and it requires a rather extensive surgical experience as to the judgment of the efficacy of the debridement. The authors' results, however, suggest that despite the potential pitfalls, allograft plus autogenous graft in conjunction with a long plate will produce a high degree of not only union but also functional forearm rotation.

The allograft itself represents a fundamental prerequisite to healing with a plate, as it provides the necessary cortex opposite the plate to limit the amount of bending stresses on the plate. This is an important fundamental mechanical principle that, at times, can be jeopardized by retention of devascularized fragments of bone in the face of open fractures which may not incorporate in sufficient time to obviate plate loosening or breakage. Whether the allograft truly incorporates completely in these cases may not be as much of an issue as its provision of mechanical stability opposite the plate to allow the autogenous graft to incorporate.

A second important principle is the use of longer plates to stabilize these complex situations. A number of investigational studies have supported the clinical impression, put forth initially by Lane in 1912, that longer plates provide more stability. One only has to look at the experience of plate failures in the upper limb to appreciate the fact that the cause is often inadequate control over the diaphyseal segment. The fact that the plates illustrated in this study in some cases were relatively flexible or were custom plates not providing compression at the bony surfaces, supports the fact that the length of the plate minimizing shear and rotation was an effective stabilizing factor.

The readers should also heed the complications identified by the authors. Where there was insufficient soft tissue or prior sepsis, the techniques illustrated by these authors may be less than optimal. There were 3 infections, which can be catastrophic with an allograft bony replacement; 2 skin break-downs; and several cases of radial or ulnar nerve palsies (or both) which, although transient, attest to the magnitude of the scar likely present in these cases.

In summary, the reader may not find it necessary to adapt these techniques for standard cases, or even cases with bony loss without associated underlying osteoporosis or other jeopardizing factors, but one should keep these techniques available for situations in which plates and screws might not provide stable fixation, with the allograft providing an opposite cortex to enhance both screw purchase and the overall stability of the bony reconstructions.

J.B. Jupiter, M.D.

Operative Treatment of Post-traumatic Proximal Radioulnar Synostosis
Jupiter JB, Ring D (Massachusetts Gen Hosp, Boston)
J Bone Joint Surg Am 80-A:248–257, 1998   3–7

Background.—Heterotopic ossification after resection for post-traumatic radioulnar synostosis substantially reduces forearm rotation. Many have advocated the use of radiation therapy and nonsteroidal anti-inflammatory drugs (NSAIDs) to prevent the recurrence of heterotopic bone. However, these authors reviewed their results for resection of proximal radioulnar synostosis without the use of these 2 therapies.

Methods.—During 8 years, 1 author performed 18 excisions for post-traumatic proximal radioulnar synostosis in 17 patients (15 men and 2 women, mean age 37 years). Average time between injury and resection was 19 months. At presentation, no rotation of the forearm was possible. Four limbs had synostosis at or distal to the bicipital tuberosity (group A); 7 had synostosis of the radial head and the proximal radioulnar joint (group B); and 7 had synostosis contiguous with heterotopic bone that extended to the distal aspect of the humerus (group C). A posterior midline skin incision was used in all surgical approaches. In groups A and B, the extensor carpi ulnaris and the supinator were elevated from the ulna, thus exposing the proximal third of the radius and the synostosis. In group C, the ulnar and radial nerves were dissected free of osseous involvement. The radial head was resected in only 2 limbs, based on whether the articular surface had any incongruity, whether radiocapitellar osteoarthrosis was present, or whether the proximal radioulnar joint was distorted. A thin layer of bone wax was applied to bleeding margins at the resection site. Each patient received physical therapy after surgery, including immediate active mobilization of the elbow and forearm. However, none received postoperative NSAIDs or radiotherapy to prevent heterotopic ossification. Follow-up averaged 34 months.

Findings.—At follow-up, the only synostosis to recur did so in the only patient who had received a closed head injury (in group C). In the other 17 limbs, an average of 139 degrees of forearm rotation was achieved (range, 65–165 degrees). Average supination was 61 degrees (range, 25–85 degrees) and average pronation was 78 degrees (range, 40–90 degrees). In groups A and B, the average total arc of ulnohumeral motion was 106 degrees (range, 75–135 degrees), and in group C it was 98 degrees (range, 60–110 degrees). Too few patients were included to determine any statistically significant relationships between postoperative forearm rotation and the size of the synostosis, but there was a trend for greater rotation in the 8 limbs that were operated on within 12 months of injury (average, 144 degrees of rotation) than in the 9 limbs that underwent resection later (average, 134 degrees of rotation). Also, patients in group A tended to have less forearm rotation (average, 126 degrees) than those in groups B or C (average, 143 degrees).

Conclusions.—Despite the absence of postoperative radiation therapy or NSAIDs, the results after resection for post-traumatic proximal radioulnar synostosis were good, with only 1 failure (5%). Thus, routine adjunctive prophylactic measures may not be necessary in these cases.

▶ This is a very important article, as it sheds significant light on, and substantially impacts our management of, proximal radioulnar synostoses. This is the largest series of patients reported by one surgeon, from which 5 conclusions can be drawn regarding resection of a proximal radioulnar synostosis. First, it is safe; no patients sustained important neurovascular injuries or serious complications. Second, it is effective; the average arch of rotation was 139 degrees, ranging from 65 to 165 degrees. Only 1 patient failed to gain motion. Third, it should probably be performed early; results were generally more favorable in those resected less than 12 months following injury than those resected later than 12 months post-injury. The general tendency currently around the elbow is to resect heterotopic bone 3 to 6 months following injury, when sequential plain radiographs stabilized with respect to the appearance of the heterotopic bone. Fourth, a posterior skin incision with a posterolateral approach to the radioulnar space is almost universally to be recommended. Fifth, postoperative radiation is not necessary; in fact, NSAIDs may not be necessary either. The rarity of recurrence of heterotopic ossification following surgical excision has been confirmed in the experience of many other elbow surgeons performing the same techniques. This has not yet come out fully in the literature. This paper should establish clearly in the minds of trauma surgeons the appropriateness of surgical excision of a post-traumatic radioulnar synostosis. The authors correctly point out that the previous pessimism regarding such treatment was based on very little data. My own personal experience would confirm the observations and recommendations found in this paper. Although I rarely use postoperative radiation in treating stiff elbows, I have used it following resection of a radioulnar synostosis, simply because of the terrible reputation that it had for recurrence, but that might not have really been necessary. One point that might merit emphasis is that the heterotopic ossification frequently involves the region of the bicipital tuberosity of the radius, and inadvertent iatrogenic release of the biceps tendon insertion is an anticipated complication to be avoided. Finally, I would concur with the recommendation that heterotopic ossification involving radioulnar synostosis as well as elbow ankylosis should be managed by complete resection and mobilization of both joints.

S.W. O'Driscoll, M.D., Ph.D., F.R.C.S.C.

Reconstruction of the Coronoid for Chronic Dislocation of the Elbow: Use of a Graft From the Olecranon in Two Cases

Moritomo H, Tada K, Yoshida T, et al (Kansai Rosai Hosp, Hyogo, Japan; Kinki Central Hosp, Osaka, Japan)
J Bone Joint Surg Br 80-B:490–492, 1998

Introduction.—It is difficult to manage patients with persistent dislocation of the elbow associated with a large fracture of the coronoid process. In the 2 cases reported here, open reductions with reconstruction of the coronoid using osteocartilaginous grafts from the ipsilateral olecranon were performed.

Case Report 1.—Man, 54, sustained a posterior dislocation of the left elbow with associated fractures of the coronoid process, the shaft of the ulna, and the head of the radius. He was initially treated by reduction, wire fixation of the coronoid fracture, plating of the ulnar fracture, and excision of the head of the radius. A radiograph obtained 3 weeks later showed posterior subluxation of the elbow. When pain and restricted movement persisted at 6 months, the patient underwent removal of extensive scar tissue around the joint and the medial collateral ligament was attached to the medial epicondyle of the humerus. Posterior subluxation, which recurred 2 weeks later, was treated by reconstruction of the coronoid process, using part of the olecranon. A plaster cast was used for 4 weeks, and radiographs at 3 months showed union was achieved. At 5-year follow-up, the patient had a range of movement from 25 to 135 degrees. The elbow was stable and painless.

Discussion.—Fractures of the coronoid process with dislocation of the elbow may result in recurrent dislocation or persistent subluxation. Use of an osteocartilaginous graft from the ipsilateral olecranon resulted in a painless, stable joint with a functional range of movement.

▶ This article merits attention for 2 reasons. The obvious reason relates to the fact that it brings to our attention a potential technical treatment for the deficient coronoid in patients with chronic sequelae from fracture dislocations of the elbow. The second, and more important, reason is that it raises our awareness of the importance of the coronoid as a biomechanical stabilizer of the elbow. This combination of elbow dislocation with fracture of the coronoid and fracture of the radial head is referred to as the "terrible triad" of the elbow because of its prognosis for terribly poor results. In a large part, this relates to our having not fully understood nor addressed the importance of the coronoid in these fractures. I have used this technique with moderate success; however, I have concern about removing a portion of the olecranon in an elbow that has already declared itself to be persistently unstable. These elbows subluxate by posterolateral rotatory mechanism, and in the acute situation, one will often observe a chondral lesion on the posteromedial aspect of the trochlea where the posteromedial olecranon has impacted it. The fulcrum or pivot point in an elbow dislocation is on the medial side, with the boney fulcrum being the contact between the olecranon and the posteromedial trochlea and the anterior bundle of the medial collateral ligament being the soft tissue tension band about which the pivoting occurs. Thus, alternatives to partial olecranon removal, including the use of an allograft or autograft (with the capsule interposed between the autograft and the trochlea) are preferable. Furthermore, 1 should attempt to reconstruct all of the constraints including the collateral ligaments if they are deficient. In these cases, the lateral collateral ligament complexes usually are attenuated or deficient. The medial collateral ligament may or may not be.

Finally, one should note that the authors recommend transplanting a piece of olecranon equal in size to the piece of coronoid that is missing, but they appear to have used larger fragments than that, creating a buttress effect anteriorly. Hopefully, reports such as this will stimulate us to learn more about the biomechanics of the coronoid and how acute and chronic injuries to this structure can be most effectively managed.

S.W. O'Driscoll, M.D., Ph.D., F.R.C.S.C.

Suggested Reading

Fahmy NRM, Kehoe N, Warner JG, et al: The "S" Quattro turbo in the management of neglected dorsal interphalangeal dislocations, *J Hand Surg [Br]* 23B:248–251, 1998.
▶ The S Quattro is an external fixator for the digits, and the turbo modification is the use of a spring to provide distraction. This report discussed 4 cases of chronic interphalangeal dislocations in which the distraction feature was used to achieve a gradual reduction before open repair was carried out. The idea of dynamic distraction in a low-profile splint is appealing; in addition, the sporty name for the device certainly catches one's attention!

P.C. Amadio, M.D.

Huber J, Bickert B, Germann G: The Mitek mini anchor in the treatment of the gamekeeper's thumb. *Eur J Plast Surg* 20:251–255, 1997.
▶ This series of cases utilizing the Mitek brand mini anchor shows that this method provides reliable fixation of the repaired ulnar collateral ligament to bone. However, the cost constraints should not be discounted. These are expensive devices. Despite the authors' preference for this method, I have not found the pull-out technique over a button to be either time-consuming or associated with complications of infection and skin necrosis. And that technique is a lot less expensive.

E.R. North, M.D.

Obert L, Garbuio P, Gérard F, et al: Recent, closed trapezio-metacarpal luxation, treated by pinning: Apropos of 7 cases with a median follow-up of 8 years [French]. *Ann Chir Main Memb Super* 16:102–110, 1997.

▶ This review of 7 patients followed for 2–13 years suggests that closed pinning can be an effective treatment for acute closed trapeziometacarpal dislocation.

P.C. Amadio, M.D.

Pellat JL, Toledano E, Fabre B, et al: External traction: An alternative treatment of articular fractures of phalanges. *La Main* 2:181–188, 1997.

▶ Articular phalangeal fractures often result in joint stiffness and may lead to arthritis. Anatomic alignment, solid fixation, and early mobilization are considered to be factors of better prognosis. The principle of articular fracture treatment by dynamic traction splints was introduced by Schenck[1] and Suzuki et al.[2] These authors have developed a small, low-cost external traction splint. It allows fracture reduction by progressive axial traction and early mobilization of the involved joint, reducing edema, joint stiffness, and tendon adhesion.

This article describes another ingenuous technique for the treatment of displaced articular fractures of the phalanges. Since the description of the banjo-splint by Robertson et al. in 1946,[3] many devices have been invented and successfully applied. These devices can be divided in 2 categories: (1) those in which traction is applied through an arcuate outrigger linked to a large short-arm cast and passive motion is performed several times a day,[1,4] and (2) those in which only pins and rubber[2,5] or pins and metallic springs[6,7] are used and immediate active motion is performed.

The device described in the study by Pellat et al. is a combination of both of these—traction is applied with pins and rubber is transmitted to a hand splint that does not include the wrist, and immediate active and passive motion are both performed. In their latter cases, the authors have further modified their technique, replacing the transosseous distal wire by an adhesive tape, thus suppressing all internal devices. Their technique is therefore the most simple and least invasive one.

When comparing the results obtained with these different techniques for proximal interphalangeal joint fractures, the final active ranges of motion are very similar, ranging from 80 degrees[2] to 95 degrees.[8] Pellat et al.'s series averages a 79-degree range of motion, thus achieving the lowest results. However, all these series are made of small numbers of patients, and they include various types of lesions (comminuted intra-articular fractures as well as fracture dislocations), thus making any comparison of results somewhat inaccurate. Larger series individualizing each type of fracture will be needed for appropriate comparisons.

C. LeClerq, M.D.

References

1. Schenck RR: Dynamic traction and early passive movement for fractures of the proximal interphalangeal joint. *J Hand Surg [Am]* 11A:850–858, 1986.
2. Suzuki Y, Malsunaga T, Sato S, et al: The pins and rubbers traction system for treatment of comminuted intraarticular fractures and fracture-dislocations in the hand. *J Hand Surg [Br]* 19B:98–107, 1994.
3. Robertson RC, Cawley JJ, Faris AM: Treatment of fracture-dislocation of the interphalangeal joints of the hand. *J Bone Joint Surg* 28:68–70, 1946.
4. Morgan JP, Gordon DA, Klug MS, et al: Dynamic digital traction for unstable comminuted intraarticular fracture-dislocations of the proximal interphalangeal joint. *J Hand Surg [Am]* 20A:565–573, 1995.

5. Agee JM: Unstable fracture dislocations of the proximal interphalangeal joint of the fingers: A preliminary report of a new treatment technique. *J Hand Surg [Am]* 3:386–389, 1978.
6. Fahmy NRM: The stockport serpentine spring system for the treatment of displaced comminuted intra-articular phalangeal fractures. *J Hand Surg [Br]* 15B:303–311, 1990.
7. Inanami H, Ninomiya S, Okutsu I, et al: Dynamic external finger fixator for fracture dislocation of the proximal interphalangeal joint. *J Hand Surg [Am]* 18A:160–164, 1993.

Seno N, Hashizume H, Inoue H, et al: Fractures of the base of the middle phalanx of the finger: Classification, management and long-term results. *J Bone Joint Surg Br* 79:758–763, 1997.

▶ These authors have presented a large series of intra-articular fractures of the base of middle phalanx. Slightly fewer than half required surgery. Extension block splinting or other closed methods might have been used instead of surgery for some of the unstable fractures that were operated. After reviewing the surgical results, the authors found that a joint space gap or step-off was associated with a worse result. If restoration of joint surface is not anticipated by open reduction, using an alternative procedure that sacrifices the excessively damaged joint surface (such as volar plate arthroplasty) can produce excellent results. I have found that upon exploration of these fractures much more joint damage is present than was previously suspected. Restoration of an anatomic surface is extremely challenging and frequently impossible.

E.R. North, M.D.

Tazaki K, Kameyama M, Satoh K, et al: Fracture of the metacarpophalangeal joint. *J Jpn Soc Surg Hand* 14(1):114–120, 1997.

▶ In this article, fractures of the metacarpal head and the proximal phalangeal base are lumped together as fractures in the metacarpophalangeal joint. Fractures of the metacarpal head are more common within the metacarpophalangeal joints of fingers than proximal phalangeal fractures, while 95% of fractures in the metacarpophalangeal joint of the thumb occur at the base of proximal phalanx. The authors analysed 39 fractures of the metacarpal head and 58 fractures of the proximal phalangeal base and classified them into 3 types. Type 1 is the avulsion fracture at the attachment of the collateral ligament, type 2 is the fracture caused by sheer force from the other bone, and type 3 is the comminuted fracture caused by axial compressive force in the joint.

The authors subdivided the types further. Of the metacarpal head, type 2 fracture is subdivided into 3 groups, namely types 2-A, 2-B, and 2-C. Of the proximal phalangeal base, type 2 and 3 fractures are subdivided into 2 groups each, namely types 2-A, 2-B, 3-A, and 3-B. Therefore, there are 5 categories in fractures of the metacarpal head and proximal phalangeal base, respectively. This classification seems very simple and useful to decide the treatment for a fracture in the metacarpophalangeal joint.

Y. Ueba, M.D., D.M.Sc.

4 Soft-Tissue Trauma and Reconstruction

Our Experience With the Use of the Dorsal Ulnar Artery Flap in Hand and Wrist Tissue Cover
Antonopoulos D, Kang NV, Debono R (St Andrew's Hosp, Patras, Greece)
J Hand Surg [Br] 22B:739–744, 1997   4–1

Objective.—Use of the dorsal ulnar artery fasciocutaneous (DUA) flap as a long flap to repair a variety of hand injuries was described, and 6 cases were discussed.

Methods.—Surface markings outline the flap, and the ulnar artery and ulnar border of the flexor carpi ulnaris tendon are identified (Fig 1). The fasciocutaneous flap is dissected, the defect is closed by grafting, a drain is inserted and the hand is elevated for 5 days (Fig 2). The fasciosubcutaneous island flap is raised over the muscle belly of the flexor carpi ulnaris. The 5- to 6-cm–wide flap is raised with the island of skin until the dorsal ulnar vessels are visible. The flap is tunnelled under the palmar skin to the primary defect. The secondary defect is closed, a drain is inserted, and the

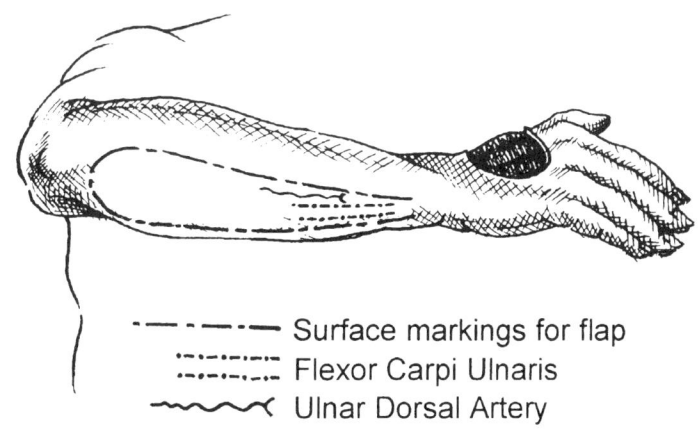

FIGURE 1.—Surface markings for the dorsal ulnar artery fasciocutaneous flap. The key landmarks are the medial epicondyle, the pisiform bone, and the tendon of flexor carpi ulnaris. (Courtesy of Antonopoulos D, Kang NV, Debono R: Our experience with the use of the dorsal ulnar artery flap in hand and wrist tissue cover. *J Hand Surg [Br]* 22B:739–744, 1997.)

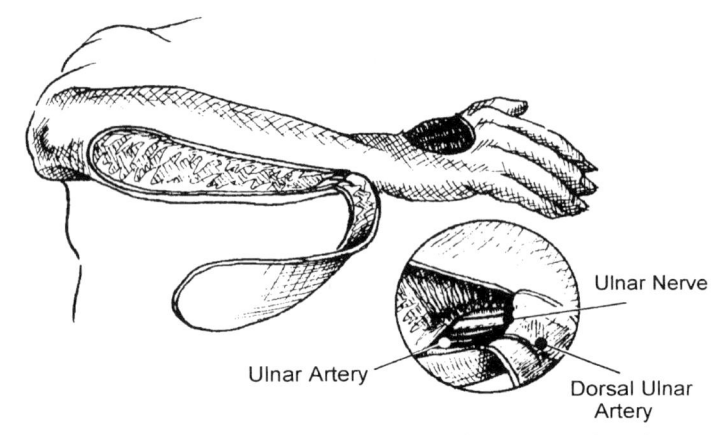

FIGURE 2.—Fasciocutaneous dorsal ulnar artery flap. The flap is raised with the fascia over flexor carpi ulnaris until the dorsal ulnar vessels are seen entering the deep surface of the flap (**inset**). (Courtesy of Antonopoulos D, Kang NV, Debono R: Our experience with the use of the dorsal ulnar artery flap in hand and wrist tissue cover. *J Hand Surg [Br]* 22B:739–744, 1997.)

hand is elevated for 5 days. The DUA flap is exposed through a Z-shaped incision on the forearm. The flap is raised, folded over, and sutured to the primary defect. The donor site is closed and a skin graft is applied to the flap.

Case studies involved repair of the dorsum of the right hand after excision of a Marjolin's ulcer, of a full thickness skin loss after extravasation of a chemotherapy agent, after excision of a nevus, and after excision of a squamous cell carcinoma; repair to the radial border of the right wrist after a circular saw injury; and repair to the ulnar border of the left palm and little finger after a circular saw injury.

Discussion.—The disadvantages of the DUA flap include required retrograde venous drainage and the small defects which can be covered. The advantages include the longer length, as used in this study (15–20 cm), that allows coverage of radial hand and wrist defects.

Conclusion.—Use of large DUA flaps is feasible, but adequate venous drainage must be conscientiously provided.

▶ The initial operative description of both the ulnar and radial forearm flap included the sacrifice of 1 or the other dominant vessel if it was to serve as the vascular pedicle for the flap. Contemporary surgeons have demonstrated that this may be unnecessary in many instances. Tissues based on the radial artery can be pedicled on just 1 of several perforators, and this article describes just how extensive a flap can be elevated on the dorsal ulnar branch of the ulnar artery. At some point, the most distally located tissues assume the status of a random flap territory, where resistance to venous outflow may exceed resistance to arterial inflow. Providing additional sources for venous outflow might extend the territory.

V.R. Hentz, M.D.

Posterior Interosseous Free Flap: Various Types
Park JJ, Kim JS, Chung JI (Kwang Myung Sung Ae Gen Hosp, Korea)
Plast Reconstr Surg 100:1186–1199, 1997

Introduction.—In some cases of soft-tissue defects of the hand or foot, the options for a flap are limited. Recent studies have examined use of the reverse posterior interosseous fasciocutaneous island flap, which consists of the skin and fascia raised from the posterior aspects of the forearm. This flap can be used to cover the dorsum of the hand and first web space, but is not reliable in cases in which the distal forearm, wrist injuries, or both are present. Three types of free flap were developed to overcome the limitations and increase the applications of the posterior interosseous free flap.

Methods.—Over a 2-year period, 23 patients underwent hand and foot reconstruction with posterior interosseous free flaps. The types of flaps used were fasciocutaneous (13 patients), fasciocutaneous-fascia (6 patients), and fascia only (4 patients). Thirteen of the free flaps were sensory flaps using the posterior antebrachial cutaneous nerve, composed of 3 fascicles. At surgery, a point is marked at the lateral epicondyle of the humerus and the distal radioulnar joint, with the forearm in full pronation. The anterior skin incision is made first, extending from the wrist to the elbow. After completion of the anterior dissection, the posterior interosseous artery in intermuscular septum and the septocutaneous perforators are identified and dissection proceeds from distal to proximal. The posterior interosseous nerve is identified, carefully dissected, and preserved. The proximal cutaneous branch of the interosseous recurrent artery is identified for inclusion in the free flap. Width of the fasciocutaneous flap should not exceed 5 cm.

Results.—Patients were 21 men and 2 women ranging in age from 19 to 48 years. Twenty-one had a hand defect and 2 had a foot defect. Duration of follow-up was 3–22 months. The length of the pedicle averaged 3.5 cm, and the external diameter of the artery averaged 2.2 mm. In all 23 patients, survival of the posterior interosseous artery free flap was complete and uneventful.

Conclusion.—Substantial soft-tissue defects of the hand and foot can be successfully covered with skin from the dorsal fore-arm, with the posterior interosseous vessel providing a good and reliable vascular supply. The flap is versatile in design and the donor site can be closed directly. Disadvantages include a short pedicle and the sometimes deep location of the posterior interosseous artery.

▶ Because the arc of rotation of the reverse posterior interosseous flap will not allow reliable coverage of soft tissue defects beyond the metacarpophalangeal joints and because the distal anastomosis between the posterior interosseous and anterior interosseous arteries can potentially be damaged in injuries involving the distal forearm and wrist, the authors have refined the posterior interosseous flap as a free flap and advocate it as being the flap of choice for reconstruction of soft-tissue defects of the hand. Whilst it has the advantage over the radial forearm flap of avoiding sacrifice of 1 of the 2 major forearm arteries and can also be used as a neurosensory flap, the posterior interosseous artery free flap has not achieved the same popularity with North American surgeons as the radial forearm flap and lateral arm flap. Dissection of the posterior interosseous artery more proximally beneath the supinator may also risk injury to the branches of the posterior interosseous nerve to the extensor muscles, leading to loss of digital extension.

N.F. Jones, M.D.

Anatomical Study of Interosseous Flaps and the Concept of Posteroanterior Interosseous Flap: Preliminary Report [French]
Roux J-L, Leandris M, Allieu Y (Hôpital Lapeyronie, Montpellier, France)
Ann Chir Plast Esthet 42:260–271, 1997   4–3

Background.—The distal posterior and anterior interosseous arteries can be used to create flaps to correct defects of the dorsum of the hand. These authors performed cadaveric studies to examine the relationships between these interosseous arteries, and their experience with the posteroanterior interosseous flap in 2 cases is discussed.

Anatomic Study.—To explore the anatomic relationship between the distal and anterior interosseous arteries, 40 cadaveric forearms were prepared. In 38 specimens there was a distal anastomosis between these arteries, at 19–32 mm (average, 25 mm) from the radiocarpal joint. In 19 specimens there was a common origin for the posterior and inferior branches, about 57 mm from the radiocarpal joint (type 1); in 21 specimens there were 2 separate branches, 1 about 49 mm and 1 about 76 mm from the radiocarpal joint (type 2). Although the fasciocutaneous artery branch of the flap was visible in all 40 specimens, its origin varied, and thus the length of the pedicle must vary.

Clinical Applications.—If the anastomosis is not found during surgical exploration, then an anterior interosseous flap is recommended. But if the distal anastomosis does exist, a posteroanterior flap can be created via classic dissection technique. The pedicle is lengthened, either proximally or distally, via the anastomosis between the distal branches of the anterior interosseous artery. Retrograde flow of the flap must be tested by clamping. This type of flap has been used in 2 patients, and results have been positive. Advantages of this technique include a greater rotational arc, the ability to create a very long pedicle, and the ability to avoid the venous problems that occur when a skin flap is created distally along the dorsal wrist.

Conclusions.—If the cutaneous area to be repaired is small, then an anterior interosseous flap is preferred. If cutaneous damage is more extensive, then a posterior interosseous flap is recommended. But for flaps that must be longer still, the posteroanterior interosseous flap should be considered. All 3 flaps give an aesthetic finish that is very similar to the skin covering the dorsum of the hand and the digits.

▶ The authors have significantly extended our knowledge of the anatomic interconnections about the distal forearm and wrist. The concept of the posteroanterior flap is unique. The potential distal range of coverage of this flap is even more interesting.

V.R. Hentz, M.D.

Role of the "Castle" Flap in the Treatment of Skin Retraction in Severe Stiffness of the Hand and Fingers [French]
Foucher G, Fehki S, Erhard L (Clinique du Parc, Strasbourg, France)
Ann Chir Plast Esthet 43:51–57, 1998　　　　　　　　　　　　　　　4–4

Background.—Often when patients are treated for severe joint stiffness in the hand, they have severe skin retraction. Skin retraction presents its own problems, and it must be addressed so that postoperative mobility is adequate and closure does not cause necrosis, disunion, or pain. The use of "castle" flaps in treating flexion and extension skin retraction and stiffness of the proximal interphalangeal (PIP) and metacarpophalangeal (MCP) joints in patients with severe joint stiffness is discussed.

Methods.—For treating stiffness with extension of the PIP, a dorsal Hueston flap was used, in which the sides of the flap were lifted and the joint was exposed to allow dorsal tenoarthrolysis. After flap advancement, the sides were sutured but the proximal part was allowed to heal by directed healing. For treating stiffness with extension of the MCP, a castle flap was used. The flap was prepared by making a transverse incision near the PIP and 2 longitudinal incisions between the PIP and MCP, leaving a skin flap that looked like the turret of a castle. The flap was then raised until there was enough skin on top of the MCP that the sides of the flap could be sutured. When more than 1 joint was being treated, the castle flap could be extended across the MCPs to allow complete visualization of the joint and tenoarthrolysis. A castle flap was also used for treating stiffness with flexion of the PIP and MCP. In these cases, the incisions were made at the level of the palmar distal interphalangeal joint (for the PIP joint) or at the palmar crease of the PIP (for the MCP joint). The flap was raised, leaving the vascular and nervous supply intact and with as much fat preserved as possible.

Findings.—The dorsal Hueston flap was used in 2 cases of stiffness with PIP extension and in 6 cases of stiffness with PIP hyperextension, with no skin complications in any case and a mean gain of 73 degrees. The palmar castle flap was used in 5 cases of PIP stiffness with flexion; at a mean of 2 years after surgery, the procedure succeeded in improving the extension deficit from 72 to 32 degrees, with complete improvement in flexion. The palmar castle flap was also used in 3 cases of MCP stiffness with flexion, and in 2 cases the mean extension deficit was improved to 15 degrees after 18 and 36 months. The third case had undergone surgery 3 times previously, and a skin graft was needed lest all MCP extension be lost. The castle flap was also used in 5 cases of MCP extension or hyperextension, with no skin problems. In 2 cases, all the long fingers were involved, and in 3 cases, only 1 finger was involved. The mean gain was 63 degrees.

Conclusions.—A castle flap can be used successfully to treat severe extension and flexion stiffness of the PIP and MCP joints. This flap has the advantages of being a local flap (which ensures the same skin color and texture), and it allows complete access to the articular and periarticular structures.

▶ The castle flap is a useful trick to mobilize fingers with tight dorsal scar. I plan to try it.

P.C. Amadio, M.D.

The Reverse Digital Artery Island Flap: Clinical Experience in 120 Fingers
Han S-K, Lee B-I, Kim W-K (Korea Univ, Seoul)
Plast Reconstr Surg 101:1006–1011, 1998   4–5

Objective.—Different methods of reconstructing fingertips after injury produce various functional and aesthetic results. The outcome after reverse digital artery island flaps for fingertip reconstruction was evaluated.

Methods.—Between July 1984 and December 1995, 120 fingertips in 110 patients (14 females), aged 9–62 years, were reconstructed using the reverse digital artery island flap at Korea University Guro Hospital. Records of patients were reviewed and analyzed for sex and age distribution, fingers involved, donor site coverage, survival rate, and sensory restoration.

Technique.—After minimal debridement, measurement of the defect, and elimination of the possibility of soft tissue injury, a flap was raised on the least-used side of the ulnar or radial side of the proximal phalanx of the finger with a digital artery as the central axis (Fig 1). The artery is separated from the digital nerve to about 5 mm from the digital palmar arch. The perivascular venules are protected by a cuff of subcutaneous tissue. The digital artery is ligated, the flap is transferred, and the dorsal branch of the digital artery is dissected and anastomosed to the digital nerve by the epineural method. The wound is closed with a skin graft.

Results.—Most injuries (75 fingers) were to the right hand, and most involved the index fingers. Most injuries were crush injuries followed by avulsion injuries and amputation. Primary surgery was performed on 93 fingers, and secondary surgery on 27 after necrosis of a composite graft. Flaps ranged from 1.5 to 3.2 cm in length and from 1.0 to 2.5 cm in width. Patients were followed up for an average of 5.4 months, and 44 fingers in 41 patients were followed up for 6 months. Twelve of these were sensate. Sensory recovery was excellent. Revision to smooth the flap edge was re-

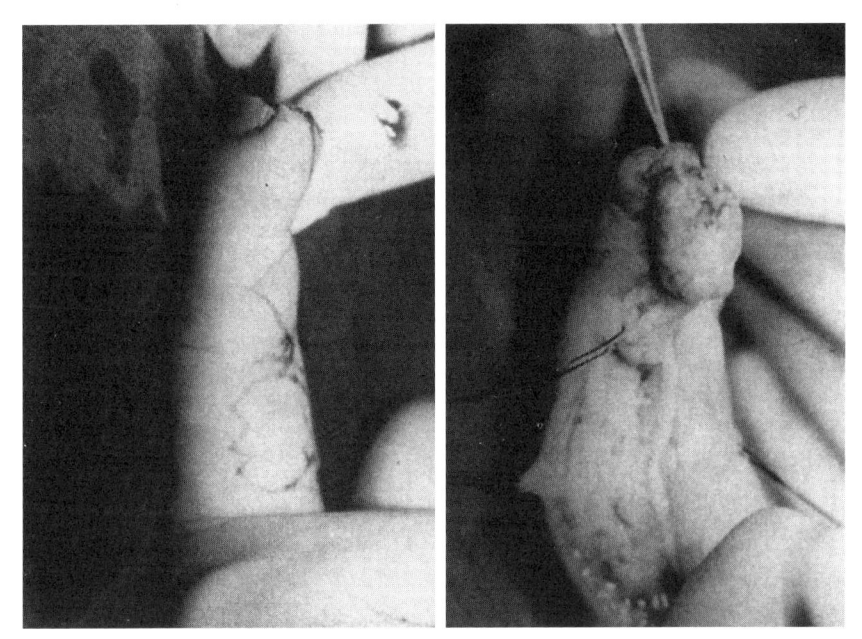

FIGURE 1.—**Left**, preoperative design of the reverse digital artery island flap on the ulnar side of the right index finger. **Right**, intraoperative view with the flap elevated. (Courtesy of Han S-K, Lee B-I, Kim W-K: The reverse digital artery island flap: Clinical experience in 120 fingers. *Plast Reconstr Surg* 101:1006–1011, 1998.)

quired for 11 fingers. Neurorrhaphy was performed in 21 fingers to restore sensation.

Conclusions.—All reverse digital artery island flaps but one survived. Sensory recovery was excellent.

▶ The authors report outstanding success with a reverse digital artery flap. In an 11-year retrospective study, 118 of 120 attempted flaps had complete survival. This technique for coverage of soft tissue defects distal to the distal interphalangeal joint has advantages of being 1 stage, maintaining finger length, and providing a good soft tissue pad. It is a flap, however, of unknown venous drainage that introduces scar throughout the length of the finger, sacrifices a digital artery, and in most cases requires a skin graft to the donor site. In particular cultures, however, the advantages of this flap outweigh the disadvantages, particularly when a success rate like this is achievable.

S.J. Finical, M.D.

The Dorsal Middle Phalangeal Finger Flap: Mid-term Results of 43 Cases

Leupin P, Weil J, Büchler U (Univ of Berne, Switzerland)
J Hand Surg [Br] 22B:362–371, 1997   4–6

Introduction.—The dorsal middle finger phalangeal finger (DMF) flap allows an area of up to 4 × 6 cm to be harvested for coverage of soft tissue defects in the hand. This new flap is based on 1 palmar proper digital artery, its venae comitantes, and the dorsal branch(es) of the palmar digital nerve. Nine variations in flap design have become available in the last decade. Forty-three DMF flap procedures performed in 41 patients were critically examined for survival, revascularization capacity, sensibility, and donor site morbidity.

Methods.—The procedures were performed from November 1985 to January 1996. All patients included in the analysis met minimum follow-up requirements (6 months for nonneurotized flaps and 36 months for neurovascular flaps). Final results of the flap were evaluated at a mean of 52 months. Patients were interviewed for pain and general satisfaction, and donor and recipient sites were examined for contour, texture, and color match.

Results.—Eighteen DMF flaps were used to cover acute multiple tissue defects caused mainly by power machinery, 19 were used in the subacute stage for defects with a variety of causes, and 6 were used to correct late posttraumatic flexion contractures or unstable scars. Most flaps were harvested within the confines of the dorsum of the middle phalanx. Three flaps showed signs of transient venous insufficiency, but there were no significant complications related to flap survival, and all DMF flap procedures achieved their goal. Some flaps required additional surgical procedures, including debulking in 4 patients and release of contracted flap margins in 3. No patients reported pain in the donor area, but 6 patients were not entirely satisfied with appearance at this site. Dissection between the proper digital nerve and the rest of the neurovascular bundle led to cold intolerance in 5% of flaps and S3+ hypesthesia in 12%. Thirty-seven recipient sites were pain free, and all flaps were perfectly integrated at the recipient site. Overall function of the affected hand was rated as normal or near normal by 16 patients, slightly or moderately impaired by 17, and significantly impaired by 5.

Conclusion.—The raising of DMF flaps is technically demanding and time consuming, but it is safe and generally eliminates the need for second stage procedures. Both palmar and digital arteries must be patent if this flap is to be used. Donor site morbidity should be weighed against the advantage of the procedure and the donor morbidity of alternative flaps.

▶ Another variety of the homodigital island flap is presented and well discussed. This flap is based on the dorsal branches of 1 of the digital arteries and its accompanying dorsal nerve branches. A series of modifications are described, including its use as a small free microvascular transfer from the opposite middle finger. The procedure, however, is technically demanding and time consuming but typically can provide definitive coverage, with or without sensibility, in 1 stage.

V.R. Hentz, M.D.

Eponychial Flap [French]
Bakhach J
Ann Chir Plast Esthet 43:259–263, 1998   4–7

Objective.—In transverse amputation of the fingertip, passing through the distal third of the nail plate, local palmar flaps allow reconstructing a good pulp, but the nail remains shorter than on neighboring fingers. A new flap is proposed to "unveil" part of the hidden nail plate.

Methods.—The eponychium is vascularized by an arterial arcade. The depth of the proximal nail fold was measured in vivo in 100 fingers and compared to the total length of the nail plate. From 28.5% to 80% (mean of 40%) of the nail plate is hidden by the eponychium.

Technique.—An eponychium flap is incised by 2 deep lateral incisions in line with the lateral fold. Then, at the level of the matrix, a rectangular flap is sectioned from the epidermis, the width being equal to the eponychium and the high point equal to the desired amount of proximal nail plate exposure. The flap is then withdrawn, and its proximal edge is sutured to the proximal edge of the flap that was removed.

Results.—Two such procedures were performed and in 1, it was necessary to incise the proximal nail fold to facilitate the migration of the flap. A thickening of the exposed proximal nail plate was noticed in both cases, without dystrophy.

Conclusion.—The eponychium flap allows increasing the visible part of the nail plate in moderate transverse distal fingertip amputations.

▶ Nail is a tool and a cosmetic appendage. A finger with a small nail is sometimes hidden by a patient concerned by its cosmetic aspect, reducing the function of the hand. This simple technique will find a place in such cases, when around 30% to 40% of the distal nail plate is amputated. In such cases, the good bone support avoids a hook deformity but not a shortening of the nail plate.

G. Foucher, M.D.

Nail Transfer: Evolution of the Reconstructive Procedure
Endo T, Nakayama Y, Soeda S (Univ of Tsukuba, Japan; St Luke's Internatl Hosp, Tokyo)
Plast Reconstr Surg 100:907–913, 1997   4–8

Objective.—There are few reports of nail reconstruction. The use of vascularized nail flaps and free nail grafts and the strategy of nail reconstruction were described. Four cases were discussed.

Methods.—Nail reconstruction was performed 24 times in 19 patients (4 males) aged 5–54 years. Thirteen had congenital defects and 6 had nail injuries. Free grafts were used for 14 defects, and vascularized nail flaps were used for 10 defects. Free nail grafts including the nail, nail bed, nail matrix, and periosteum were inserted into a skin flap. For vascularized nail flaps, a nail flap from the big toe was transferred, and the dorsalis pedis vessels and the dorsal cutaneous veins of the foot were anastomosed to the radial vessels and the cutaneous veins of the hand. The nail flap with intact cutaneous veins was transferred, and arteriovenous and venovenous anastomoses were performed. The short-pedicled flap is transferred, and the donor digital artery of the toe is anastomosed to the digital artery of the involved finger.

Results.—There was 1 failure, a free nail graft. Good nail growth was observed in all other cases. Free nail grafts are useful for congenital nail defects but not for defects caused by trauma. The long-pedicled vascularized nail flap is the treatment of choice for traumatic nail defects. The surgery is lengthy (more than 7 hours) and leaves scarring at the donor and recipient sites. The venous flap is fast and easy, but the possible presence of venous valves can be dangerous. The short-pedicle vascularized nail flap combines the advantages of the free nail graft and the vascularized nail flap.

Conclusions.—The short-pedicle vascularized nail flap transfer is the procedure of choice for nail reconstruction.

▶ The authors present a spectrum of experience with fingernail reconstruction. Their experience is presented as a critique of procedures ranging from free nail grafts to sophisticated, short-pedicled nail bed flaps. At present, the authors recommend the short-pedicled nail bed flap as the procedure producing the most favorable reconstruction and donor site.

W.C. Lineaweaver, M.D.

Composite Graft Replacement of Digital Tips: 2. A Study in Children
Moiemen NS, Elliot D (St Andrew's Centre for Plastic Surgery, Billericay, England)
J Hand Surg [Br] 22B:346–352, 1997   4–9

Objective.—There is substantial disagreement on the success of composite grafting. Fifty consecutive children with 50 digital tip amputations treated by composite grafting during a period of 3 years and 6 months were studied, to establish when, if at all, this procedure might be expected to work.

Methods.—In 50 children (12 girls) aged 1–14 years, 50 digital tips that were completely amputated by crush injury were minimally debrided and reattached. Levels of amputation (modified Ishikawa classification) were 4 zone Ia, 17 zone Ib, 21 zone II, and 8 zone III.

Results.—There were 11 complete graft takes, 13 total failures, and 26 partial takes. Of the 18 tips reattached within 5 hours, 11 (61%) survived completely, 4 (22%) survived partially, and 3 (17%) failed. Of the 32 tips reattached after 5 hours, 22 (69%) survived partially and 10 (31%) failed. The survival differences before and after 5 hours were significant. The average time elapsed between injury and reattachment in successful procedures was 3.9 hours, whereas the time elapsed between injury and reattachment in unsuccessful procedures was significantly longer, 7.8 hours. Healing time was 28 days in the successful group, 40 days in the partial survival group, and 44 days in the failure group. According to the children's mothers, 95% of children with partial survival and 73% of children with successful reattachment were using the hand normally.

Conclusions.—Composite graft replacement of the digital tip in children was significantly more successful if the tip was replaced within 5 hours of injury. Successful reattachment and partial reattachment resulted in normal functional use.

▶ The authors asked and answered an important question using a simple retrospective study. They showed that composite graft tips replaced within 5 hours are likely to completely survive, and those replaced after 5 hours do not survive (at least not completely). They also note that the appearance of a "partial take" improves with time, and based on this finding, they recommend that the surgeon delay débridement of necrotic tissue (in other words, don't pick at the scab, just let it fall off).

Although they specify the age of their patients (1–14 years; mean, 5.7 years), they do not state whether age was associated with composite graft take. This information would also be useful.

M.A. James, M.D.

Upper Limb *Escherichia coli* Cellulitis in the Immunocompromised
Brzozowski D, Ross DC (Univ of Western Ontario, London)
J Hand Surg [Br] 22B:679–680, 1997   4–10

Objective.—Because patients with acute lymphoblastic leukemia have a low neutrophil count, they are at risk of infection from gram-negative organisms. A case of rapidly ascending cellulitis of the arm caused by *Escherichia coli* was reported.

Case Report.—Man, 21, who was receiving reinduction chemotherapy for relapse of acute lymphoblastic leukemia, had a high fever on day 5. His neutrophil count was zero. He was given IV tobramycin and cefazolin followed by vancomycin, but severe sudden pain developed in the web space of his left hand. Blood cultures grew *E. coli*. He was given piperacillin in place of cefazolin. Ultrasound showed fluid collected in the web space, and duplex Doppler revealed a subclavian vein thrombosis. The wound was drained, but the cellulitis spread to the level of the axilla, and forequarter amputation was performed. Diffuse fibrosis found in the area of the subclavian vein was thought to be the result of a previous line insertion. His neutrophil count began to return to normal 5 weeks later. He was admitted, 3 weeks after discharge, for a bone marrow transplantation but had severe abdominal pain. Gram-negative rods were isolated from blood samples, and the patient died of cardiorespiratory and renal failure.

Discussion.—Characteristic signs and symptoms of cellulitis are blunted in neutropenic patients, and the source of infection is usually not obvious in patients receiving chemotherapy.

Conclusion.—Progression of cellulitis in neutropenic patients is rapid. Signs and symptoms of infection, except for severe pain, are usually blunted and may contribute to fatal outcomes. Early antibiotic therapy is crucial and débridement is recommended.

▶ This case illustrates the aggressive surgery necessary to control progressive extremity infection in an immunocompromised patient.

W.C. Lineaweaver, M.D.

Suggested Reading

Bertelli J, Nogueira C: Treatment of recurrent digital scar contracture in paediatric patients by proximal phalangeal island flap. *Ann Chir Main Memb Super* 16:310–315, 1997.
▶ The authors describe a flap of skin and subcutaneous tissue harvested as an island from the skin of the dorsum of the finger near the proximal interphalangeal joint. This flap is then rotated to cover the volar skin defect that is the consequence of releasing a contracture of the proximal interphalangeal joint. The dorsal skin in these cases has been overstretched as a consequence of the contracture. The authors base this small flap on a relatively constant branch off the digital artery that arises about 10 mm proximal to the proximal interphalangeal joint.

V.R. Hentz, M.D.

El-Khatib HA: Island fasciocutaneous flap based on the proximal perforators of the radial artery for resurfacing of burned cubital fossa. *Plast Reconstr Surg* 100:919–925, 1997.
▶ This is a report of a fasciocutaneous flap for coverage of a burned cubital fossa after excision of scar and release of contracture. The author reports the

results from his cadaveric dissection of 10 fresh cadaver upper extremities and from 18 of his clinical cases. This study supports the use of burned tissue for coverage of the defect based on the fact that the injury may not involve the deeper fascia and its vasculature. This technique does afford the use of local tissue without the morbidity of a free flap or compromise of the vasculature to the extremity. Unfortunately, this flap seems to have limited applications. As the extent of the injury at the donor site may be equivocal, the surgeon may be transferring marginal tissue to an already compromised area.

N.F. Jones, M.D.

Giddins GEB, Hill RA: Late diagnosis and treatment of crush injuries of the fingertip in children. *Injury* 29:447–450, 1998.
▶ This is a useful reference for hand surgeons who deal with emergency room staff on a regular basis. The combination of pediatric distal phalanx fracture and nailbed injury still goes unrecognized in many settings.

P.C. Amadio, M.D.

Kostakoğlu N, Keçilc A: Upper limb reconstruction with reverse flaps: A review of 52 patients with emphasis on flap selection. *Ann Plast Surg* 39:381–389, 1997.
▶ These authors review their experience with 52 patients who had reconstruction of variously located and variously sized defects by means of reversed or retrograde flaps, typically island flaps. Their message is that the anatomy of the upper limb, with its multiple longitudinal arterial systems, lends itself particularly well to flaps of this design. The use of these flaps has significantly reduced the need for microvascular free tissue transfer. For palmar loss, the authors most frequently used radial forearm flaps, and for dorsal loss, posterior interosseous flaps. Their place on the reconstructive ladder deserves readjustment. Perhaps they should be the first thought.

V.R. Hentz, M.D.

5 Tendon Trauma and Reconstruction

Controlled Active Motion Following Primary Flexor Tendon Repair: A Prospective Study Over 9 Years
Kitsis CK, Wade PJF, Krikler SJ, et al (Coventry and Warwickshire Hosp, England)
J Hand Surg [Br] 23B:344–349, 1998   5–1

Background.—In patients undergoing flexor tendon repair, postoperative immobilization can lead to adhesions, and unrestricted motion can raise the risk of rupture. Recent approaches have tried to balance the need for active motion with the need to protect against excessive motion. The results of a high-strength suture technique followed by a more aggressive regimen of postoperative motion are reported.

Methods.—The 8-year prospective study included 130 patients undergoing repair of 339 flexor tendons affecting 208 fingers, including 87 fingers in zone 2. In each case, primary repair was performed by a multistrand technique using a modified Kessler core stitch of 4/0 braided polyester and a strong peripheral running suture of a Halsted or Lembert configuration using 5/0 braided polyester. The patients went through an early active motion regimen, with protection by a modified Kleinert dynamic traction splint. Follow-up evaluations were performed at 6 months and 1 year postoperatively.

Results.—The results, as expressed by Strickland grade, varied among zones. The results in zone 2 were excellent in 56% of the cases, good in 33%, fair in 9%, and poor in 2%. These results were not strongly affected by the experience of the operating surgeon. There were a total of 43 complications, including 17 moderate joint contractures, 5 tendon ruptures in zone 2, and 1 rupture in zone 5.

Conclusions.—A flexor tendon repair technique of high-strength suture repair followed by controlled active motion with protection by a Kleinert-type splint requires high-quality physical therapy and splint-construction ability. However, the approach provides very good results, with low rates of rupture and reoperation.

▶ This article accurately summarizes the current state of early active mobilization after primary flexor tendon repair. The authors describe a regimen using a single modified Kessler suture of 4/0 polyester and a running peripheral suture of 5/0 polyester. Early active motion under daily therapy supervision is encouraged. Active finger flexion and extension are permitted with the wrist in a neutral position, as are blocking exercises. Only stretch and resistance are avoided. Despite this aggressive protocol, and less-than-aggressive repair technique (many others are more sturdy), the results were impressive, with 90% good or excellent results at 6 months. Only 10% fair or poor results were recorded for zone 2, but they were assessed after any rerepairs for rupture (6%) or tenolysis (13%). Nonetheless, these results are certainly comparable to those of other series, and might be improved further with less stressful active programs, such as the place-and-hold or synergistic regimens, or with a stronger repair, or both—all this without even beginning to address biological therapies to improve tendon healing and to reduce tendon friction. We have truly come a long way in tendon surgery.

P.C. Amadio, M.D.

Double Armed Reinsertion Suture (DARS) of the Profundus Flexor Tendon With Immediate Active Mobilization of the Finger: 63 Cases
Messina A, Messina JC (Clinica Fornaca, Torino, Italy)
Ann Chir Main Memb Super 16:245–251, 1997   5–2

Objective.—Profundus flexor tendon repairs often fail as a result of trauma or technical problems. The double-armed reinsertion suture (DARS) technique allows immediate active mobilization of the finger, thereby overcoming problems with adhesions and tendon disruption during early mobilization.

Technique.—The repair can be performed immediately or within 1 or 2 weeks of injury. The technique, performed under regional anesthesia, preserves the blood supply to the posterior section of the tendon (Figs 1 and 2).

Methods.—Between 1982 and 1994, the DARS technique was performed on 63 patients. Of these, the cases of 40 patients (5 females), aged 7–75 years, were reviewed in December 1995. Digits repaired included 13 thumbs, 9 index fingers, 6 long fingers, 5 ring fingers, and 7 small fingers.

Results.—There were 8 excellent outcomes (full active and passive motion), 28 good (full passive and possibility of full active motion), and 4 poor (joint stiffness, adhesions, or tendon shortening). Total active motion scores were 8 excellent, 24 good, 4 fair, and 4 poor.

Conclusion.—The DARS "lost thread" technique is an effective tendon repair method that permits early active mobilization and results in a satisfactory functional outcome with no risk of tendon rupture.

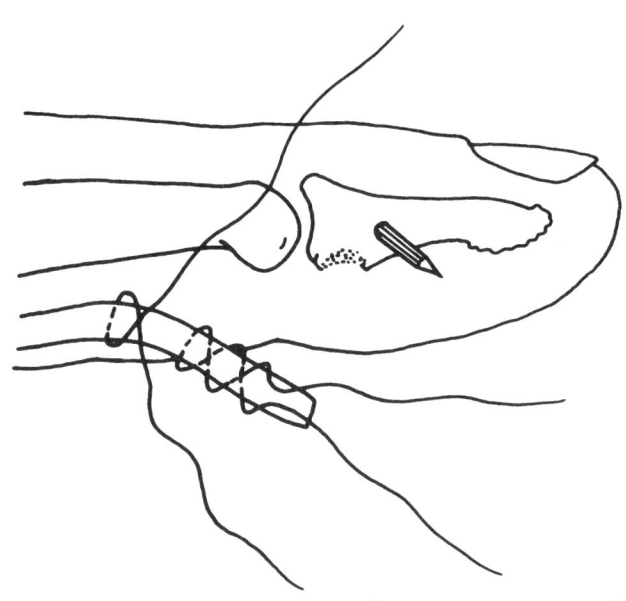

FIGURE 1.—The double-armed reinsertion suture. A first nylon suture is crisscrossed through the tendon stump; a second nylon suture is inserted 1 cm more proximally and then crisscrossed in the lateral and median lines of the tendon thickness. Both nylon sutures are passed through the hole of the metaphysis of P3 and tied laterally and left in situ as a lost thread. (Courtesy of Messina A, Messina JC: Double armed reinsertion suture [DARS] of the profundus flexor tendon with immediate active mobilization of the finger: 63 cases. *Ann Chir Main Memb Super* 16:245–251, 1997.)

▶ In 1992, the authors published their experience with a double-suture technique to repair flexor tendons lacerated within the digital sheath.[1] In this article, the authors describe a double-suture technique that anchors the profundus tendon to the bone, using a nonpullout technique for zone 1 profundus tendon injuries. The results, as determined by the total active motion method, are very respectable. However, it is difficult to understand the authors' preference for the Bunnell crossing suture when so much research has demonstrated that it is less effective than later-described methods.

V.R. Hentz, M.D.

Reference

1. Messina A: The double armed suture: Tendon repair with immediate mobilization of the fingers. *J Hand Surg [Am]* 17A:137–142, 1992.

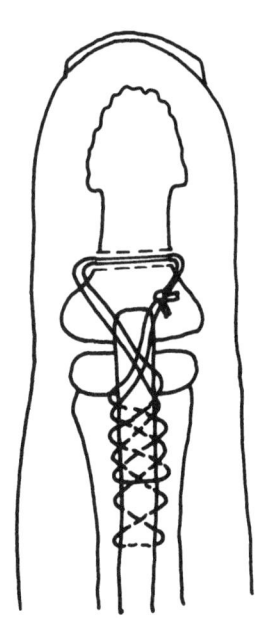

FIGURE 2.—Nylon sutures in the double-armed reinsertion suture are strongly anchored to the metaphysis of P3. This allows immediate active mobilization of the finger without any risk of rupture of the suture or tendon disruption. (Courtesy of Messina A, Messina JC: Double armed reinsertion suture [DARS] of the profundus flexor tendon with immediate active mobilization of the finger: 63 cases. *Ann Chir Main Memb Super* 16:245–251, 1997.)

The Range of Excursion of Flexor Tendons in Zone V: A Comparison of Active vs Passive Flexion Mobilisation Regimes
Panchal J, Mehdi S, Donoghue JO, et al (Cork Univ, Ireland)
Br J Plast Surg 50:517–522, 1997   5–3

Background.—Flexor tendon repair is associated with adhesion formation, which can limit the excursion range of the repaired tendon. Postoperative early mobilization regimens have been instituted in an effort to minimize the formation of adhesions. Recently, active flexion mobilization regimens have begun to replace early passive flexion mobilization regimens. The outcome after repair of multiple flexor tendons in zone V (spaghetti wrist) has not been well studied. To determine the range of excursion of flexor tendons in zone V and to compare the excursion range between active and passive flexion mobilization regimens, both cadaveric and patient wrists were assessed.

Methods.—Two cadaveric wrists and the wrists of 2 patients with multiple flexor tendon divisions in zone V were studied. Active (Belfast) flexion mobilization was compared to passive (modified Duran) flexion mobilization regimens in cadavers and in patients, intraoperatively and postoperatively, at 10 days, 3 weeks, and 6 weeks.

TABLE 3.—Mean Excursion of Flexor Tendon in the Postoperative Period

		10 days (mm) Passive	10 days (mm) Active	21 days (mm) Passive	21 days (mm) Active	42 days (mm) Passive	42 days (mm) Active
FDS:	Mean Patient (A,B)	1 (0, 2)	3 (2, 4)	1 (0, 2)	5 (4, 6)	9 (8, 10)	12 (13, 11)
FDP:	Mean Patient (A,B)	4 (5, 3)	10 (8, 12)	2 (2, 2)	15 (13, 17)	7 (8, 6)	33 (35, 31)
FPL:	Mean Patient (A,B)	4 (3, 5)	12 (10, 14)	1 (1, 1)	21 (19, 23)	4 (5, 3)	20 (19, 21)

(Courtesy of Panchal J, Mehdi S, Donoghue JO, et al: The range of excursion of flexor tendons in zone V: A comparison of active vs passive flexion mobilisation regimes. *Br J Plast Surg* 50:517–522, 1997.)

Results.—In cadaveric wrists with passive flexion, the mean tendon excursion in zone V was 1 mm for flexor digitorum superficialis (FDS), flexor digitorum profundus (FDP), and flexor pollicis longus (FPL) tendons. With simulated active flexion, the mean tendon excursion was 14 mm for FDS, 10 mm for FDP, and 11 mm for FPL. Intraoperatively, the mean tendon excursion with passive flexion was 2 mm for FDS, FDP, and FPL. After simulated active flexion, it was 10 mm for FDS, 11 mm for FDP, and 11 mm for FPL. Ten days postoperatively with passive flexion, the mean excursion of FDS was 1 mm, of FDP was 4 mm, and of FPL was 4 mm. On active flexion, the mean excursion of FDS was 3 mm, of FDP was 10 mm, and of FPL was 12 mm. After 3 weeks with passive flexion, the mean excursion of FDS was 1 mm, of FDP was 2 mm, and of FPL was 1 mm. On active flexion, the mean tendon excursion was 5 mm for FDS, 15 mm for FDP, and 21 mm for FPL. Six weeks postoperatively with passive flexion, the mean tendon excursion was 9 mm for FDS, 7 mm for FDP, and 4 mm for FPL. With active flexion, the mean tendon excursion was 12 mm for FDS, 33 mm for FDP, and 20 mm for FPL (Table 3).

Conclusions.—In both cadaveric and clinical studies and in both intraoperative and postoperative studies, both active and simulated active flexion produced greater tendon excursion in zone V than passive flexion. The active flexion regimen appears to be the superior option for avoidance of adhesion after tendon repair of zone V injuries.

▶ The authors have performed a valuable study on the range of excursion of flexor tendons in zone V in both a cadaveric model and in 2 patients who sustained zone V wrist laceration, which resulted in a division of the FPL, FDS, and FDP to the index, middle, ring, and little fingers. The authors are to be congratulated for including a cadaveric study, as well as a dynamic postoperative study, in the design of their work. This study also addresses a deficit in the literature, as no prior work has investigated the range of excursion of flexor tendons in zone V either in cadavers or postoperatively. The authors have shown convincingly that both in cadavers and postoperatively, there is a significant excursion of repaired flexor tendons in zone V after active flexion mobilization as compared to a passive flexion regimen (see Table 3).

They suggest that this significant range of excursion may reduce formation of adhesions.

As the authors point out, there have been very few studies on the outcome of zone V injuries. One report[1] suggests excellent or good outcome in 87% of cases with passive mobilization, whereas another work[2] notes only half of the patients in their series had good to excellent results using early controlled passive mobilization. No doubt the outcome of these injuries will depend on the number of tendons injured and repaired, as well as the type and extent of nerve and vascular injuries requiring repair.

The constant debate about when and how to apply either active or passive mobilization regimens after flexor tendon repair applies to this work as well. The authors have clearly shown increased excursions with active motion and have indeed initiated very early (10-day) active motion postoperatively. The study, however, was performed in only 2 patients, which does not constitute a series. Therefore, there is no indication regarding the rates of rupture of the repairs after initiating early active motion. Many authors have noted rapid loss of muscle elasticity in zone V injuries, which may add to the forces on tendon repair(s) at the wrist in causing increased rupture rates either with active or passive flexion.

The authors have provided good data and insight into "spaghetti wrist" injuries and flexor tendon excursions with both active and passive motion. The ultimate outcome of their suggestion that initiating active early motion postoperatively is a reasonable course to prevent adhesions will await their future results on rates of tendon rupture after such a regimen.

M.A. Badalamente, Ph.D.

References

1. Puckett CL, Meyer VH: Results of treatment of extensive volar wrist lacerations: The spaghetti wrist. *Plast Reconstr Surg* 75: 714–719, 1985.
2. Hudson DA, de Jager LT: The spaghetti wrist: Simultaneous laceration of the median and ulnar nerves with flexor tendons at the wrist. *J Hand Surg [Br]* 18B: 171–173, 1993.

Early Active Mobilization for Extensor Tendon Injuries: The Norwich Regime
Sylaidis P, Youatt M, Logan A (West Norwich Hosp, England)
J Hand Surg [Br] 22B:594–596, 1997   5–4

Background.—After extensor tendon repair, dynamic splinting has been found to provide better results than static splinting, but involves clumsy splints and complicated protocols. A controlled, active mobilization protocol without dynamic splinting, the Norwich regimen, was evaluated prospectively in a series of 27 consecutive patients.

Study Group.—All patients who had primary finger extensor tendon repair for complete division between the proximal half of the proximal phalanx and the wrist were eligible for the study. The 27 patients in this

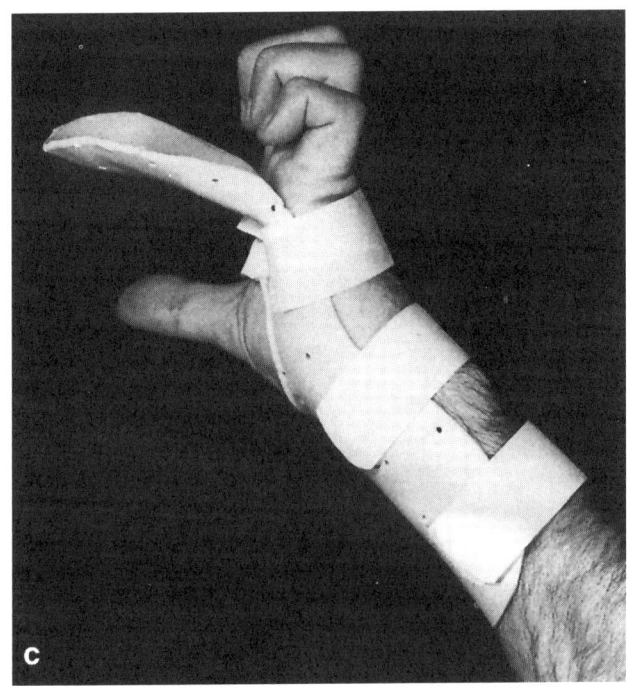

FIGURE 1, C.—Interphalangeal flexion exercise. (Courtesy of Sylaidis P, Youatt M, Logan A: Early active mobilization for extensor tendon injuries: The Norwich regime. *J Hand Surg [Br]* 22B:594–596, 1997.)

series were all male, aged 19–81 years; 17 had simple tendon injuries and 10 had complex injuries.

Methods.—After extensor tendon repair, tension was controlled by wrist extension and avoidance of composite metacarpophalangeal and interphalangeal flexion. The hand was rested on a palmar splint with the wrist at 45 degrees extension, metacarpophalangeal joints flexed to at least 50 degrees, and interphalangeal joints extended. Controlled active mobilization was initiated on the first day after surgery. The patients performed 2 exercises: combined interphalangeal and metacarpophalangeal extension and metacarpophalangeal joint extension with interphalangeal joint flexion (Fig 1, C). These exercises were performed no more than 4 times per session for 4 sessions daily for 4 weeks. Then, the splint was worn only at night, and the exercises were replaced with gentle flexion of the metacarpophalangeal and interphalangeal joints, increasing over time to full flexion and power grip. Progress was evaluated at 4 and 6 weeks after surgery with the Dargan criteria. The average time to return to work was also noted.

Results.—Among those patients with simple tendon injuries, 2 were unavailable for follow-up between the fourth and sixth postoperative week. Of the remaining patients, there were 14 excellent, 8 good, and 2 fair results at 6-week follow-up. Of the patients with complex fractures, 2 were unavailable for follow-up between the fourth and sixth postoperative week. Of the remaining patients, there were 9 excellent, 2 good, and 2 fair results. The average time to return to work was 6.5 weeks for simple tendon injuries and 8.5 weeks for complex injuries.

Conclusions.—Early active mobilization of extensor tendon injuries using the Norwich regimen leads to results that are comparable with those after dynamic splinting. The Norwich regimen does not require complicated splintage and exercise protocols to achieve these results.

▶ This is an extremely simple protocol compared with those using dynamic extensor splinting. Therapy is initially limited to a single visit at 1 day after surgery for fabrication of an intrinsic-plus flexion-blocking splint and instruction for a basic home exercise program. Follow-up is at 4 weeks with gradual weaning from the splint and progressive flexion and strengthening. The initial home program consists of active extension of the digits and claw maneuvers, 4 sets, 4 times a day. The authors' experience with 27 patients with zone IV–VII injuries is similar to published results for other popular protocols.

It surprises me that this protocol—which seems to do little to protect stretching of the extensor repair—has no higher incidence of extension lags than those that carefully maintain extension of the digits at all costs. This regimen offers cost saving with less therapy time and simpler splints. It also may improve patient compliance because of simpler exercises and splinting. If, indeed, further experience confirms the efficacy of this protocol, I would imagine that dynamic extension splints, with their cumbersome outriggers, will lose favor in extensor tendon repair.

K.A. Bengtson, M.D.

Simplified Functional Splinting After Extensor Tenorrhaphy
Slater RR Jr, Bynum DK (Univ of California–Davis, Sacramento; Univ of North Carolina, Chapel Hill)
J Hand Surg [Am] 22A:445–451, 1997   5–5

Background.—It has recently been suggested that extensor tendon repair would benefit from dynamic splinting similar to that used for flexor tendon rehabilitation. Whether good functional results could be achieved using simpler, cheaper, and less labor-intensive functional static splinting was studied retrospectively.

Methods.—A computerized search of the medical records of the University of North Carolina identified 22 patients who were treated for lacerations of finger extensor tendons in zones V–VIII and/or thumb extensor tendons in zones TIII–TV from 1983 to 1995. These patients composed the study group. There were 21 male patients and 1 female patient, with an average age of 32.7 years. Splints were applied 3–7 days after surgery to either the dorsal or volar extremity surface (Fig 1). All wrists were immobilized with approximately 30 degrees of extension. In

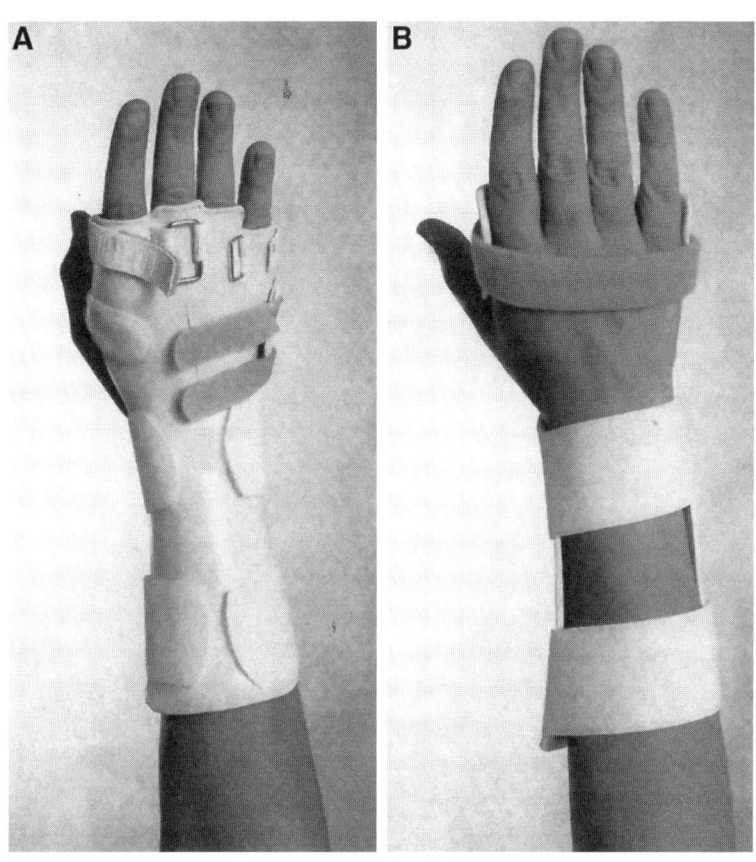

FIGURE 1.—Splints may be applied to either the dorsal (A) or volar (B) surface of the forearm/wrist, as dictated by associated wounds, soft-tissue injuries, and surgeon's preference. (Courtesy of Slater RR Jr, Bynum DK: Simplified functional splinting after extensor tenorrhaphy. *J Hand Surg [Am]* 22A:445–451, 1997.)

cases without thumb extensor tendon involvement, finger metacarpophalangeal (MP) joints were flexed 20–30 degrees and the thumb MP joints and finger interphalangeal joints were left free. When thumb extensor repairs were involved, the thumb carpometacarpal and MP joints were held in neutral extension. Patients were instructed to wear their splints full time and to perform active interphalangeal joint range-of-motion exercises. Patients wore their splints for an average of 6 weeks. The average follow-up was 4.5 months.

Results.—Excellent results were achieved in 10 cases, good results in 9, and fair results in 3 cases. No differences in outcome were related to differences in suture material or technique. All patients were able to return to preinjury work status. There were no impairments that interfered with activities of daily living. Complications were rare. There were no ruptures of the repaired extensor tendons in this patient series.

Conclusions.—A review of extensor tendon repairs in zones V–VIII and TIII–TV using functional static splinting found that good to excellent results were achieved in 86% of patients. None of the 22 patients had problems with hand function. All returned to preinjury work status and activities of daily living. The technique was well tolerated. Functional static splinting is cheaper, easier, and less labor-intensive than dynamic splinting and appears to achieve good results. A prospective, controlled clinical trial comparing functional static splinting and dynamic splinting in the rehabilitation of extensor tendon repairs has yet to be performed.

▶ The results of this study are convincing, and this splinting routine (in some cases without supervised therapy) may be an effective solution as we struggle to work within managed care restraints. However, splinting that rests the MP joints in 20–30 degrees of flexion between exercise sessions will often result in an extensor lag in zones V and VI, and resting the proximal interphalangeal (PIP) joint in flexion with a splint cut away at the PIP level, particularly if the digit is swollen, may result in PIP joint flexion contracture, especially if the patient is reluctant to move the digits through the prescribed range of motion. I would guess that the patients in this study with a mean age of 32.7 years were not reluctant to move, and most likely were actively moving at the MP joint level from the 20–30 degrees of flexion to full extension, thereby ensuring some proximal migration of the repair site in zones V–VII.

Motion at the MP level is required to obtain adequate excursion for tendon repairs on the dorsum of the hand and be more proximal. Moving the MP joint through 1 radian will glide the tendon the distance of its moment arm at the MP joint ". . .approximately 30 degrees of MP joint flexion for the index and long fingers and 40 degrees flexion for the ring and small fingers creates about 5 mm of excursion for the respective extensor tendons," according to Brand[1] whose work has been verified intraoperatively by Evans and Burkhalter.[2] The extensor pollicis longus glides 5 mm through the retinacular level and at the level of Lister's tubercle with 60 degrees of interphalangeal motion.[2] Immobilizing the MP joints in the digits as described with this technique may not ensure adequate excursion of the repair site and may result in extension contracture at the MP joints, especially for the ulnar digits. This design does, however, allow for adequate excursion of the extensor pollicis longus.

It has been demonstrated that modest MP flexion of just 15 degrees significantly reduces or eliminates proximal extensor activity[3]; therefore, this splint design may not allow for transmission of active tension to the repair site unless the MP joint moves into some extension with the exercise.

Extensor tendon injuries are best managed with formal therapy programs where the hand can be removed from the splint for some wrist tenodesis motion, and for active place-and-hold exercise for the digits—both exercises designed to ensure adequate tendon excursion at the repair site. Internal tendon forces are increased with active exercise as the wrist is placed in increased increments of extension and may exceed the tensile strength of some extensor tendon repairs.[4] The position of least internal tendon tension for the extensor system in zones V–VII is with the wrist positioned at 10–20 degrees of flexion for place and hold with all digital joints positioned in extension. This should be a consideration in the determination of wrist position when designing the protective splint if the digital joints are allowed to move actively.

With regard to the cost of the splint, the static splint offers savings only if time in therapy and time lost from work are minimal. This information is not provided in the study. Although dynamic splints made with prefabricated components can be expensive, dynamic splints made with spring steel wire add only pennies to the cost of the material and take about 10 minutes to fabricate. Digital motion is most often reestablished by 6 weeks postoperatively in patients who are referred to therapy within a few days of surgery and who are treated with programs that ensure adequate excursion at the repair site(s).

R.B. Evans, O.T.R./L., C.H.T.

References

1. Brand PW: Transmission, in Brand PW, Hollister A (eds): *Clinical Mechanics of the Hand*, ed 2. St Louis, Mosby, 1993, p 67.
2. Evans RB, Burkhalter WE: A study of the dynamic anatomy of extensor tendons and implications for treatment. *J Hand Surg [Am]* 11A:774–779, 1986.
3. Newport ML, Shukla A: Electrophysiologic basis of dynamic extensor splinting. *J Hand Surg [Am]* 17A:272–277, 1992.
4. Evans RB, Thompson DE: The application of force to the healing tendon. *J Hand Ther* 6:266–284, 1993.

Mallet Deformity of the Finger: Five-Year Follow-up of Conservative Treatment
Okafor B, Mbubaegbu C, Munshi I, et al (Queen Elizabeth II Hosp, Welwyn Garden City, England)
J Bone Joint Surg Br 79-B:544–547, 1997   5–6

Objective.—The long-term course of mallet deformity of the finger is unknown because of the paucity of studies. A review is presented of 31 patients at an average of 5 years after treatment of mallet deformity of the finger with a thermoplastic splint.

Methods.—Pain on a visual analogue scale, functional impairment, patient satisfaction, extension deficit, arc of flexion, presence of a swan-neck deformity, and radiologic changes were assessed at an average of 66 months in 31 patients (15 women), aged 32–71 years, with mallet deformity of the finger.

Results.—Eleven (35%) patients had a fracture of the distal phalanx. The mean distal interphalangeal joint extension lag averaged 8.9 degrees in patients with a fracture and 8 degrees in patients without a fracture. The mean distal interphalangeal joint arc of flexion averaged 42.7 degrees in patients with a fracture and 55.6 degrees in patients without a fracture. There was degeneration in 10 digits in patients with a fracture and in 5 digits in patients without a fracture. Swan-neck deformity occurred in 6 digits in patients with a fracture and in 3 digits in patients without a fracture. Fifteen (48%) patients had radiologic evidence of degeneration. Eleven (35%) patients experienced a loss of extension greater than 10%.

Conclusion.—Despite the presence of degeneration, patient satisfaction was high, probably because of mobility of the proximal interphalangeal and metacarpophalangeal joints. Treatment of mallet deformity with a thermoplastic splint results in few complications.

▶ It is commonly held that closed treatment of mallet deformity yields good results, and indeed this paper confirms that. However, good is not perfect; although function is satisfactory, significant anatomical problems often persist. Further, it is not clear that this series is consecutive. The outcome measures used are not well defined and may not all be valid. Finally, it is not clear who did assessment. Observer bias is a notorious problem in surgical series; patient self-report often discloses problems that the surgeon's interrogation fails to detect, probably because our patients do not wish to disappoint us. Better outcome studies, using better measures, are needed for this and many other conditions.

P.C. Amadio, M.D.

Suggested Reading

Levadoux M, Carli P, Gadea JF, et al: Repeated rupture of the extensor tendons of the hand due to fluoroquinolones: Apropos of a case [French]. *Ann Chir Main Memb Super* 16:130–133, 1997.

▶ This case report describes extensor tendon rupture associated with the use of norfloxacin and perfloxacin. Although hand surgeons may not commonly use those antibiotics (which are used for urinary tract infections), hand surgeons may use ciprofloxacin, a drug from the same fluoroquinolone family. This class of drugs is associated with a risk of tendinopathy, including tendon rupture. Most commonly, the Achilles tendon is affected. Ciprofloxacin appears to be less tendon-toxic than some of the other drugs in this class.[1] Although this side effect is uncommon, it can occur even with short-term therapy.[2]

P.C. Amadio, M.D.

References

1. Kashida Y, Kato M: Characterization of fluoroquinolone-induced Achilles tendon toxicity in rats: Comparison of toxicities of 10 fluoroquinolones and effects of anti-inflammatory compounds. *Antimicrob Agents Chemother* 41:2389–2393, 1997.
2. Wilton LV, Pearce GL, Mann RD: A comparison of ciprofloxacin, norfloxacin, ofloxacin, azithromycin and cefixime examined by observational cohort studies. *Br J Clin Pharmacol* 41:277–284, 1996.

Soucacos PN, Beris AE, Malizos KN, et al: Two-stage treatment of flexor tendon ruptures: Silicon rod complications analyzed in 109 digits. *Acta Orthop Scand* 68:48S–51S, 1997.

▶ This is a nice and readable review of the complications of 2-stage flexor tendon grafting using a silicon or other pseudo-tendon-sheath–producing implant. The authors discuss complications that can occur after stage 1 (rod insertion) such as buckling or migration, as well as complications occurring after stage 2. The uniqueness of this article is in its contrast to most articles about staged flexor tendon grafting in which complications might be mentioned as part of a discussion of results but not discussed to any great extent. There is a deeper message in this article. Staged flexor grafting, while an important adjunct to tendon reconstruction in difficult circumstances, requires careful attention to operative and postoperative details to be successful. It should be an adjunct, not a first choice for all flexor tendon injuries that cannot be directly repaired. However, for too many hand surgeons, there are only 2 procedures applicable for the lacerated or ruptured flexor tendon, either primary repair or 2-stage flexor tendon grafting. This is unfortunate.

V.R. Hentz, M.D.

6 Nerve Trauma and Reconstruction

Reconstruction of Upper-Extremity Peripheral-Nerve Injuries With ePTFE Conduits
Stanec S, Stanec Z (Univ of Zagreb, Croatia)
J Reconstr Microsurg 14:227–232, 1998   6–1

Introduction.—Despite the development of microsurgical techniques, reconstruction of peripheral nerve injuries remains a challenging problem in hand surgery. A study of 43 patients was designed to evaluate the role of a new synthetic conduit for the clinical repair of median and ulnar nerves in the upper extremities. The new conduit consists of an expanded polytetrafluoroethylene (ePTFE) tube.

Methods.—Twenty-one (49%) patients had injuries to the median nerve, and 22 (51%) had ulnar nerve injuries. Causes of injury were gunshot or explosives in 58.1% of the patients and sharp nerve transections in 41.9%. Patients were categorized into 2 groups according to nerve-gap lengths. Twenty-eight patients (group 1) had gaps from 1.5 to 4 cm; 15 (group 2) had gaps from 4.1 to 6 cm. Sterile ePTFE tubes of lengths exceeding the gap length by 1 cm and with 4- to 8-mm diameters were used. Nerve stumps were pulled into the tube to a length of 5 mm on either end (Fig 2). All surgical procedures were secondary reconstructions, with an average delay from injury to repair of 4.2 months.

Results.—In group 1, 78.6% of patients exhibited functional motor and sensory recovery (15 [88.2%] of 17 reconstructed median nerves and 7 [63.6%] of 11 reconstructed ulnar nerves). Grip strength and pinch strength was 73% and 53%, respectively, of the uninjured hand. Useful, functional results were achieved in only 13.3% of group 2 patients (1 of 4 reconstructed median nerves and 1 of 11 reconstructed ulnar nerves). Statistically significantly better results were obtained after repair of clean, sharp lacerations than gunshot or explosive injuries. Only 1 patient required tube removal because of slight discomfort at the site of injury.

Conclusion.—The ePTFE is a reliable and successful procedure for nerve repair in the upper extremities when used in reconstruction of nerve gaps up to 4 cm between the ends of the median and ulnar nerves. Compared

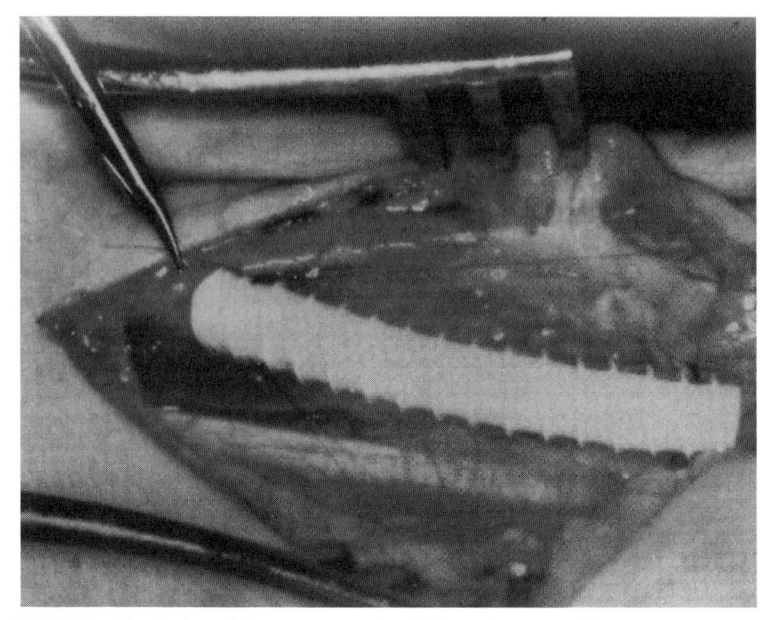

FIGURE 2.—Two horizontal U-sutures are used to facilitate placement of the 5-mm nerve stump into the tube at each end. (Reprinted with permission from the *Journal of Reconstructive Microsurgery*, from Stanec S, Stanec Z: Reconstruction of upper-extremity peripheral-nerve injuries with ePTFE conduits. *J Reconstr Microsurg* 14:227–232, 1998. Copyright Thieme Medical Publishers, Inc.)

with other synthetic tubes, the ePTFE has advantages in promoting nerve regeneration.

▶ This manuscript introduces the use of a new synthetic conduit to manage nerve gap following peripheral nerve injury. The ability to restore motor and sensory function effectively across gaps in damaged peripheral nerves without the use of autologous graft material is exciting. Unfortunately, the inability of the ePTFE conduits to provide good results in longer gaps (4.1–6 cm) negates the major clinical value of this device. The management of small gaps (1.5–4 cm) can be managed by a variety of techniques with comparable results. Although this manuscript is an important preliminary report, it does not support the unrestricted use of this product in patients. Additional studies, including age- and injury-matched patients, which compare alternative grafts (including autograft nerve) with conduits, is necessary. At this point, the use of ePTFE conduits should be reserved for experimental protocols.

L.A. Koman, M.D.

Primary Epineural Repair of the Median Nerve in Children
Hudson DA, Bolitho DG, Hodgetts K (Red Cross Children's Hosp, Cape Town, South Africa; Univ of Cape Town, South Africa)
J Hand Surg [Br] 22B:54–56, 1997
6–2

Objective.—Primary epineural repair of the median nerve in children was studied retrospectively to assess results of the surgery.

Methods.—Between 1982 and 1993, primary epineural repairs after acute transectional lacerations in 18 children (6 girls), aged 14 months to 13 years, were reviewed. Repairs were performed within 24 hours of injury in 16 children and within 1 week of injury in 2 children. Injuries were sustained in 17 children by falling on broken glass. The level of injury was at the wrist in 10 patients, above the elbow in 2, below the elbow in 2, and in the palm in 4. Patients were followed for an average of 52 months. Fifteen children had associated injuries.

Results.—Average return of opponens pollicis function was 4.5 and ranged from 3 to 5. The power grip of the injured hand was within 85% of that of the uninjured hand in 17 children. The static 2-point discrimination averaged 5 mm and ranged from 2 to 10 mm. No child who injured the dominant hand changed dominance. Those with dominant hand injury had dominant hand function within 90% for their age group. The nondominant hand functioned within 10% of the dominant hand.

Conclusion.—Primary epineural repair of the transected medial nerve in children results in satisfactory function and motor recovery.

▶ The result of simple epineural repair of the median nerve in the children reported in this series is equivalent to the results reported for more complex (fascicular) repair. Loupes and 8-0 sutures gave results similar to repair with 10-0 sutures and the surgical microscope. Some elements of postoperative care deserve mentioning. All children were immobilized with the limb in flexion for 6 weeks. This was followed by a period of joint mobilization. We do not worry so much about residual stiffness in children and, therefore, the children tend to be protected longer in a cast than adults. Careers are made on outcomes of surgery in children.

V.R. Hentz, M.D.

Pain Relief After Nerve Resection for Post-Traumatic Neuralgia
Yamashita T, Ishii S, Usui M (Sapporo Med Univ, Japan)
J Bone Joint Surg Br 80-B:499–503, 1998
6–3

Introduction.—The definition and mechanism of posttraumatic neuralgia are controversial. Effective treatment for this disorder can be challenging. Reported are outcomes of treatment in 20 patients who underwent local resection of part of the injured peripheral nerve for prolonged posttraumatic neuralgia.

Methods.—Mean time from onset of symptoms to surgery was 55.7 months. Mean follow-up was 91.2 months. All patients had paresthesias and burning pain in the area innervated by the damaged nerve, with cutaneous dysesthesias so severe that they could not tolerate contact with clothing. Five and 7 patients, respectively, had complete motor palsy and incomplete paralysis in the area innervated by the injured nerve. The remaining 8 patients had no motor function in the area innervated by the affected nerve. The nerve was resected from 3 cm proximal to 3 cm distal to the site of injury. After surgery, pain disappeared in the area from which the nerve was excised but continued in the distal innervation of the injured nerve. The area of nerve resection was extended step by step in subsequent surgical procedures. Disappearance of pain corresponded to the region of the portion of the nerve removed. For distal pain, only the peripheral nerve within the area in which the patient felt pain was dissected; this included a 3-cm normal portion proximal to the injury site. If involved, motor and sensory branches were resected to the area peripheral to the injured site. Resected nerves underwent histologic and immunohistochemical study.

Results.—Local pain was completely or markedly relieved in all patients. The areas of pain relief and nerve resection were in complete agreement in 17 patients, and they were in partial agreement in 3 patients. Patients rated results as 5 excellent, 11 good, 4 fair, and 0 poor. Histologic evaluation of resected nerves revealed wallerian degeneration. Immunohistochemical study showed that substance P (a polypeptide that could contribute to nociceptive transmission) was present in the tissue around the degenerated nerves.

Discussion.—It is likely that a positive feedback system of nociceptive signals due to axon reflexes may be formed in the peripheral nervous system and have a key role in the persistence of burning pain. Further study is needed to assess endogenous algogenic substances in the degenerated nerve and substance P around adjacent intact nerves.

▶ The distal end of a divided nerve is not a "dead and inert structure," rather, after axonotomy the distal nerve will upregulate for trophic factors, such as nerve growth factor. As such, it will be a "sensory lure" to adjacent cutaneous nerves, which may spontaneously sprout into the distal nerve. Although clinically this is not usually a problem in the management of painful neuromas, my approach to the distal nerve is to treat it with the same aggression as I do the proximal nerve.[1] I will locate the proximal nerve in a muscle environment well away from overlying skin and scar and coagulate the distal end of the proximal segment before placing the nerve in this environment. Similarly, the *distal* end of the divided nerve will be treated with resection for as reasonable a distance as possible, coagulation of the nerve end, and location of this distal nerve in an environment away from overlying skin and scar. It has been only within the last decade that we have been aware of the importance of the *distal* end of the nerve when treating neuromas. The recent literature on collateral sprouting supports the contention that this distal nerve is important in influencing adjacent nerve activity and regeneration.[2] Manipulation of the *distal* end of the involved nerve in management of neuroma may offer improvement in the overall results of management of this difficult problem.

S.E. Mackinnon, M.D., F.R.C.S.C.

References

1. Mackinnon SE: Evaluation and treatment in painful neuroma, in Weiland A (ed): *Techniques in Hand and Upper Extremity Surgery,* vol 1. Philadelphia, Lippincott-Raven, 1997, pp 1–19.
2. Tarasidis G, Watanabe O, Mackinnon SE, et al: End-to-side neurorrhaphy resulting in limited sensory axonal regeneration in a rat model. *Ann Otol Rhinol Laryngol* 106:506–512, 1997.

Treatment of Painful Neuromas of the Hand and Wrist by Relocation Into the Pronator Quadratus Muscle
Sood MK, Elliot D (St Andrew's Centre for Plastic Surgery, Billericay, England)
J Hand Surg [Br] 23B:214–219, 1998   6–4

Introduction.—Pain and limited activity levels observed with end neuromas may be diminished when nerves are relocated to an appropriate site. Use of the pronator quadratus muscle as a site for relocation of resected end neuromas of nerves is described.

Patients.—Ten patients with 13 neuromas had previously undergone a total of 50 surgical procedures on affected hands. Twenty-three of these procedures on the 13 neuromas had failed.

Surgical Technique.—Neuromas were identified preoperatively and marked on the overlying skin. During surgery, the neuroma was exposed and dissected proximally to the level of the pronator quadratus muscle. Intraneural dissection of the part of the nerve ending in the neuroma from the uninjured remainder of the median nerve, ulnar nerve, or its dorsal branch was performed, except when the palmar cutaneous branch of the median nerve was involved. The neuroma was excised with a variable length of its feeding nerve. Sufficient length was left to allow comfort and loose passage of the nerve through the flexor tendons at the wrist to the pronator quadratus muscle. Tension on the nerve was avoided in all positions of the wrist and forearm (Fig 2). The nerve ending was buried in the pronator quadratus muscle at a depth of about 0.5 cm. The epineurium of the nerve was sutured to the epimysium of the pronator quadratus at the site of entry of the nerve into the muscle. An intravenous cannula was situated just proximal to the site of separation of the buried nerve or nerve part from the main body of its nerve of origin, and a 0.125% bupivacaine solution was continuously infused onto the parent nerve over, a period of 2–7 days until pain was controlled adequately with oral analgesics.

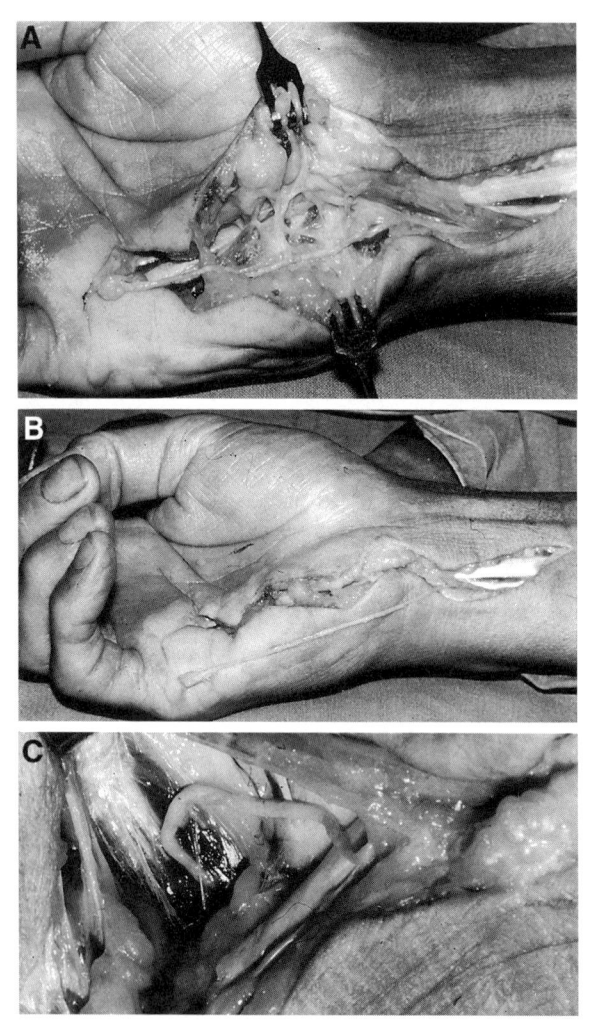

FIGURE 2.—A, surgical exposure of an end neuroma of the ulnar digit nerve of the little finger in a patient referred from elsewhere for treatment of neuroma pain after removal of the whole of this nerve beyond the distal palm during a fasciectomy for Dupuytren's disease. B, dissection of the nerve fascicles giving rise to the ulnar digital nerve of the little finger from the main trunk of the ulnar nerve proximally to the level of the pronator quadratus muscle. C, the proximal end of the dissected nerve has been buried in the pronator quadratus muscle after excision of the neuroma and the excess of nerve length but leaving sufficient length of proximal nerve to avoid tension in all positions of the wrist and forearm. The proximal forearm is on the right, and the dissected nerve crosses the anterior aspect of the main ulnar nerve to be inserted into the pronator quadratus muscle radial to the main ulnar neurovascular bundle. (Courtesy of Sood MK, Elliot D: Treatment of painful neuromas of the hand and wrist by relocation into the pronator quadratus muscle. *J Hand Surg [Br]* 23B:214–219, 1998.)

Results.—All 10 patients reported either total relief or marked improvement in affected hands. The 5 patients for whom the neuroma was the only significant cause of hand dysfunction were able to achieve sufficient improvement to return to work.

Conclusion.—The pronator quadratus muscle was a suitable site for relocating sensory nerve endings after resection of painful neuromas in the proximal part of the hand and wrist.

▶ With only 10 patients and a follow-up as short as 4 months, the reader is wise to be skeptical of the simplistic suggestion for management of neuromas in the 3 zones of the hand and wrist, as described by Sood and Elliot in Figure 1 of their manuscript. However, review of Figure 2 provides the reader with many important "tips" for the management of recalcitrant painful neuromas in the hand. If the distal nerve is available, then resection of the neuroma and reconstitution of the nerve injury with a nerve graft or nerve conduit is appropriate. However, in patients in whom such procedures have failed, proximal transposition of the involved nerve out of the hand and into an innervated muscle environment will routinely give patients good relief from their discomfort.[1] In Figure 2, B, the involved cutaneous nerve has been identified and will be transferred proximally out of the hand. In Figure 2, C, the authors demonstrate relocation of the involved nerve into the pronator quadratus. It is important that there is no tension on the nerve and that it is located in an area well away from the overlying skin and scar. By contrast, if the nerve is placed in the pronator quadratus under any amount of tension, then movement of the wrist will increase patients' symptoms. My location of choice for transposition of the neuromas involving the median or ulnar nerves is in the interval between the superficialis and profundus muscles, so that the distal end of the involved nerve lies well up in the mid-forearm, under no tension, and out of the contact zone of the hand. The radial sensory nerve (plus or minus the lateral antebrachial cutaneous nerve) is treated with transposition into the brachioradialis muscle.[2]

S.E. Mackinnon, M.D., F.R.C.S.C.

References

1. Novak CB, van Vliet D, Mackinnon SE: Subjective outcome following surgical management of upper extremity neuromas. *J Hand Surg [Am]* 20A:221–226, 1995.
2. Mackinnon SE: Evaluation and treatment in painful neuroma, in Weiland A (ed): *Techniques in Hand and Upper Extremity Surgery*, vol 1. Philadelphia, Lippincott-Raven, 1997, pp 1–19.

Prevention of the Formation of Neuromas in Nerves Implanted in Bone [Spanish]
Fernández AD, Rosales RS, Sicilia HF, et al (Unidad de Cirugía de la Mano y Microcirugía; Universidad de La Laguna)
Rev Esp Cirugía Mano 24:9–14, 1997   6–5

Introduction.—Among the techniques used for the prevention of neuroma formation is that of inserting the cut nerve into the bone marrow of adjacent bone. This study documents the morphological features that explain why a transected nerve does not develop a neuroma under this procedure.

Methods.—In 20 adult Sprague-Dawley rats, the sciatic nerve was cut, and the transected end was inserted into the bone marrow of the adjacent femur. The animals were sacrificed at different time intervals, and the specimens were excised and examined under light and electron microscopy.

Results.—Three different phases were observed. Between days 2 and 4, degenerative changes in nerve fibers and most of the hematopoietic elements were observed. In a second phase, between days 5 and 6, osteoblasts and osteoid material were observed surrounding the nerve fibers, which had diminished in number, together with some strands of Schwann cells, macrophages, and fibroblasts. Finally, between days 7 and 30, osteoblasts incorporated the nerve fibers, leaving the degenerated axons trapped inside the cells, which were surrounded by the new osteoid material. No regeneration signs were observed in these nerve fibers.

Conclusion.—Neuroma formation of a severed nerve inserted into bone is prevented not only by a mechanical effect, but also by a histochemical reaction from the bone marrow.

▶ Prevention of neuroma formation by mechanical means such as by using silicone or acrylic caps has not proved to be effective. By using an electron microscope, this article shows evidence for the first time, that axons are trapped inside the cytoplasm of an osteoblast, and later surrounded by newly formed bone. This may isolate them from neurotrophic factors responsible for their regeneration, which happens when they are in contact with muscle or other connective tissues. However, a definite statement that nerve growth is prevented solely on a biochemical basis from the bone marrow environment should not be drawn from this study. It would be interesting to observe the nerve fiber behavior inside a bone marrow chamber large enough so that it would not cause a mechanical restraint to nerve regeneration.

A. Lluch, M.D., Ph.D.

Clinical Features and Management of Traumatic Posterior Interosseous Nerve Palsy
Hirachi K, Kato H, Minami A, et al (Hokkaido Univ, Sapporo, Japan)
J Hand Surg [Br] 23B:413–417, 1998   6–6

Introduction.—Although several different causes of nontraumatic posterior interosseous nerve (PIN) palsy have been documented, few reports have addressed traumatic PIN palsy. Seventeen patients with traumatic PIN palsies are reported.

Patients.—The study included 13 males and 4 females, age range 8–54 years. Only patients with isolated PIN palsies were included. Twelve patients had complete PIN palsy, including weak wrist extension with radial drift, loss of extension at all metacarpophalangeal joints, and weak thumb adduction. The other patients had partial palsies of varying types. Seven patients had dislocation of the radial head, 6 had forearm fracture, 2 had forearm contusion, and 2 had forearm laceration. When the injury occurred at the level of the elbow joint, complete PIN palsy was always present. For patients with forearm injuries, the characteristics of PIN palsy varied. These variations depended on the presence of injury to the recurrent vs. descending branch of the PIN.

Outcomes.—Neurolysis was performed in 7 patients and tendon transfer in 2. The remaining 8 patients were treated conservatively. In all patients but 1, recovery started within 6 weeks after injury. At last follow-up, these 16 patients all had greater than M4 motor power.

Conclusions.—Patients with various types of injuries to the elbow and forearm may experience traumatic PIN palsy. The patients with radial head dislocations will have complete PIN palsy. The authors recommend conservative treatment of closed injuries to the PIN. When open injuries are present, the nerve should be exposed for immediate repair.

▶ This useful article details the results in traumatic PIN injury. I agree with the recommendation that closed injuries be observed with electromyography at 6 weeks and exploration thereafter, if no sign of recovery is evident. Depending on the findings, neurolysis or tendon transfer can be done at that point. Open wounds should, of course, be explored immediately, and the nerve repaired, if possible; if nerve repair is not possible, plans should be made for later tendon transfer. The main benefit of this article is its recommendation for earlier electromyography in closed injury—at 6 weeks instead of 3 months if there is no clinical sign of recovery. This timing is practical for the PIN because the motor points are so close to the likely injury point (the radial neck). For other nerves, such as the radial nerve more proximally, the 3-month dictum may still be more appropriate.

P.C. Amadio, M.D.

Cold Intolerance Following Peripheral Nerve Injury: Natural History and Factors Predicting Severity of Symptoms
Irwin MS, Gilbert SEA, Terenghi G, et al (Queen Victoria Hosp, East Grinstead, England; Northwick Park Hosp, Harrow, England)
J Hand Surg [Br] 22B:308–316, 1997   6–7

Background.—Hand injury can lead to severe, debilitating cold intolerance. Little is known about the natural history of cold intolerance or the factors predicting symptom severity. Cold intolerance was studied in a large group of patients who had had surgical repair of a peripheral nerve in the upper limb.

Methods and Findings.—Questionnaires were sent to all 814 patients with upper-limb peripheral nerve injuries occurring in a 12-year period. Patient records were also reviewed. Three hundred ninety-one patients completed the first questionnaire, for a response rate of 57%. Eighty-three percent reported cold intolerance. Of this subgroup, 23% reported that their symptoms were mild; 41%, moderate; 15%, severe; and 4%, extreme. Symptom onset was within 1 month of the initial injury in 48%. Fifty-nine percent of the original group responded to the second questionnaire. At a mean follow-up of 51 months, 21% reported improved symptoms and 18% reported deterioration. Cold intolerance was more likely to develop in smokers and less likely to develop in patients sustaining a sharp injury. Symptom severity was significantly increased with complete nerve division, median and ulnar nerve division, and an associated vessel injury. Improvement in symptoms was significantly more likely to occur in nonsmokers. Deterioration was most likely in patients with a high severity score.

Conclusion.—This study provides insight into the natural history of cold intolerance after peripheral nerve injury. Several factors, such as smoking, were associated with the development and severity of symptoms.

▶ This manuscript shows the complexity of the pathophysiology of cold intolerance after peripheral nerve injury. Unfortunately, this retrospective study had only a 57% response rate to the initial questionnaire and 59% of those responded to the second questionnaire. Nevertheless, important information is available. A high incidence of cold intolerance is expected in at least half of the patients who sustain a peripheral nerve injury, and cold intolerance, if present, persists for many years. These data provide risk factors: complete nerve injury, major mixed nerve injury, associated vessel injury in digital nerves, and smoking. Unfortunately, there are no data to evaluate the effects of the quality of nerve recovery after neurorrhaphy or cold sensitivity.

L.A. Koman, M.D.

Anterior Interosseous Nerve Palsy: A Review of 16 Cases
Sood MK, Burke FD (Derbyshire Royal Infirmary, Derby, England)
J Hand Surg [Br] 22B:64–68, 1997   6–8

Objective.—There is debate about whether surgical release of the arcuate ligament or conservative management is the better treatment for paralysis of the anterior interosseous nerve (AIN). Some investigators have reported that patients with partial, rather than complete, lesions have a more favorable outcome. Results for 16 patients treated expectantly or surgically for AIN were reviewed retrospectively, and 3 cases were presented.

Methods.—In 16 patients (7 women), aged 32–75 years, with AIN paralysis of 19 limbs were treated expectantly (11 limbs in 9 patients) or surgically (8 limbs). Patients were followed for 2–14 years and examined for return of power, range of motion, pinch and grip strength, and scar quality.

Case 1.—Woman, 68, with sudden right forearm pain and inability to bend the tips of her fingers was revealed by electromyography to have complete denervation of the muscle supplied by the right AIN. With conservative treatment, she improved at 4 months and recovered completely at 10 months.

Case 2.—Man, 36, with severe forearm pain could not move the tips of his fingers because of complete denervation of muscle supplied by the left AIN. Surgery to relieve compression distal to the reflection of the fascia of the flexor digitorum superficialis resulted in disappearance of pain at 2 weeks, partial recovery at 3 months, and complete recovery at 18 months.

Case 3.—Woman, 26, who was pregnant, had right wrist and shoulder pain and could not straighten her arm. Her condition worsened after delivery but had spontaneously improved by 4 months, although an electromyogram revealed a lesion of the AIN. She was fully recovered at 3 years but experienced similar pain in her left wrist and shoulder on the day after delivery after a second pregnancy. Surgical exploration revealed no abnormalities. Her pain resolved immediately and function was completely restored at 8 months.

Results.—At follow-up, there were good results in 15 patients, fair results in 1, and poor results in 3. Seven of 8 limbs treated surgically had a good result and 1 had a poor result, with full recovery ranging from 6 to 18 months. Of 11 patients treated conservatively, 8 had good results, 1 had fair results, and 2 had poor results, with full recovery times ranging from 1 to 24 months. The 7 patients with partial lesions recovered regardless of the type of management.

Conclusion.—Outcome for patients with AIN palsy was similar regardless of type of management, although surgery is indicated for patients with complete lesions who fail to make a recovery in 6 months.

▶ The authors make a strong case for the conservative management of all patients seen with sudden onset of weakness or paralysis of AIN-innervated muscles, especially when the palsy is incomplete. Like the authors, I believe that almost all of these patients have a neuritis and are no different from patients with a Bell's palsy of the facial nerve. Few of these patients demonstrate muscle atrophy. Without convincing intraoperative conduction studies, it is likely that the improvement seen after surgery may be unrelated to the surgery.

V.R. Hentz, M.D.

Suggested Reading

Reznik M, Thiry A, Fridman V: Painful hyperplasia and hypertrophy of pacinian corpuscles in the hand: Report of two cases with immunohistochemical and ultrastructural studies, and a review of the literature. *Am J Dermatopathol* 20:203–207, 1998.

▶ Painful hypertrophy of Pacini's corpuscles is rare, with only 29 cases reported to date. The findings are those of a painful, tender mass along the course of a nerve in the finger or palm. They may develop spontaneously or after trauma. Excision is curative.

P.C. Amadio, M.D.

Ruch DS, Poehling GG: Anterior interosseous nerve injury following elbow arthroscopy. *Arthroscopy* 13:756–758, 1997.
▶ Elbow arthroscopy offers a unique opportunity to perform intra-articular surgery through small incisions, respecting capsular integrity and speeding postoperative recovery. The risk of nerve injury is, however, real. A thorough understanding of relevant anatomy is necessary to avoid inadvertent nerve injury. Injury may occur during establishment of arthroscopic portals or, as in this case, as the result of aggressive synovectomy violating the anterior capsule.

P.C. Amadio, M.D.

Schoeller T, Otto A, Wechselberger G, et al: Distal nerve entrapment following nerve repair. *Br J Plast Surg* 51:227–230, 1998.
▶ Two cases are reported in which radial nerve repair in the arm was followed by excellent regeneration, which stopped abruptly at the arcade of Frohse. The tip-off was the presence of reinnervation of the extensor carpi radialis, and progression of Tinel's sensory sign, with arrest of motor recovery at the elbow. Decompression permitted regeneration to continue to progress distally. It seems likely that a similar problem could occur for other nerves at other locations, such as the median nerve at the wrist.

P.C. Amadio, M.D.

7 Compression Neuropathy

A New Provocative Test for Carpal Tunnel Syndrome: Assessment of Wrist Flexion and Nerve Compression
Tetro AM, Evanoff BA, Hollstien SB, et al (State Univ of New York at Buffalo; Washington Univ, St Louis; Orthopaedic Surgical Med Group of Santa Barbara, Calif)
J Bone Joint Surg Br 80-B:493–498, 1998   7–1

Background.—The clinical diagnosis of carpal tunnel syndrome (CTS) is typically based on history, physical signs, and the results of provocative tests. The value of median nerve compression with wrist flexion as a provocative test for CTS was assessed.

Methods.—Sixty-four patients with electrodiagnostically confirmed CTS and 50 healthy subjects were included in the prospective study. The subjects underwent Tinel's percussion test, Phalen's wrist flexion test, and

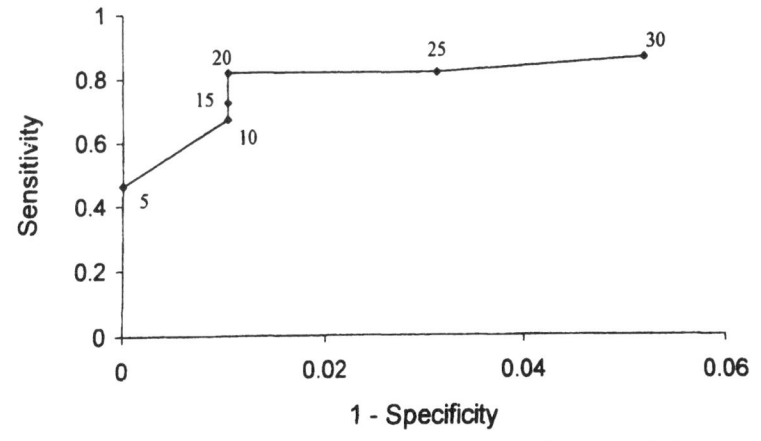

FIGURE 1.—A graph of the receiver operating characteristic curve for the wrist-flexion and nerve-compression test showing sensitivity vs. 1−specificity at 5-second intervals. A time for 20 seconds gives the optimal combination of sensitivity and specificity. (Courtesy of Tetro AM, Evanoff BA, Hollstein SB, et al: A new provocative test for carpal tunnel syndrome: Assessment of wrist flexion and nerve compression. J Bone Joint Surg Br 80-B:493–498, 1998.)

the carpal compression test as well as the new test, which combined wrist flexion and median nerve compression.

Findings.—A receiver operating characteristic curve showed that the optimal cutoff time for the wrist-flexion and median-nerve compression test was 20 seconds, resulting in a sensitivity and specificity of 82% and 99%, respectively. These values were significantly better than those of Phalen's wrist-flexion, which were 61% sensitivity and 83% specificity, and Tinel's test, which had a sensitivity of 74%. The positive predictive values of the wrist-flexion and median-nerve compression test were 99% at a population prevalence of 50%, 95% at 20%, and 81% at 5%, significantly better than the positive predictive values of the other 3 provocative tests (Fig 1).

Conclusions.—Provocative tests continue to be important in the diagnosis of CTS. Wrist flexion combined with the median-nerve compression test at 20 seconds is significantly better than the other methods tested. Thus, this new test may be of clinical value.

▶ This timed combination of the carpal tunnel compression test and Phalen's test seems to be far more sensitive and specific than either alone. I believe it should replace both of those less sensitive tests in the hand surgeon's diagnostic tool kit.

P.C. Amadio, M.D.

Value of the Carpal Compression Test in the Diagnosis of Carpal Tunnel Syndrome
González del Pino J, Delgado-Martínez AD, González González I, et al (Virgen de la Torre Hosp, Madrid)
J Hand Surg [Br] 22B:38–41, 1997   7–2

Objective.—Diagnostic tests for carpal tunnel syndrome (CTS) vary in their accuracy, depending on range of motion, pain, and changes in electrophysiologic parameters. There is a need to develop a clinical provocative test that is highly sensitive and specific, easy to perform, and applicable to all wrists. The usefulness of Durkan's test of carpal compression in diagnosing CTS was evaluated prospectively.

Methods.—Three tests—the Phalen, Tinel, and carpal compression test (CCT)—were performed in 200 hands (144 dominant) of 180 patients (34 men), aged 16–84 years, treated conservatively and unsuccessfully for CTS for 6 months. Also tested were 200 hands of 100 healthy volunteers (78% women), aged 37–67 years. Sensitivity and specificity for the 3 methods were compared statistically.

Results.—The CCT was positive in 87% of patients' hands and negative in 13%, for a sensitivity of 87%, and positive in 4.5% of the control hands and negative in 95.5%, for a specificity of 95%. The sensitivity and specificity of Phalen's test were 87% and 90%, respectively. The sensitivity and specificity of Tinel's test were 33% and 97%, respectively. Whereas the CCT and Phalen's test were equally sensitive, the CCT was significantly more sensitive than Tinel's test. The CCT and Tinel's test were equally specific, but the CCT was significantly more specific than Phalen's test. The CCT can be used to evaluate wrists with a limited range of motion or pain that cannot be assessed by Phalen's test. Rates of positivity for examiners were similar.

Conclusion.—The CCT is significantly more sensitive than Phalen's test and significantly more specific than Tinel's test for diagnosing CTS. The CCT is also easy to use, fast, and reliable.

▶ I have used the CCT in patients who could not easily, or would not, flex their wrists. Based on the results of these authors, I will use this test more often, especially because it is not too critical to exert a uniform pressure from case to case.

V.R. Hentz, M.D.

Preliminary Evaluation of a Sensory and Psychomotor Functional Test Battery for Carpal Tunnel Syndrome: Part 1. Confirmed Cases and Normal Subjects
Jeng O-J, Radwin RG, Fryback DG (New Jersey Inst of Technology, Newark; Univ of Wisconsin—Madison)
Am Ind Hyg Assoc J 58:852–860, 1997   7–3

Background.—Carpal tunnel syndrome (CTS) is usually diagnosed based on clinical and electrophysiologic signs. However, many patients are unwilling to undergo electrodiagnostic methods because of the discomfort. The development of 2 new functional tests for the diagnosis of CTS is reported, and the results of the tests in control subjects and patients with confirmed CTS are compared.

Methods.—The 2 tests, collectively known as the Wisconsin test battery, consist of a gap detection sensory test and a pinch/release psychomotor test and are computer controlled. The gap detection sensory test uses an aesthesiometer to measure both dynamic (the finger moves toward the gap) and static (the gap moves toward the finger) stimulus thresholds for areas of the hand innervated by the median nerve (Fig 1, A). The pinch/release psychomotor test uses a dynamometer to measure upper- and lower-force levels of muscles innervated by the motor branch of the median nerve (Fig 1, B). The battery was used with 10 patients (18 hands; mean age, 42.3 years) with CTS, as confirmed by physical examination and nerve conduction studies, and with 8 control subjects (16 hands; mean age, 41.9 years). The battery required 1 hour 15 minutes to perform, which included practice trials with both tests (the tactile test was always first) and completion of a demographics questionnaire.

Findings.—Both the tactile and psychomotor tests showed that patients with CTS had significant functional deficits compared with the control subjects. With the tactile test, on average, patients with CTS had 104%

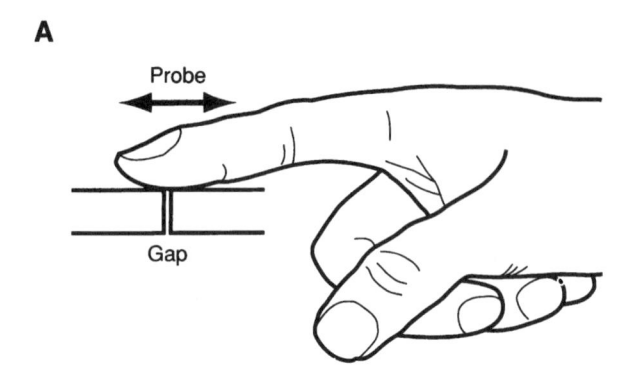

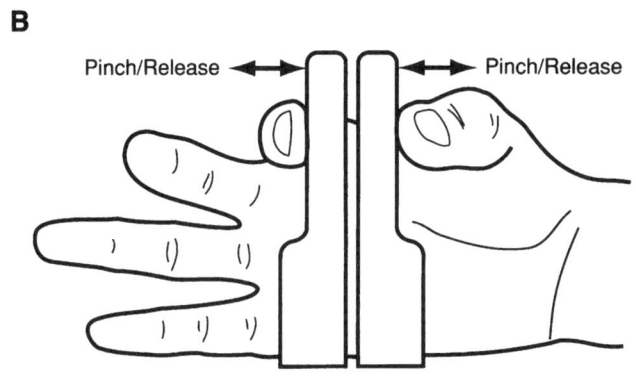

FIGURE 1.—Schematic drawings for the gap detection sensory test (**A**) and the rapid pinch-and-release psychomotor test (**B**). (Courtesy of Jeng O-J, Radwin RG, Fryback DG: Preliminary evaluation of a sensory and psychomotor functional test battery for carpal tunnel syndrome: Part 1. Confirmed cases and normal subjects. *Am Ind Hyg Assoc J* 58:852–860, 1997.)

greater thresholds for dynamic stimulation and 51% greater thresholds for static stimulation than the normal subjects. All participants experienced a decrease in the sensory threshold when the contact force was increased from 25 to 50 g, but patients with CTS had a significantly larger decrease (24% vs. 16%). With the psychomotor test, on average, patients with CTS had 28% less pinch strength and a 24% slower average pinch rate than the control subjects. Patients with CTS also had 76% greater overshoot than control subjects. Cutoff points for normal values were determined to assess the usefulness of the 2 tests to identify patients with CTS. Either test alone was not sufficiently useful, but their combination resulted in a sensitivity of 78% and a specificity of 81%. For patients with well-differentiated CTS, the battery's usefulness increased to a specificity of 94% and a sensitivity of 72% (Fig 3). Furthermore, the results of the tactile and psychomotor tests correlated significantly with the results of nerve conduction studies.

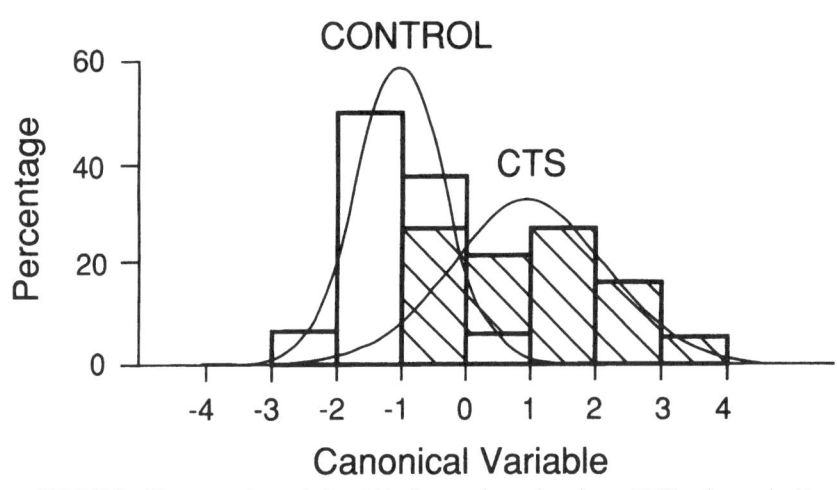

FIGURE 3.—Histogram of canonical variables for carpal tunnel syndrome (CTS) and normal subject samples. Canonical variable = $-1.07 + 32.23 \times (\Delta R_p/\Delta F_{upper}) + 0.04 \times T_{lower}$, where R_p is the pinch rate, F_{upper} is the upper-force level, and T_{lower} is the time spent below the lower-force level. (Courtesy of Jeng O-J, Radwin RG, Fryback DG: Preliminary evaluation of a sensory and psychomotor functional test battery for carpal tunnel syndrome: Part 1. Confirmed cases and normal subjects. Am Ind Hyg Assoc J 58:852–860, 1997.)

Conclusions.—When taken together, the gap detection sensory test and the rapid pinch/release psychomotor test are useful in identifying CTS. Although a larger study is required to confirm this result, these findings hold the promise of offering a more patient-acceptable method of assessing median nerve function.

Preliminary Evaluation of a Sensory and Pyschomotor Functional Test Battery for Carpal Tunnel Syndrome: Part 2. Industrial Subjects
Jeng O-J, Radwin RG, Moore JS, et al (New Jersey Inst of Technology, Newark; Univ of Wisconsin—Madison; Univ of Texas, Tyler; et al)
Am Ind Hyg Assoc J 58:885–892, 1997   7–4

Background.—Carpal tunnel syndrome (CTS) is more common in some industries, and tests that could detect CTS would help in its early identification and management. In this study, the Wisconsin test battery was used to test employees of industries in which CTS is more common.
Methods.—Nerve conduction studies (NCS) and the 2 components of the Wisconsin test battery, the tactile gap detection test and the psychomotor pinch/release test, were performed in 27 employees (54 hands; mean age, 40.2 years) of a food processing plant. Hands were rated on the basis of symptoms and NCS results as symptom negative, NCS negative (symp⁻/NCS⁻) (16 subjects, 23 hands); symptom negative, NCS positive (symp⁻/NCS⁺) (5 subjects, 6 hands); symptom positive, NCS negative (symp⁺/NCS⁻) (11 subjects, 14 hands); and symptom positive, NCS positive (symp⁺/NCS⁺) (9 subjects, 11 hands). Then the results of the physical

examination and NCS studies were compared with those of the Wisconsin test battery.

Findings.—For most of the tests, Wisconsin test battery performance in the symp⁻/NCS⁻ hands was significantly better (between 15% and 60%) than performance in the symp⁺/NCS⁺ hands. Battery performance did not differ between symp⁺ and symp⁻ hands, however, which indicates a good correlation between battery results and NCS regardless of symptoms. NCS⁺ hands had a significantly better gap detection threshold than NCS⁻ hands. However, gap detection thresholds did not differ in symp⁺ and symp⁻ hands. Symp⁻ hands had a significantly better pinch rate and significantly less overshoot than symp⁺ hands. NCS⁻ hands also had a significantly better pinch rate, plus a better change in pinch rate with respect to the upper-force level and a better change in time spent below the lower-force level, than NCS⁺ hands. The single best discriminator between NCS⁺ and NCS⁻ hands was the change in pinch rate with respect to the upper-force level (sensitivity, 71%; specificity, 68%). This same variable was also the single best discriminator between symp⁻/NCS⁻ hands and all other hands (sensitivity, 74%; specificity, 85%). To discriminate symp⁺/NCS⁺ hands from the others, the pinch rate was the best measure (sensitivity, 82%; specificity, 81%). When both tests were combined, they could discriminate symp⁻/NCS⁻ hands from symp⁺/NCS⁺ hands with a sensitivity of 91% and a specificity of 87%.

Conclusions.—Regardless of symptoms, the Wisconsin test battery correlated well with NCS results. Thus, it can be a useful, noninvasive tool in the surveillance of employees in industries prone to CTS.

▶ These 2 excellent articles (Abstracts 7–3 and 7–4) are recommended to all those who would like to understand the science of clinical epidemiology as it relates to CTS. The authors clearly show the problem with any gold standard attempts—there is a significant overlap between the normal and symptomatic groups using any examination or test criterion, even in combination. To some extent, any case definition will be arbitrary, and there will be cases where the diagnosis may be debated. Nevertheless, physical examination criteria can perform useful screening, as shown in the second article.

P.C. Amadio, M.D.

Median Nerve Compression Can Be Detected by Magnetic Resonance Imaging of the Carpal Tunnel
Horch RE, Allmann KH, Laubenberger J, et al (Albert Ludwigs Universität, Freiburg, Germany)
Neurosurgery 41:76–83, 1997
7–5

Introduction.—Interest in the anatomical correlation of median nerve compression has surged since the introduction of minimally invasive techniques for the surgical decompression of carpal tunnel syndrome. A new diagnostic tool was studied to determine therapeutic options in patients without measurably impaired nerve conduction values. Little is known about dynamic morphological changes in patients with carpal tunnel syndrome, and there has never been a direct comparison with healthy volunteers. Static and dynamic changes in the carpal canal in patients with carpal tunnel syndrome were analyzed and compared with asymptomatic volunteers.

Methods.—Twenty patients with carpal tunnel syndrome and pathologic nerve conduction values had MRI performed, and these patients were matched to 20 healthy volunteers. In patients, T2-weighted signal intensity of the median nerve was measured preoperatively and postoperatively.

Results.—Healthy volunteers tend to have larger cross-sectional areas of the carpal tunnel than patients with carpal tunnel syndrome. At the pisiform and hamate levels, the cross-sectional area of the carpal tunnel decreases. At the level of the pisiform, the cross-sectional area decreases during wrist extension. It increases at the level of the hamate during extension. In 94% of the patients, the distal flattening of the median nerve recovered postoperatively. The motor latency recovered in only 39% of patients, despite the signal intensity of the median nerve on T2-weighted images decreasing by 67%.

Conclusion.—The space available for the median nerve narrows during flexion and extension, which may lead to potential median nerve compression. For diagnosis and postoperative follow-up of carpal tunnel syndrome, MRI is accurate and reliable and may help in making a decision regarding surgical decompression.

▶ The authors add to the growing body of knowledge regarding the CT and MRI of the carpal tunnel in the symptomatic and asymptomatic population. Although the authors contend that the tunnel volumes in symptomatic patients are smaller than those in the normal population, the numbers don't quite achieve statistical significance, except at 1 location (level of the pisiform) and only in 1 direction (flexion).

The current expense of MRI will surely preclude its general use as a screening tool or a tool to provide confirmation of a diagnosis. I would choose to explain to the rational patient, with appropriate signs and symptoms of carpal tunnel syndrome whose conduction studies were still within normal parameters, that the probability is that the symptoms are from median nerve compression and that a relatively simple procedure will alleviate the symptoms; on the other hand, normal conduction study results indicate that insignificant damage is occurring, so it is safe for the patient to "live" with the symptoms for the time being. Of additional interest are the 3 commentaries that follow the article.

V.R. Hentz, M.D.

The Relationship of Vitamin B₆ Status to Median Nerve Function and Carpal Tunnel Syndrome Among Active Industrial Workers

Franzblau A, Rock CL, Werner RA, et al (Univ of Michigan, Ann Arbor)
J Occup Environ Med 38:485–491, 1996   7–6

Introduction.—Reports vary regarding the effectiveness of vitamin B₆ status and carpal tunnel syndrome (CTS). The relationship between vitamin B₆ status and CTS was evaluated in a series of 125 active industrial workers using a large number of randomly selected research subjects, standardized electrophysiologic assessments of nerve function, and multiple complementary measures of vitamin B₆ status.

Methods.—Participants underwent a self-administered questionnaire; physical examination focused on the upper extremities, bilateral ulnar and median sensory nerve conduction studies, anthropometric measures, and venipuncture for blood samples. Vitamin B₆ status was determined using the erythrocyte glutamic-pyruvic transaminase assay and quantification of plasma pyridoxal-5'-phosphate.

Results.—Most research subjects were female (67%) and the mean age was about 37 years. Of 125 participants, 31 (24.8%) met the criterion for median mononeuropathy. There was no significant relationship between measurements of vitamin B₆ status and self-reported symptoms potentially consistent with CTS, electrophysiologically determined median or ulnar nerve function, and CTS as defined by self-reported symptoms and electrophysiologic measurements.

Conclusion.—There was no clear indication of a relationship between CTS and vitamin B₆ status. On the basis of these findings, use of vitamin B₆ in the treatment of CTS is unwarranted.

▶ The authors correctly criticize previous studies that demonstrate an association between vitamin B₆ status and CTS on several points, notably, that they include small numbers of nonrandomly selected subjects, that they rely on nonstandard or entirely subjective measures of outcome, and that they suffer from serious design flaws, including providing little information about the source of patients and other criteria for the diagnosis of CTS and not controlling for other pre-existing and potentially confounding medical conditions. The same criticisms can be made for the majority of the literature that tries to establish a causal relationship between repetitive motion and CTS. The population studied here were workers from automotive plants. The self-administered questionnaire, nerve conduction studies, and physical examination, as well as a blood specimen for vitamin B₆ formed the study parameters. The authors, however, found a prevalence for median mononeuropathy equal to 25% in this population of patients, which they claim is comparable with results of similar industry-based studies; however, all the studies referenced were those of the author. In a widely quoted study by Silverstein et al.[1] trying to establish a relationship between CTS and repetitive forceful motion, the authors could identify only 14 cases of CTS out of 652 active workers in 39 jobs from 7 different industrial sites (prevalence =

2%), and the criteria for diagnosis in fact were much more lenient. In the final analysis, I do agree with the authors that treatment for CTS syndrome with vitamin B_6 supplementation is unwarranted. Their sensitivity for diagnosing CTS was very high, and it is unlikely that they missed any cases; however, in view of the 25% prevalence of case patients by their definition, none of whom were noted to be seeking medical care, the specificity of diagnosis was probably rather low. It is equally important not to accept "cases" by several independent criteria as this process overestimates the "true cases." The power of this study with regard to vitamin B_6 was increased with this misclassification error; however, the statements regarding prevalence of work-relatedness of CTS were very misleading.

R.M. Szabo, M.D., M.P.H.

Reference

1. Silverstein BA, Fine LJ, Armstrong TJ: Occupational factors and carpal tunnel syndrome. *Am J Ind Med* 11:343–358, 1987.

Influence of Body Mass Index and Work Activity on the Prevalence of Median Mononeuropathy at the Wrist
Werner RA, Franzblau A, Albers JW, et al (Univ of Michigan, Ann Arbor; Veterans Affairs Med Ctr, Ann Arbor, Mich)
Occup Environ Med 54:268–271, 1997   7–7

Introduction.—The risk for carpal tunnel syndrome (CTS) is thought to be increased among individuals whose work involves repetition, awkward posture, high force, vibration, and local pressure. Some studies, however, suggest that personal factors, particularly obesity, have the greatest influence on the development of CTS. A cross-sectional study of workers examined the importance of work activity, body mass index (BMI), and other demographic factors on the prevalence of median mononeuropathy at the wrist.

Methods.—Workers were drawn from 5 different settings, 4 industrial and 1 clerical, in the midwestern United States. Industrial sites included manufacturers of car parts, furniture, and paper containers; the clerical site was an insurance company. Of the 527 workers, 363 were industrial and 164 were clerical. The industrial jobs were rated for frequency of hand repetition. Although the clerical work involved some repetitive handwork, it did not require extremely high rates of hand exertion or movement. The presence of a median mononeuropathy in either hand was measured by electrodiagnostic techniques; BMI was calculated from the measured height and weight.

Results.—The median age of the 527 workers was 34; women had greater representation in clerical work (87%) than in industrial work (49%). The overall prevalence of an abnormality of the median sensory nerve at the wrist was 30%. Among industrial workers, the adjusted risk for median mononeuropathy was twice that of clerical workers. Workers who were obese (BMI > 29) were 4 times more likely than those who were normal or slender (BMI < 25) to have a median mononeuropathy identified. The logistic regression model found that BMI, age, and work site were the only significant factors related to the prevalence of median mononeuropathies.

Conclusion.—The risk for median mononeuropathy at the wrist among active workers appears to be increased among individuals with a higher BMI, in industrial settings, and for older workers. The prevalence of median mononeuropathy in clerical workers is increased over that of a normal healthy population, but lower than that of industrial workers.

▶ This study shares a common problem with the previous work concerning median mononeuropathy. The authors lack a nonworking matched controlled cohort. They also lack knowledge of the patients' activities away from work. Work composes a small part of life, and must not be the only hand use factor evaluated.

M.L. Kasdan, M.D.

The Association Between Different Patterns of Hand Symptoms and Objective Evidence of Median Nerve Compression: A Community-based Survey
Ferry S, Silman AJ, Pritchard T, et al (Univ of Manchester, England; Manchester Royal Infirmary, England; Univ of Keele, Stroke-on-Trent, England)
Arthritis Rheum 41:720–724, 1998   7–8

Background.—The association of hand symptom pattern and objective evidence of delayed nerve conduction in the general population is unknown. Determining this association is important to help clinicians decide which patients with hand symptoms should be referred for additional assessment.

Methods.—Six hundred forty-eight persons were surveyed about the presence of hand symptoms. Two hundred twelve reported hand symptoms. One hundred fifty-five persons, including 40 reporting no hand symptoms, underwent testing for nerve conduction of sensory and motor median nerve latencies. Patterns of hand symptoms were compared with nerve conduction findings. Associations were then weighted back to the general population.

Findings.—The presence of any hand symptoms was 40% sensitive for delayed nerve conduction on latency testing. The sensitivity for the presence of typical symptoms of carpal tunnel syndrome (CTS) was much lower.

Conclusions.—The distribution of hand symptoms in a community setting is not usefully correlated with delayed nerve conduction in the median nerve. However, hand symptom patterns may be more strongly associated with delayed conduction among symptomatic persons seeking primary care.

▶ This interesting study shows that the hand diagram is not very helpful by itself in identifying members of the general population who are likely to have nerve conduction changes consistent with CTS. This is in contrast with patients prescreened for CTS, where the hand diagram does correlate with electrodiagnostic findings. As these authors point out, these data confirm the importance of disease prevalence in determining the predictive value, and therefore the clinical value, of a given diagnostic test. Even a tiny false positive rate can produce hordes of false negative results if the true positive rate in the population is low. As this study shows, both false positives and false negatives are an issue with the hand diagram when used alone. Of course, that is also true for Phalen's test, Tinel's sign, etc. For such circumstances, a case definition requiring the presence of a combination of findings is often the answer. For example, a case definition of hand diagram, night pain, and positive Phalen's sign may prove far more reliable than any one of the 3 alone. Finally, this study also points out that symptom diagrams and other patient self-report items may be very useful for outcome assessment, but they are not very useful at making diagnoses. Do not turn in your brain yet. Your patients still have need of it, even in the brave new world of outcomes research.

P.C. Amadio, M.D.

Carpal Tunnel Syndrome in the Mucopolysaccharidoses and Mucolipidoses
Haddad FS, Jones DHA, Vellodi A, et al (Hosp for Sick Children, London)
J Bone Joint Surg Br 79-B:576–582, 1997   7–9

Background.—Children with mucopolysaccharidosis or mucolipidosis experience progressive disability of the hand in relation to dysfunction of the median nerve. Bone marrow transplantation has significantly improved survival but does not seem to change the musculoskeletal symptoms. Some authors recommend decompression, but there is little objective information on cause, natural history, neurophysiology, and functional outcome after such surgery. Carpal tunnel syndrome is different in these children than in adults and can cause decreased sweating, pulp atrophy, thenar wasting, and manual clumsiness.

Methods.—Evaluations were done in 48 consecutive children with mucopolysaccharidosis or mucolipidosis who required carpal tunnel decompression. All patients were between the ages of 8 months and 16 years at the most recent review. Clinical, radiologic, and neurophysiologic assessments were performed. Symptoms, signs, radiologic, electrophysiologic and operative findings, histology, and upper-limb function were analyzed.

Results.—At the time of surgery, the flexor retinaculum was thickened and a mass of white tenosynovium engulfed the flexor tendons. Most of the children had nerve constriction with a thickened epineurium. After early decompression, functional improvement was seen. Simultaneous tendon release also benefited some patients. Improved hand movement was maintained by regular physiotherapy.

Conclusion.—The authors recommend early surgery to lower the risk of irreversible damage.

▶ Bone marrow transplants in patients with previously fatal metabolic disorders (such as Hurler's syndrome) have allowed the patients to lead reasonably comfortable lives. The effect of the disorder on peripheral nerves remains, however. One of the common manifestations of this is median nerve compression, or carpal tunnel syndrome. The presentation is unique in these patients. They complain of few symptoms, such as nocturnal paresthesias, but instead exhibit more functional evidence of involvement (e.g., clumsiness) or anatomic evidence (e.g., thenar wasting). Hand surgeons need to be aware of these differences if we are going to act appropriately before irreversibility of symptoms occurs.

V.R. Hentz, M.D.

Nerve and Tendon Gliding Exercises and the Conservative Management of Carpal Tunnel Syndrome
Rozmaryn LM, Dovelle S, Rothman ER, et al (Rockville, Md)
J Hand Ther 11:171–179, 1998
7–10

Introduction.—Release of the carpal tunnel ligament is 1 of the 10 most commonly performed surgical procedures in the United States. Results of surgical intervention are not always satisfactory. Described is a series of nerve and tendon gliding exercises for the conservative management of carpal tunnel syndrome.

Methods.—One hundred ninety-seven patients (240 hands) were treated by standard conservative methods and placed in 1 of 2 groups: a group that participated in a program of nerve and tendon gliding exercises (93 patients) and a control group that did not perform these exercises (104 patients). The exercises were created to maximize the excursion of the digital flexors and the median nerve through the carpal tunnel. For tendon gliding exercises, the fingers were positioned in 5 discrete positions: straight, hook, fist, tabletop, and straight fist. The median nerve was mobilized by placing the hand and wrist through 6 other positions. All patients were evaluated at 4 months.

Results.—Significantly more patients in the control group than in the experimental group underwent surgery (71.2% vs. 43%). Fifty-three patients in the experimental group who did not have surgery were interviewed at an average follow-up of 23 months (range, 14–38 months). Of these, 47 (89%) responded to a detailed interview. Of the 47 respondents, 70.2% reported good or excellent outcomes, 19.2% still had symptoms, and 10.6% were noncompliant.

Conclusion.—A program of nerve and tendon gliding exercises coupled with traditional nonsurgical approaches decreases symptoms. A significant proportion of patients who would have otherwise undergone surgery were spared the morbidity and expense of surgical carpal tunnel release.

Clinical Significance.—Effective nonsurgical treatment could have a significant impact on the number of patients undergoing carpal tunnel release nationwide. With more than 200,000 of these operations performed annually at an estimated cost of $3.5 billion and the expensive loss of productive work time, it is important to develop more efficient methods of nonsurgical treatment for this growing epidemic.

▶ This study reports on patients with carpal tunnel syndrome who were treated with and without nerve gliding exercises. The exercise group had carpal tunnel surgery less often. Unfortunately, the 2 groups were not treated concurrently, nor was assignment randomized. Thus, any differences noted may simply be due to the fact that the exercise group was treated some years after the no-exercise group. For example, it is possible that the surgeon's indications had changed in the meantime, that the patients had changed in some way (we know that the occupational mix was different, with more clerical workers in the later-exercise group), or simply that patient, surgeon, and therapist shared a belief that the exercises were useful and thus eschewed surgery more often. This report underlines the need for prospective, randomized trials of any new therapy. This was no experiment. It was simply a comparison of 2 case series. It is my opinion that the conclusion that the exercises were beneficial is only one of many possible explanations supported by the data.

P.C. Amadio, M.D.

Ultrasound Treatment for Treating the Carpal Tunnel Syndrome: Randomised "Sham" Controlled Trial
Ebenbichler GR, Resch KL, Nicolakis P, et al (Univ of Vienna; Univ of Exeter, England)
BMJ 316:731–735, 1998

Background.—Ultrasound treatment has the potential to induce various types of biophysical effects within tissue. It has been suggested that ultrasound might help to enhance recovery from nerve compression, although few studies have tested ultrasound treatment for carpal tunnel syndrome under clinical conditions. The efficacy of pulsed ultrasound for the treatment of idiopathic carpal tunnel syndrome was assessed.

Methods.—The randomized, double-blind controlled trial included 45 patients with mild-to-moderate bilateral carpal tunnel syndrome, as demonstrated by electroneurographic studies. The patients received 20 sessions of active ultrasound treatment to 1 wrist and an identical-appearing sham treatment to the other (Fig 1). Ultrasound was delivered in 15-minute sessions at a frequency of 1 MHz, an intensity of 1.0 W/cm^2, and pulsed mode 1:4 using a 5-cm^2 transducer. Treatment was daily for the first week, then twice weekly for 5 weeks. The results between wrists were compared by subjective symptom ratings and by electroneurographic measures.

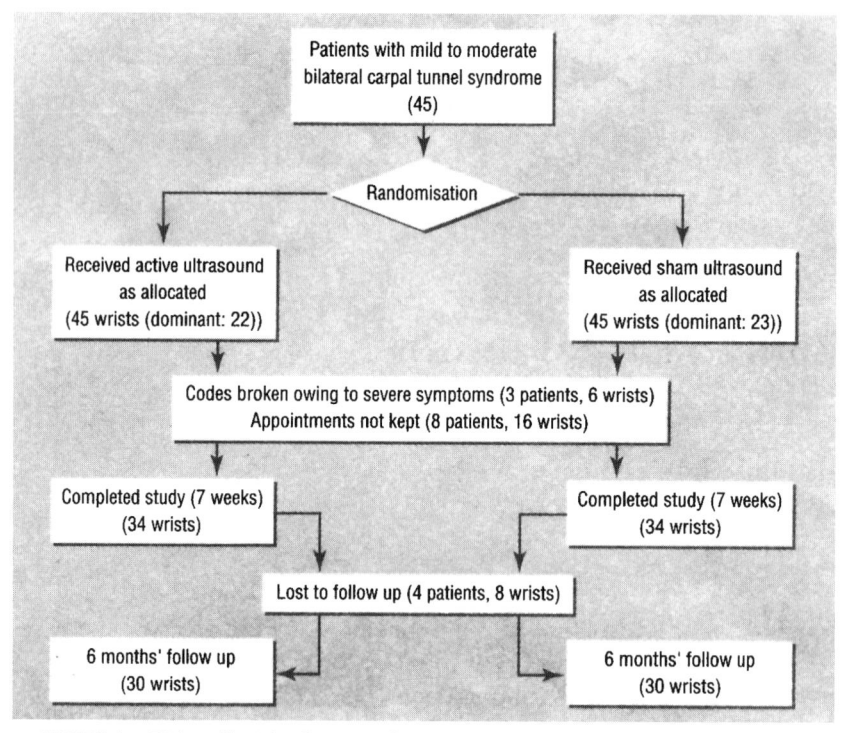

FIGURE 1.—Trial profile. (This figure was first published in the *BMJ*, courtesy of Ebenbichler GR, Resch KL, Nicolakis P, et al: Ultrasound treatment for treating the carpal tunnel syndrome: Randomised "sham" controlled trial. *BMJ* 316:731–735. Copyright 1998, with permission of the *BMJ*.)

Results.—By both subjective and objective assessment, wrists receiving ultrasound treatment showed significantly greater improvement than those receiving the sham treatment. The improvements were sustained at 6 months' follow-up. At 6 months, satisfactory improvement in symptoms was noted in 74% of ultrasound-treated wrists vs. 20% of placebo-treated wrists. Ultrasound also achieved significant and lasting changes in motor distal latency and the velocity of sensory nerve conduction.

Conclusions.—For patients with mild-to-moderate carpal tunnel syndrome, ultrasound therapy produces good short- to medium-term subjective and objective effects. Further studies are need to confirm these results, to identify optimal treatment schedules, and to assess possible combinations of ultrasound with other nonsurgical treatments.

▶ This fascinating study shows a beneficial effect in 30 randomly allocated, electromyogram-documented patients with carpal tunnel syndrome who were treated with 20 ultrasound treatments over a period of 7 weeks. The effect lasted up to 6 months, although the electromyogram changes at 6 months showed some tendency to return to initial values.

Why this should work is unclear. The authors postulate an anti-inflammatory effect, but multiple studies have failed to show a significant component of inflammation in most cases of carpal tunnel syndrome. Nonetheless, the results are promising and deserve a further look.

P.C. Amadio, M.D.

Carpal Tunnel Syndrome With Normal Electrodiagnostic Study [Spanish]
Romón MV, del Pino JG, Lovic A (Hosp Virgen de la Torre, Madrid)
Rev Ortop Traum 41:350–356, 1997   7–12

Introduction.—The purpose of this article is to determine the incidence of normal electrodiagnostic studies in patients suffering from compression of the median nerve in the carpal tunnel.

Methods.—One hundred nineteen patients with a clinical diagnosis of carpal tunnel syndrome (CTS) underwent decompression of the median nerve. All of them had electrodiagnostic studies before the surgery was done. In 18 (15%) of 120 hands, the results of electrodiagnostic studies were normal. All patients were followed up for a minimum postoperative period of 6 months.

Results.—Sixteen (88.9%) of the 18 hands with negative findings from electrodiagnostic studies were relieved from the preoperative symptoms after median nerve decompression.

Conclusion.—Electrodiagnostic studies should not be used routinely for the diagnosis of CTS as such studies have demonstrated 15% negative results.

▶ There is no doubt that the diagnosis of CTS should be done on a clinical basis, as some negative results after electrodiagnostic studies have been reported. One explanation for this is that the nerve conduction studies are done in many patients at a time when the nerve fiber has recovered its neurophysiology. A higher percentage of positive results would be obtained if the electrodiagnostic studies were done in the early morning, at the bedside of the patient, when the symptoms are more manifest, from swelling of the paratenon of the digital flexor tendons. Another way to obtain a positive diagnosis with electrodiagnostic studies would be to perform "dynamic" studies with the patient holding a small weight with the wrist in flexion. In recent years, more refined techniques of sensory conduction studies have yielded a higher percentage of positive results.

A. Lluch, M.D., Ph.D.

Suggested Reading

Grundberg AB: Carpal tunnel decompression in spite of normal electromyography. *J Hand Surg [Am]* 8A:348–349, 1983.

Lluch A: Thickening of the synovium of the digital flexor tendons: Cause or consequence of the carpal tunnel syndrome? *J Hand Surg [Br]* 17B:209–212, 1992.

Endoscopic Carpal Tunnel Release: A Review of 208 Consecutive Cases
Armstrong AP, Flynn JR, Davies DM (Charing Cross Hosp, London)
J Hand Surg [Br] 22B:505–507, 1997   7–13

Introduction.—Carpal tunnel release, first reported in 1933, is now one of the most frequently performed operations. Endoscopic techniques have been used since 1987 and appear to lessen scar discomfort and provide an earlier return of strength. The patients reported here underwent endoscopic carpal tunnel release using the Chow 2-portal technique.

Methods.—Over a 30-month period (1992 to 1995), 176 patients underwent 254 endoscopic releases; 149 responded to a follow-up questionnaire on the subjective results of surgery. Ninety of these patients had unilateral and 59 had bilateral procedures. The mean age of the group was 50.5 years and the male-to-female sex ratio was 1:3.3. Follow-up ranged from 3 to 34 months.

Results.—The procedure was performed in a day surgery unit. Patients had a local anesthetic block of the median and ulnar nerves at the wrist, and a forearm tourniquet was used in all cases. Eighteen hands were excluded from analysis because the patients were converted from endoscopic to open release when the flexor retinaculum was not adequately visualized. The operation was considered successful by 67% of patients; they reported freedom from the preoperative symptoms of carpal tunnel syndrome. Symptoms persisted, however, in 32% of patients, and 6 hands (2.9%) had postoperative numbness that was not present before surgery. In 2 of these 6 hands, the iatrogenic nerve complication was permanent. There were no other serious complications.

Discussion.—The overall permanent nerve injury rate in this series of endoscopic releases was 0.9% (2/208). Potential causes of this complication include intraneural injection of local anesthetic and stretching, compression, or division of the communicating branch between the median and ulnar nerves in the palm. The persistence of symptoms in one third of patients may be attributed to the fact that most patients in the series had experienced symptoms of median nerve compression for more than 1 year.

▶ There is no real argument that endoscopic carpal tunnel release can be performed in a safe manner by a surgeon with appropriate skills. More central to the issue is whether the surgeon can apply these appropriate skills without doing unnecessary harm. The same is obviously true for the open technique.

                                                        V.R. Hentz, M.D.

Sensory Function After Median Nerve Decompression in Carpal Tunnel Syndrome: Preoperative vs Postoperative Findings
Rosén B, Lundborg G, Abrahamsson SO, et al (Lund Univ, Sweden; Malmö Univ, Sweden)
J Hand Surg [Br] 22B:602–606, 1997   7–14

Objective.—Recovery of sensory function after carpal tunnel release depends on the stage of the disease, intraneural microvascular dysfunction, and nerve fiber injury. The recovery of sensory functions was monitored for as long as 1 year after median nerve decompression in patients with carpal tunnel syndrome in a prospective, consecutive study. Rate of recovery, importance of constant or intermittent symptoms, and influence of sex were assessed.

Methods.—Between March 1992 and April 1994, 69 patients (18 men, 71 hands), aged 24–82 years, were followed up at 10, 21, 42, 84, and 365 days after carpal tunnel release. Before surgery, 41 patients experienced intermittent numbness/paresthesia, and 30 patients had constant numbness/paresthesia. Conventional open surgery was performed on 36 hands and endoscopic release on 35. The influences of preoperative status and sex were analyzed statistically.

Results.—Subjective symptoms had resolved completely in 41 hands. Most patients recovered a sense of touch and vibration within 3 weeks. Patients with abnormal nerve conduction and sensory amplitude recovered slowly during the follow-up. Patients with preoperative intermittent numbness/paresthesia were significantly more likely than patients with constant numbness/paresthesia to recover normal nerve conduction and perception of touch. Women were more likely than men to recover nerve conduction and perception of touch. Men and women with matched preoperative symptoms improved significantly and similarly.

Conclusion.—Patients with carpal tunnel syndrome who are treated earlier have improved recovery of normal nerve conduction and perception of touch.

▶ This article provides useful information for our own patients who are to undergo carpal tunnel surgery. Interestingly, the authors were able to correlate certain differences in outcome with whether preoperative symptoms were intermittent or constant. These findings reinforce a long-standing personal bias, in that I have frequently left it up to the patient to decide "yes" or "no" regarding proceeding to surgery if his or her symptoms were intermittent. In contrast, I have typically urged surgery when symptoms became more or less constant.

V.R. Hentz, M.D.

Ligament Lengthening Compared With Simple Division of the Transverse Carpal Ligament in the Open Treatment of Carpal Tunnel Syndrome

Karlsson MK, Lindau T, Hagberg L (Lund Univ, Malmö, Sweden)
Scand J Plast Reconstr Surg Hand Surg 31:65–69, 1997   7–15

Introduction.—A simple incision into the carpal ligament is recommended for carpal tunnel syndrome, but postoperative results are reported to be poor in 20% of patients. Some authors suggest that reconstruction of the transverse carpal ligament can prevent weakness of the hand, an important problem after release of the carpal tunnel. A retrospective study followed up patients who underwent open release of the carpal tunnel with or without a simultaneous lengthening of the transverse carpal ligament.

Methods.—All patients were operated on at the same university-affiliated hospital. Sixty-seven underwent only section of the transverse carpal ligament and 32 had the ligament lengthened (Fig 1). Patients with other operations on the hand were excluded, leaving 50 patients in the section group and 24 in the lengthening group. Mean duration of follow-up was 5 years in the section group and 6 years in the lengthening group. The 2 groups were similar in median age, number of associated diseases, type of conservative treatment received, and duration of symptoms before opera-

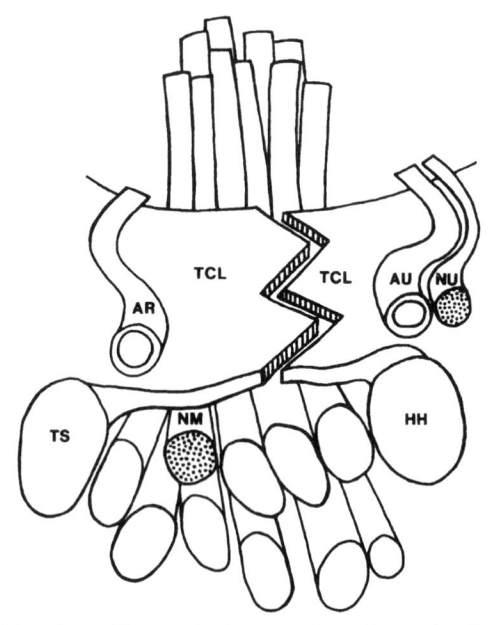

FIGURE 1.—Incision of carpal ligament in the group that underwent lengthening of the ligament. *Abbreviations:* TCL, transverse carpal ligament; TS, scaphoid tuberosity; HH, hook of the hamate bone; AR, radial artery; AU, ulnar artery; NU, ulnar nerve; NM, median nerve. (Courtesy of Karlsson MK, Lindau T, Hagberg L: Ligament lengthening compared with simple division of the transverse carpal ligament in the open treatment of carpal tunnel syndrome. *Scand J Plast Reconstr Surg Hand Surg* 31:65–69, 1997.)

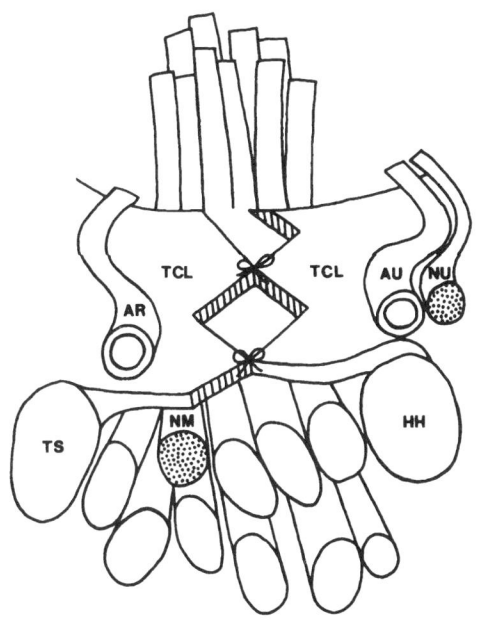

FIGURE 2.—After lengthening of the ligament. *Abbreviations: TCL,* transverse carpal ligament; *TS,* scaphoid tuberosity; *HH,* hook of the hamate bone; *AR,* radial artery; *AU,* ulnar artery; *NU,* ulnar nerve; *NM,* median nerve. (Courtesy of Karlsson MK, Lindau T, Hagberg L: Ligament lengthening compared with simple division of the transverse carpal ligament in the open treatment of carpal tunnel syndrome. *Scand J Plast Reconstr Surg Hand Surg* 31:65–69, 1997.)

tion. In the lengthening group, the transverse carpal ligament was explored more thoroughly and incised in a zigzag fashion. The ligament was lengthened, and the tips of the 2 triangular flaps created were sutured together after completion of the release (Fig 2).

Results.—The 2 groups did not differ in the number of postoperative complications, patients' subjective opinions about the results, grip strength, or wrist extension. The lengthening group exhibited superior wrist flexion but required significantly longer sick leave than the section-only group.

Conclusion.—Long-term follow-up in this group of patients with carpal tunnel syndrome indicates that treatment by simple section is as effective as a widening ligament-lengthening operation. The lengthening technique may not actually result in a better widening of the carpal arch or displacement of the median nerve and tendons.

▶ The transverse carpal ligament serves primarily as a retinaculum or pulley, maintaining the moment arms of the flexor tendons as they cross the wrist joint. There is much evidence that some of the loss of strength following release of this ligament is secondary to induced changes in the length-tension relationships of the flexor tendons. Many hand surgeons advocate disturbing the mechanics of these tendons as little as possible while still accomplishing the primary goal, which is to release nerve compression. This interesting article tells us that there is little or no long-term difference in outcome, whether or not one makes an attempt at reapproximating the edges of the transverse carpal ligament. The fact that the patients with ligament elongation didn't return to work sooner might indicate that little immediate gain was experienced as well. The study does not address this key point, however.

V.R. Hentz, M.D.

Predictors of Return to Work Following Carpal Tunnel Release
Katz JN, Keller RB, Fossel AH, et al (Harvard Med School, Boston; Univ of Massachusetts, Lowell; Maine Med Assessment Found, Augusta)
Am J Ind Med 31:85–91, 1997   7–16

Introduction.—Hand pain is now more prevalent than back pain among workers in the United States, and carpal tunnel syndrome (CTS) accounts for approximately 14% of work-associated upper-extremity disorders in industry. One study reported a high rate of long-term work absence associated with CTS. A prospective, community-based study evaluated predictors of return to work after surgery for CTS.

Methods.—Data were obtained from the Maine Carpal Tunnel Study that recruited patients from July 1992 through October 1993. Eligible study participants had paresthesia involving 2 of the first 4 fingers, were symptomatic for at least 1 month, and were employed or out of work because of CTS. Most patients who underwent nerve conduction tests had positive results. A questionnaire and physical examination were administered at study entry, and patients completed a mailed questionnaire 6 months postoperatively.

Results.—Of 184 patients eligible for analysis, 135 completed all required questions at the 6-month follow-up. Thirty-one (23%) of these patients reported being out of work at 6 months because of CTS. Patients who were out of work preoperatively because of CTS, those who received workers' compensation, and those who hired a lawyer had significantly greater work absence at 6 months. Work absence at 6 months varied considerably by work category, from 9% of professionals and managers to 40% of laborers and machine operators. Patients who ultimately remained out of work also had significantly worse baseline symptom severity and functional status and less improvement after surgery than those who had returned to work. In logistic regression analyses, workers' compensation, preoperative work absence, and worse mental health status had the greatest influence on postoperative work absence.

Conclusion.—A variety of economic and psychosocial variables can influence return to work and the extent of symptom relief in patients who have undergone surgery for CTS. When both postoperative and preoperative variables were included in the models, the major correlate of return to work was the degree of clinical improvement.

▶ This study offers some interesting perspectives, and confirms some information that appears to be obvious. That is, there is significant influence of the psychosocial environment in the determinant of return to work. The paper is weak in that the diagnosis of median neuropathy is not confirmed.

M.L. Kasdan, M.D.

Touch Allodynia Following Endoscopic (Single Portal) or Open Decompression for Carpal Tunnel Syndrome
Povlsen B, Tegnell I, Revell M, et al (Univ of Linköping, Sweden; St Thomas' Hosp, London)
J Hand Surg [Br] 22B:325–327, 1997   7–17

Introduction.—Because single-portal endoscopic techniques for treatment of carpal tunnel syndrome leave the palmar skin intact, postoperative touch allodynia may be reduced compared with open surgical treatment. A study of patients who underwent either open or endoscopic decompression was conducted to determine whether the Agee single-portal instrument causes increased carpal tunnel pressure during the release and whether endoscopic release reduces postoperative touch allodynia.

Methods.—Initial studies of 13 cadavers measured pressure changes during maximal range of motion and during introduction of the endoscope into the carpal tunnel of the wrist. Fifty of 100 patients with carpal tunnel syndrome were treated by the open technique and 50 by the endoscopic method. All had the wrist immobilized in plaster for 2 weeks after the procedure. Pressure pain thresholds were assessed with a featherweight instrument designed to measure the pressure generated on a scale of 0 to 50 newton. Patients were asked to indicate when the pain reached a value of 5 on a scale of 0 (no pain) to 10 (unbearable pain). Three measurements were obtained on each test point.

Results.—Cadaver studies showed that introduction of the endoscope into the carpal canal led to a mean pressure increase of 59 mm Hg. Higher pressures for considerably longer periods would be required to cause a conduction block in the nerve. Observed pressures were similar to those produced during maximal range of motion. Compared with controls, both endoscopic and open treatment groups had significant postoperative touch allodynia at 1 month, but allodynia was significantly less in the endoscopic technique group than in the open method group. Thresholds in the endoscopic group were similar to those of controls at 3 months.

Conclusion.—The Agee endoscope does not appear to increase carpal pressure sufficiently during release to cause a disturbance of nerve function. Use of the Agee endoscopic release may be of particular benefit to patients who would be seriously disadvantaged by the development of postoperative touch allodynia.

▶ This is an interesting study of touch allodynia after either single portal or open release of the carpal tunnel. Although the authors do not use the term "pillar pain," it seems as though this postoperative effect is what they are measuring. The thresholds are in the range of 20–40 newton, which represents more than just a "touch" of pressure. This effect was found to be less in the endoscopic group over the duration of the study. The authors make the argument that this might play a role in selecting 1 technique over another, i.e., the patient's job or hobby might be resumed sooner if the presence of this side effect were diminished.

I cannot put much faith in the intracarpal pressure part of the study. I have never faced any difficulty in introducing the Agee device in a cadaver wrist, but I have abandoned the approach on more than 1 occasion in a living hand because I believed I was having to push too hard.

V.R. Hentz, M.D.

Pillar Pain as a Postoperative Complication of Carpal Tunnel Release: A Review of the Literature
Ludlow KS, Merla JL, Cox JA, et al (London Health Sciences Centre, Ont; Univ of Western Ontario, London)
J Hand Ther 10:277–282, 1997   7–18

Introduction.—Pillar pain, a potential complication of surgery for carpal tunnel syndrome, has not been consistently defined, but most authors distinguish pillar pain from scar tenderness. This study reviews the literature on open surgery vs. endoscopic carpal tunnel release (CTR), focusing on pillar pain.

Endoscopic vs. Open Carpal Tunnel Release.—Postoperative complications associated with the open technique, including persistent weakness, delayed return to work, scar tenderness, and pillar pain, are well known. The endoscopic approach is recommended as a means of minimizing postoperative morbidity; yet, complications can occur, and the method is prone to technical errors. Currently, the choice of an open or endoscopic procedure is based on surgeon and/or patient preference.

Pillar Pain.—Pillar pain can significantly delay recovery after CTR. Theories place its etiology fall into 4 categories: ligamentous or muscular causes, alteration of the structure of the carpal arch, neurogenic causes, and edematous causes. One author proposes that pillar pain results from cutting the ligament and occurs whether the incisions are short, long, or endoscopic. Other authors suggest that pillar pain can be prevented by leaving the superficial fascia intact. Pillar pain has also been attributed to changes in the pisotriquetral joint alignment, to division of cutaneous nerve branches, and to swelling at the base of the palm superficial to the carpal tunnel.

Incidence and Significance of Pillar Pain.—Estimates of the incidence of pillar pain are difficult to obtain because there is no recognized assessment technique or grading system. Some authors report pillar pain in approximately one third of cases, whereas others do not mention it as a complication. Pillar pain generally appears to subside by 12–16 weeks after surgery, but hand use and return to work can be considerably delayed. It is not known whether postoperative splinting might be helpful in preventing pillar pain. Treatments include immobilization, heat, ice, and massage.

Conclusion.—There is little definite knowledge about the origin of pillar pain or about the means to prevent this complication of CTR. None of the surgical techniques designed to prevent pillar pain has been completely successful, and it has not been possible to predict occurrence, severity, or responsiveness to treatment.

▶ In this article on pillar pain, the authors have brought to our attention an important issue that needs further investigation and research. There are not any clear definitions of pillar pain, its etiology, and its surgical post-operative management. It is very challenging for therapists to treat these patients, because of the lack of predictive indicators of occurrence, severity, or responsiveness to the treatment of pillar pain. It has been recognized as a frequent complication of carpal tunnel surgery and can significantly delay the patients' functional recovery.

In today's cost-containment environment, and with the high incidence of carpal tunnel syndrome, it is worthwhile to look into this important issue, so physicians and allied health groups can come to some consensus over surgical and postoperative management.

P. Lalwani, O.T.R., C.H.T.

Open Carpal Tunnel Release: Does a Vascularized Hypothenar Fat Pad Reduce Wound Tenderness?
Jones SMG, Stuart PR, Stothard J (Middlesbrough Gen Hosp, England)
J Hand Surg [Br] 22B:758–760, 1997   7–19

Background.—Although full release of the tight flexor retinaculum provides good symptom relief in 85% to 90% of patients with carpal tunnel syndrome (CTS), many patients report postoperative scar tenderness and pain, which delay the return to normal hand use. Loss of the normal median nerve movement of longitudinal sliding during wrist flexion and extension because of scar adhesion, which results in shear trauma of the nerve, may be responsible for these postoperative problems. The efficacy of mobilizing and rotating a vascularized pad of hypothenar fat to lie over the median nerve in reducing these symptoms was reported.

Methods.—Patients with bilateral CTS undergoing a total of 102 procedures were included in the study. In each patient, a vascularized hypothenar fat pad flap was laid over the median nerve in 1 hand. The flap was held by 2 or 3 fine Vicryl sutures to the radial side of the divided flexor retinaculum. The free edge of the pad was mobilized from the hypothenar skin and flexor retinaculum by sharp dissection just enough to permit tension-free placement across the gap in the flexor retinaculum. Mean tourniquet time was 6 minutes. Neither the patient nor the evaluator knew which hand had undergone this additional procedure.

Findings.—Overall, 87% of the patients reported improvement, and 55% said they had no symptoms (although only 23% denied having any problems on direct questioning). The use of the hypothenar flap was not correlated with improved surgical outcomes. The presence of wound pain, pillar pain, and the presence or distribution of neurologic symptoms were unassociated with the use of a hypothenar fat pad.

Conclusions.—The use of a hypothenar fat pad flap does not significantly relieve pain or other symptoms postoperatively in patients with CTS. This additional technique is not recommended.

▶ Hypothenar fat pad flaps do not reduce palm tenderness in the routine case of CTS, according to this study. No confidence limits are provided, however, and the paper does nothing to tell us whether there are subsets of CTS patients where a hypothenar fat pad flap might be helpful, such as in certain reoperations. Stay tuned for further developments.

P.C. Amadio, M.D.

Safe Carpal Tunnel Release via a Limited Palmar Incision
Lee WPA, Strickland JW (Harvard Med School, Boston; Indiana Univ, Indianapolis)
Plast Reconstr Surg 101:418–426, 1998   7–20

Objective.—Whereas endoscopic carpal tunnel release results in greater grip and pinch strength, less scar and pillar tendencies, and an earlier return to activities of daily living and to work, the technique is expensive, has a steep learning curve, and sometimes leads to nerve injury. The safety and efficacy of a technique of carpal tunnel release through a small palmar incision with a new carpal tunnel "tome" was evaluated over a 29-month period.

Technique.—Performed after the induction of local anesthesia, the procedure involves making a 1.0- to 1.5-cm incision along the third web space, excising the palmar aponeurosis, and dividing the distal edge of the transverse carpal ligament. The ligament is elevated and, with the wrist in mild extension, the tome is inserted under the ligament, which is then divided from the distal antebrachial fascia. The incision is closed and dressed. The patient is instructed to move the digits. The sutures and dressing are removed in 10–14 days.

Results.—Between November 1992 and April 1995, 694 procedures were performed on 525 patients (74.4% women), aged 21–88 years, of whom 21% were insured by workers' compensation. Patients were followed up for an average of 8.3 weeks after surgery. There were 2 early complications—a 20% median nerve laceration and a complete nerve laceration, with the latter occurring in a patient with altered carpal anatomy after a second pass of the tome, a procedure that has subsequently been abolished. Complete or nearly complete resolution of symptoms was achieved in 92.2% of the patients. Patients with significant residual symptoms were considerably older. Patients' rating of scar and pillar tenderness on a scale of 1 (not tender) to 4 (very tender) scored scar, radial pillar, and ulnar pillar tenderness at 1.4, 1.2, and 1.1, respectively, at 6–8 weeks.

Conclusion.—Carpal tunnel release using the limited pillar incision produced results that were as good as or better than endoscopic techniques. Recovery was faster, and patient satisfaction was high.

▶ Drs. Lee and Strickland have reported the results of a limited-incision carpal tunnel release with a sharp instrument through the distal palm. It would appear to this reviewer that the technique is associated with a high potential for soft-tissue injury because of the retrocut technique against the "grain of the median nerve." It would remain questionable whether the safety of this procedure, with 2 divided median nerves, is acceptable. The achievement of perfect results in 72% of the patients, even with limited follow-up, appears low. Nonetheless, with many techniques of carpal tunnel syndrome now available, I would believe strongly that all specialized techniques can be performed satisfactorily and safely in the appropriate hands of those who advocate them. Problems seem to occur when adapted techniques are developed by individuals who make minor changes that result in higher levels of complications. Although this device undoubtedly is reasonable and safe in the hands of these authors, it may not be in the hands of others attempting to copy this technique.

R.D. Beckenbaugh, M.D.

Three Ulnar Nerve Conduction Studies in Patients With Ulnar Neuropathy at the Elbow
Kothari MJ, Heistand M, Rutkove SB (Pennsylvania State Univ, Hershey; Beth Israel Hosp, Boston)
Arch Phys Med Rehabil 79:87–89, 1998   7–21

Background.—Although ulnar neuropathy at the elbow is common, localizing the site of entrapment is a challenge. The sensitivities of motor conduction studies and mixed nerve conduction studies across the elbow in localizing the site of nerve entrapment were compared.

Methods.—The participants were 21 patients with ulnar neuropathy and 20 healthy subjects. For the ulnar motor conduction studies, recording electrodes were placed over the muscle belly and the distal tendinous insertion. For the first dorsal interosseous muscle (FDI), the electrodes were placed over the base of the thumb. With the elbow flexed at 90 degrees, the ulnar nerve was stimulated at 3 locations: the wrist, below the elbow 3–4 cm from the medial epicondyle, and 10–14 cm above that site. Conduction velocities were calculated for the segment from below the elbow to the wrist (BE-WR) and for the segment from above the elbow to below it (AE-BE). For the ulnar sensory studies, recording electrodes were placed over the metacarpophalangeal joint and the distal interphalangeal joint of the fifth digit. Then the wrist was antidromically stimulated and sensory nerve action potentials were recorded.

For the mixed nerve conduction studies, potentials were recorded above and below the elbow. With the elbow flexed at 90 degrees, the ulnar nerve was stimulated at the wrist and BE-WR and AE-BE conduction velocities were measured. All participants underwent mixed nerve studies, but only the patients underwent the motor studies. Patients also underwent electromyography with concentric needle electrodes placed on the abductor digiti quinti (ADQ), FDI, flexor carpi ulnaris muscle, and the flexor digitorum profundus to the fourth and fifth digits.

Findings.—Conduction velocities in the control subjects were 73.9 m/sec for the BE-WR segment and 64.6 m/sec for the AE-BE segments. The mean difference between segments was 9.3 ± 3.9 m/sec; thus, 17.1 m/sec was set as the upper limit of normal (mean + 2SD). For the patients, mean BE-WR segment velocities were 55.2, 54.6, and 65.3 m/sec as measured at the ADQ, at the FDI, and in the mixed nerve studies, respectively. Mean AE-BE segment velocities were 47.2, 40.9, and 45.8 m/sec, measured at the same points, respectively. Mean differences in velocities between the 2 segments were 14.1, 13.6, and 17.4 m/sec, respectively. In 15 of 21 (71%) patients, motor conduction to the ADQ was abnormal; in 17 of 21 (81%), motor conduction to the FDI was abnormal; and in 12 of 21 (57%), the mixed nerve study was abnormal. All 3 tests were abnormal in 8 of 21 (38%) patients, and both motor studies were abnormal in 12 of the 21 (57%) patients. Four of the 21 (19%) patients had normal conduction to the ADQ, but abnormal conduction to the FDI, and in 2 of the 21 (10%), this situation was reversed. In only 1 of the 21 (5%) patients was the mixed nerve study abnormal but motor studies were normal. Twelve of the 21 (57%) had an abnormal ulnar sensory study. Needle electromyography results were abnormal in all cases.

Conclusions.—Motor studies with the FDI were slightly more sensitive than studies with the ADQ. The mixed nerve study was less sensitive than either motor study. Motor studies with both the FDI and ADQ may be needed if the ulnar neuropathy at the elbow is very mild.

▶ The article presents a useful comparison of some of the techniques now available for assessing suspected ulnar neuropathy at the elbow. The study suggests that recording from the FDI would be helpful in a small number of patients when an ulnar neuropathy is suspected and not identified with routine studies.

It should be noted that conduction to the FDI is more difficult than to the hypothenar muscles, because of the much more common occurrence of anomalous innervation. If unrecognized, this may lead to the incorrect conclusion that there is a localized conduction block.

The report does not indicate whether the abnormalities that were found localized the lesion to the elbow or the recordings just found nonlocalized changes. It would be of little clinical help if the FDI recordings identified only nonlocalized abnormalities.

Finally, the study tested ulnar mixed nerve action potentials, but did not compare them with the standard antidromic sensory nerve action potentials. The latter might, in fact, have demonstrated greater sensitivity than the mixed nerve technique.

J.R. Daube, M.D.

Splinting and Local Steroid Injection for the Treatment of Ulnar Neuropathy at the Elbow: Clinical and Electrophysiological Evaluation
Hong C-Z, Long H-A, Kanakamedala RV, et al (Univ of California, Irvine; VA Med Ctr, Orange, Calif)
Arch Phys Med Rehabil 77:573–577, 1996

Introduction.—After carpal tunnel syndrome, ulnar neuropathy at the elbow is the second most common entrapment neuropathy of the upper extremity. It may be treated with surgery or conservatively with an elbow splint alone or with local steroid injection. The outcome of splinting alone was compared with splinting plus local steroid injection.

Methods.—Ten males with 12 ulnar nerve lesions at the elbow were randomly assigned to 1 of 2 groups: group A, 5 nerves treated with elbow splinting alone; or group B, 7 nerves treated with local steroid injection (40 mg of triamcinolone plus 1 mL of 1% lidocaine) in addition to splinting. Patients were evaluated for clinical signs and symptoms and underwent ulnar and sensory nerve conduction studies at baseline and 1 and 6 months after treatment.

Results.—Both groups had significant improvements in symptoms at 1 and 6 months after treatment. At 1-month evaluation, patients in group A had improvement in ulnar motor nerve conduction velocity across the elbow. Significant improvement in this measure was observed in both groups at 6-month follow-up.

Conclusions.—Splinting alone was sufficient for improvement of symptoms and ulnar nerve conduction across the elbow. Local steroid injection did not provide any additional benefit.

▶ This is a nice small study with useful clinical implications. The main drawback is its small-sample size.

P.B.J. Wu, M.D., M.P.H.

Pain After Surgery for Ulnar Neuropathy at the Elbow: A Continuing Challenge

Antoniadis G, Richter H-P (Univ of Ulm, Guenzburg, Germany)
Neurosurgery 41:585–591, 1997   7–23

Background.—Ulnar nerve entrapment at the elbow is a common upper-extremity compression neuropathy. More than half of the patients undergoing surgery for this condition continue to have pain and paresthesias or have a recurrence of these symptoms after temporary improvement, regardless of the surgical procedure performed. Outcomes of subsequent surgery for ulnar neuropathy have not been well documented. One study of various surgical techniqnes and their outcomes is reviewed.

Methods.—Twenty-five patients underwent 28 operations for ulnar nerve entrapment at the elbow in a 5.5-year period. All had had excruciating pain after initial surgery. Ten patients had had a simple decompression, and 15, a nerve transposition. Subsequent surgery included external or internal neurolysis, epineurectomy, anterior transposition, and subsequent transfer of the nerve back into the sulcus. Mean follow-up after the last procedure was 17 months.

Findings.—All 5 patients undergoing subsequent transfer of the ulnar nerve into the sulcus were pain free after surgery. Only 2 of 5 patients undergoing secondary IM transposition for subluxation were pain free postoperatively. The outcomes of internal neurolysis were unsatisfactory, with only 1 of 6 patients pain free after the subsequent procedure. After 3 or 4 procedures, outcomes were comparable to those after the first repeated procedure.

Conclusions.—In this series, simple, less extensive methods used for subsequent surgery yielded relatively good outcomes. The less the nerve is manipulated during the initial operation, the less likely painful sequelae are to occur.

▶ This review of reoperation for failed ulnar nerve surgery turns up the usual suspects; that is, failure to resect the medial intermuscular septum in cases of transposition, instability after in situ decompression, and perineural fibrosis. Also usual is the lack of improvement after neurolysis. What is interesting is the observation that reposition of the nerve in its original bed can work, particularly in cases where the intermuscular septum had not been excised. Nevertheless, submuscular transposition remains for me the mainstay of revision surgery, particularly for revision of prior subcutaneous or IM transposition.

P.C. Amadio, M.D.

Cheiralgia Paresthetica—Entrapment of the Superficial Branch of the Radial Nerve: A Report of 15 Cases
Stahl S, Kaufman T (Israel Inst of Technology, Haifa)
Eur J Plast Surg 20:57–59, 1997

7–24

Background.—Cheiralgia paresthetica or Wartenberg's syndrome is a rare condition caused by entrapment of the superficial sensory branch of the radial nerve (SBR) of the forearm. Because of its anatomical location, this nerve is susceptible to trauma and neuroma, which can be debilitating by causing pain, paresthesia, and numbness. The outcomes of 15 patients who were treated for superficial radial neuropathy were assessed.

Methods.—The study group consisted of 15 patients with neuropathy of the SBR, conforming to the description of Wartenberg's syndrome, who were treated from 1988 to 1995. Their symptoms had persisted from 2 months to 2 years. All patients complained of pain, burning, and numbness or tingling over the styloid process of the radius, radiating to the first web and the base of the thumb and index fingers. In 2 patients, precipitating factors could not be determined, whereas the neuropathy was related to external compression in 5, job-related activities in 5, and blunt trauma in 3 patients (Table 1). There was a positive Tinel's sign over the SBR after tapping in all patients. Grip and pinch strength were weakened. Conservative treatment consisted of splinting, restriction of activities, and physiotherapy, such as soft-tissue mobilization, ultrasound, and electric analgetic modalities. Five patients received methylprednisolone injections. Five patients, with an average symptom duration of 13 months, had SBR neurolysis.

Results.—Of the 15 patients in this study group, 10 experienced a complete recovery over an average of 5 months of treatment. In 2 patients with job-related dynamic compression neuropathy, job modification resulted in early symptom resolution. The 5 patients who did not respond to treatment had SBR neurolysis, which resulted in complete symptom resolution in 4 patients. One patient had persistent mild discomfort.

Conclusions.—Physicians should be aware of entrapment of the superficial sensory branch of the radial nerve, which is relatively rare, but may

TABLE 1.—Precipitating Causes

Causes	No. of patients
Tight plaster	2
Hand cuffs	1
Watch strap	2
Job-related habitual movements	5
Blunt indirect trauma to forearm	3
Unknown	2
Total	15

(Courtesy of Stahl S, Kaufman T: Cheiralgia paresthetica—Entrapment of the superficial branch of the radial nerve: A report of 15 cases. *Eur J Plast Surg* 20:57–59. Copyright 1997, Springer-Verlag.)

be debilitating. It can be caused by job-related activities. Treatment should be consistent with the cause and pathophysiology of the SBR injury.

▶ We cannot be reminded too often of the importance of this small superficial sensory nerve subject to acute or chronic injury because of its location and anatomical relationships. Cheiralgia paresthetica can be truly disabling and may even precipitate a dreaded sympathetic dystrophy. The authors judicially advise a thorough trial of conservative, nonsurgical measures before exploration for neurolysis, repair, or deep placement of the proximal nerve end and its inevitable neuroma. Precipitating causes for the 15 patients whose neuropathy confirms to the original Wartenberg's syndrome are listed in Table 1.

R.A. Chase, M.D.

The Posterior Interosseous Nerve and the Radial Tunnel Syndrome: An Anatomical Study
Portilla Molina AE, Bour C, Oberlin C, et al (Universite Catholique de Louvain, Brussels, Belgium; Clinique Sainte Croix, Le Mans, France; Université de Paris V)
Int Orthop 22:102–106, 1998   7–25

Background.—Some authorities believe that radial tunnel syndrome is caused by compression of the posterior interosseous nerve in the radial tunnel, which is formed by the musculoaponeurotic septa of the distal part of the arm and the proximal part of the forearm. Others believe that this syndrome results from intermittent and dynamic compression of the nerve in the proximal part of the forearm associated with repeated pronation and supination. The relationship between the nerve distal to the supinator and the radial tunnel syndrome is not well understood. An anatomical study was performed to study the possible connection between the posterior interosseous nerve and the radial tunnel syndrome.

Methods and Findings.—Twenty anatomical specimens were examined. Various structures could compress the posterior interosseous nerve distal to the supinator muscle. These structures included the distal border or the supinator muscle, the ramifications of the anterior and posterior interosseous vessels, and the septum between the extensor carpi ulnaris and extensor digitorum minimi. The posterior interosseous was also stressed during passive supination and passive pronation.

Conclusions.—The posterior interosseous nerve is subjected continuously to dynamic stresses and passive compression. Other sites of compression in the more distal regions may be responsible for some treatment failures. The effects of dividing the superficial layer of the supinator muscle and of exploring the area of the nerve where most of its motor branches originate will be studied in the future.

▶ This is an excellent anatomical study. I agree with the authors' observations. Although they go on to say that there have been no reports of decompression of the posterior interosseous nerve by dividing the superficial layer of the supinator, William Sanders, M.D., of San Antonio, Texas, described just such an approach at the 1990 meeting of the American Society for Surgery of the Hand. That work was never published, but I have since used the technique in about 20 patients and have been highly satisfied with the results. The exposure, through a Thompson approach extended proximally, is easier than one might suppose, and by freeing the nerve through the supinator, one also addresses the proximal radial tunnel and even the lateral epicondylar region, thus addressing all possible culprits of refractory lateral elbow pain.

P.C. Amadio, M.D.

Anterior Interosseous Nerve Syndrome: Literature Review and Report of 11 Cases
Vrieling C, Robinson PH, Geertzen JHB (Univ Hosp Groningen, The Netherlands)
Eur J Plast Surg 21:189–195, 1998   7–26

Background.—Anterior interosseous nerve syndrome (AINS) is a neuropathy of the proximal forearm that causes weakness of the flexor pollicis longus and flexor digitorum profundus of the index finger. Reports in the orthopedic literature suggest that compression of the anterior interosseous nerve is the cause, and thus surgery is required. Reports in the neurologic literature suggest that neuritis or neuralgic amyotrophy is the cause, and thus nonoperative treatment is indicated. Both approaches with up to 10 years of a follow-up study are compared.

Methods.—Eleven patients (mean age, 44 years) with AINS were retrospectively studied. Ten of the 11 patients had pain and muscle weakness, and 1 had pain alone. Four patients also experienced sensory changes. Eight patients underwent surgery, typically between 3 and 8 months after the onset of symptoms. Fibrous bands in the pronator teres were compressing the nerve in 2 of the surgical patients, and the fibrous arch of the flexor superficialis was causing compression in 2 others. The nerve was an empty sheath in 2 patients, the nerve was swollen in 1 patient (no compression was evident), and operative findings were not recorded in 1 patient. Three patients refused surgery and underwent immobilization and/or physiotherapy. Follow-up ranged from 2 weeks to more than 10 years after surgery and from 3 to 6 years after conservative management. Results were graded as excellent (grade 5 motor power and/or complete pain relief), good (grade 4 motor power and/or slight elbow pain if the arm was used heavily), fair (grade 3 motor power and/or pain on moderate exertion), or poor (basically unchanged from baseline).

Findings.—In the surgical group, improvements occurred 1 day to 10 months after surgery (i.e., 3–42 months after symptom onset). One year after surgery, a plateau occurred, although 1 patient did report improvement even at 8 years. One patient had excellent results, 3 had good results, 1 had fair results, and 2 had poor results. The 1 patient with pain only was not graded, and pain relief occurred within 2 months postoperatively. However, 3 years later pain recurred, but symptoms resolved without treatment. In the conservatively treated group, improvements occurred 6 months to 1 year after symptom onset. Three months after the initial improvements, a plateau occurred, although 2 patients did report improvements even at 24 and 34 months. One patient had excellent results, 1 had good results, and 1 had fair results.

Conclusions.—Overall, the long-term results after surgery and conservative management did not differ substantially. The results indicate that, when patients have neurologic symptoms not caused by AINS (e.g., weakness of muscles not innervated by the anterior interosseous nerve, or sensory changes), then compression is not likely, and surgery would not be recommended. When the symptoms are caused by AINS alone, then a waiting period of at least 8 months to 1 year is warranted, to allow the neuropathy to resolve spontaneously before surgery is performed.

▶ It seems increasingly clear that the vast majority of cases AINS should be managed nonoperatively. Compression neuropathy does not appear to be a frequent cause in most cases, the cause is probably vascular or viral. Like the carpenter with a hammer, to whom everything looks like a nail, the hand surgeon with a scalpel needs to be doubly sure that the initial clinical impression is not colored by the availability of the tools at hand.

P.C. Amadio, M.D.

Suggested Reading

Al-Qattan MM, Thomson HG, Clark HM: Carpal tunnel syndrome in children and adolescents with no history of trauma. *J Hand Surg [Br]* 21B:108–111, 1996.
▶ The authors alert us to the existence of carpal tunnel syndrome in children with several types of conditions, including mucopolysaccharidoses such as Hurler-Scheie syndrome, mucolipidoses of various types, as well as symptoms of median nerve compression associated with lipofibromatous enlargement of the median nerve. I have seen carpal tunnel syndrome in 2 children with collagen disorders including Ehlers-Danlos syndrome. The etiology in these cases may be secondary to excessive wrist laxity combined with abnormal neural connective tissues. This is a useful article to reference.

V.R. Hentz, M.D.

Atroshi I, Johnsson R, Sprinchorn A: Self-administered outcome instrument in carpal tunnel syndrome. *Acta Orthop Scand* 69:82–88, 1998.
▶ For those who have Swedish patients, take heart: the Brigham carpal tunnel questionnaire[1] has now been successfully translated, with similar reliability and responsiveness.

P.C. Amadio, M.D.

Reference

1. Levine DW, Simmons BP, Koris MJ, et al: A self-administered questionnaire for the assessment of severity of symptoms and functional status in carpal tunnel syndrome. *J Bone Joint Surg Am* 75:1585–1592, 1993.

Donahue JE, Raynor EM, Rutkove SB: Forearm velocity in carpal tunnel syndrome: When is slow too slow? *Arch Phys Med Rehabil* 79:181–183, 1998.
▶ When median nerve conduction is slowed at the wrist alone, a diagnosis of carpal tunnel syndrome is likely. When slowing extends to include the median nerve in the forearm, roughly half of the time some other pathology (e.g., axonopathy, radiculopathy, plexopathy) will be found after further testing.

P.C. Amadio, M.D.

Mondelli M, Della Porta P, Zalaffi A, et al: Carpal tunnel syndrome in amyotrophic lateral sclerosis and late onset cerebellar ataxia. *J Hand Surg [Br]* 21B:553–558, 1996.
▶ The authors caution against operating on patients with amyotrophic lateral sclerosis and late-onset cerebellar ataxia because most of their patients did not experience symptomatic relief and had short life spans from the time of diagnosis of the principal disease.

V.R. Hentz, M.D.

Tada H, Hirayama T, Katsuki M, et al: Long term results using a modified King's method for cubital tunnel syndrome. *Clin Orthop* 336:107–110, 1997.
▶ These authors review 40 patients with ulnar nerve entrapment at the elbow, treated by medial epicondylectomy and splitting of the fibrous bands bridging the 2 heads of the flexor carpi ulnaris. If the patients' preoperative symptoms and signs were not severe, all did well postoperatively. Tada et al. determined that, in the patients with more severe compression, good symptom relief was obtained only when an aggressive epicondylectomy was performed, although this predisposed the elbow to medial instability. Symptoms tended to recur probably secondary to impingement of the nerve on the residual epicondylar elements. They advocate repair of the medial collateral ligament after aggressive epicondylectomy for these patients.

V.R. Hentz, M.D.

8 Wrist

General

Wrist Arthroscopy: A Prospective Analysis of 53 Post-Traumatic Carpal Injuries
Sennwald GR, Zdravkovic V (Berit Paracelsus-Klinik, Teufen, Switzerland; Univ of Zürich, Switzerland)
Scand J Plast Reconstr Hand Surg 31:261–266, 1997   8–1

Objective.—Clinical and anatomic findings are not always correlated in injured wrists. The location and degree of ligamentous ruptures necessary to alter the position of the carpal tunnel bone are unknown. Whether specific torn ligaments can be correlated with radiologic alterations was investigated prospectively.

Methods.—Arthroscopy was performed in 53 consecutive patients (24 women), with an average age of 30 years, with serious wrist injuries. Application of transverse pressure and shear stresses resulted in ratings of positive or negative depending on whether it caused pain. The location of the pain was recorded. Bilateral radiographic examinations were performed. All ligaments were evaluated at arthroscopy. The contralateral wrist was used as the control.

Results.—Patients were unable to explain the mechanism of injury in sufficient detail to allow evaluation. In both men and women, the radiolunate angle of the injured wrist was significantly smaller than that of the contralateral wrist. Arthrography revealed 13 communications between the radiocarpal and midcarpal joint on the radial side and 20 on the ulnar side, as well as 12 leaks around the triangular fibrocartilage complex. Ligamentous tears at the triquetrum significantly affected the positioning of the proximal carpal row because of clustering with the radiolunate and scapholunate angles. Arthroscopy detected 26 tears not found on arthrography, and arthrography showed 14 leaks not revealed by arthroscopy.

Conclusion.—Arthroscopy is a valuable tool for helping to determine the function of the ligaments of the wrist.

▶ Sennwald and Zdravkovic, in this analysis, have shown us the benefit of wrist arthroscopy as a sensitive research tool to better define the effects of injury on wrist pathomechanics. This study correlated ulnar midcarpal ligament injury with radiographic changes in the radiolunate angle. This confirms my own observation of increased laxity with the Schuck test when triquetral-capitate and triquetral-hamate ligament injuries are identified arthroscopically. There are many variables with wrist injuries, including extent and combination of ligaments injured, articular cartilage damage, and extra-articular injury.

Using arthroscopy to identify injury, followed by careful analysis of variables, we can better understand the pathomechanics of the injured and painful wrist and the response to treatment. The more sensitive the data we use in analysis, the more meaningful the results. I make a plea that when performing wrist arthroscopy, a full assessment of all the ligaments and articular cartilage be included in the operative report.

E.R. North, M.D.

Carpal Stability: A Mechanical Reality Well Defined [French]
Sennwald GR, Zdravkovic V (Handchirurgie, Saint-Gallen, Switzerland)
La Main 3:101–108, 1998

Background.—When describing carpal function, the terms *stable* and *unstable* are misnomers, based on subjective determinations rather than on joint mechanics. Because these terms are often used to mean different things in different studies, a standardized descriptive system based on mechanics is sorely needed. Such a system and its application to the scapholunate joint is described.

Methods.—In mechanical systems, an object is described as stable if, when subjected to an external force, it returns to its original position. It is described as neutral if it remains in its new position after the force stops, and it is described as unstable if it continues to move after the force stops. This same concept can be applied to intercalated systems, with 1 component being stable while the other component is either stable, neutral, or unstable. Furthermore, 2 intercalated systems can coexist, such that their interaction maintains the equilibrium of their articulation. This maintenance of equilibrium applies to the scapholunate joint, in which the scapholunate ligament binds the scaphoid and lunate bones and keeps them stable, the articular angles represent the area where the movement occurs, and the external force is applied by the muscles. The scapholunate joints of 10 normal cadaveric forearms were analyzed to confirm this concept. The radius and ulna were fixed in neutral pronation and supination. The thumb was fixed by wire and 2 wires were inserted on the scaphoid and the lunate so that their ranges of motion during flexion and extension could be measured. A force was then applied to each of the flexor and extensor carpal tendons. Infrared images were taken first with the wrist bones intact and then with the scapholunate ligament removed.

Findings.—The kinematics of the scaphoid, lunate, and triquetrum were normal when the scapholunate ligament was still in place. During flexion and extension, the bones in the proximal carpal row changed position smoothly and in a coordinated manner. However, once the scapholunate ligaments were sectioned, the proximal row no longer moved in a coordinated manner. The flow of movement became chaotic, particularly in the midrange of flexion-extension. This deformed pattern of movement was reproducible and evident in all specimens tested.

Conclusions.—Sectioning of the scapholunate ligament disrupts normal flexion and extension. The forces can no longer be transferred in a coordinated manner because the bones have moved. Thus, premature wear and tear is inevitable once the stability of the first carpal row is compromised, resulting in a change to the dynamics of the scapholunate joint. This situation leads to a precise, mechanical definition of stability: a joint is stable if movements between the articulating surfaces are continuous, harmonious, coordinated, and reproducible, regardless of the forces transferred or the position of the articulation. The current vocabulary of *stability, instability, dissociated, static,* and *dynamic* must be revisited and the conditions they describe must be formulated in mechanical terms.

▶ This article discusses the concept of carpal stability, and provides a single experimental example. Briefly, the authors' thesis is that stability is defined as that state which produces identical joint positions before and after a destabilizing force is applied. This homing concept of stability is useful but incomplete. It presupposes a black and white world, where a joint fits neatly into a single category: stable, unstable, or neutral-indifferent. Two important issues are not discussed: (1) whether a joint might be stable under certain loading conditions but not others (e.g., a joint might return to a neutral position after low loads but not higher ones); and (2) how to consider a joint that might be stable in an abnormal position or arc of motion in cases of malunion or arthrosis. They also do not address the case of an injury, such as a partial SL ligament tear seen arthroscopically, without instability (the so-called predynamic injury).

The authors are correct that prior schemes have often confused instability with malalignment, and that prior schemes have mixed anatomy, etiology, severity, and mechanics in various ways in classification schemes. The authors argue that terms such as *static, dynamic, predynamic, dissociative* and *nondissociative* are either neologisms, or are used in ways not intuited by their dictionary definitions. Clarity of expression is certainly important. But clinical carpal instability comprises more than a simple mechanical concept. To be useful to clinicians, a true understanding must include not only mechanical principles, but also the clinical features, such as severity and the anatomical nature of the condition. A useful classification scheme likewise must cover these concepts, and others, such as *etiology* and *duration*. This in turn will, of necessity, lead to a plethora of terms, often with the name assigned before the concept is clear. Currently we have terminology that literally describes effects, but is now being used to identify causes. For example, the terms *dissociative* and *nondissociative* were coined initially to describe the radiographic appearance of certain injuries, in which proximal row bones either were widely separated (dissociated) or not. Now we know that these 2 types of observation relate to the nature of the anatomical lesion, and the terms are used to cluster anatomically related families of pathology (intercarpal and capsular, respectively). Similarly, the terms *static, dynamic* and *predynamic* originally referred to x-ray examination, and whether malposition was noted at rest or only with movement or stress. Now these terms describe the degrees of injury severity that often produce that x-ray appearance. It is true that the English terms in common usage are not always well chosen in terms of dictionary meanings and do not translate well. Yet if the concept they convey is clearly understood, perhaps a new definition can be added in the dictionary. It is well-established usage to use a part or an attribute to refer to the whole (e.g., when we say we have so many head of cattle, the bodies are understood to be included). Even for larger stretches of meaning, it would not be the first time the meaning of an English word has changed, as my children, confused by Shakespeare's usage, constantly point out. And, unlike French, English speakers do not need the permission of a linguistic Academy to make such changes. Common usage is sufficient. Twenty years later, the words are there. If we can find better words, we should use them. What was reflex sympathetic dystrophy is now complex regional pain syndrome. Maybe a new set of names will be adopted for carpal instability. Until then, let us make sure that the concepts of mechanics, severity, and anatomy are well understood through the names they have been given.

P.C. Amadio, M.D.

The Influence of Joint Laxity on Periscaphoid Carpal Kinematics
Freedman DM, Garcia-Elias M (Roosevelt Hosp, New York; Institut Kaplan for Surgery of the Hand and Upper Extremity, Barcelona)
J Hand Surg [Br] 22B:457–460, 1997
8–3

Introduction.—Differences in scaphoid motion can explain variations in wrist laxity. Other kinematic parameters such as lunate and hamate motion may vary in proportion to the degree of soft tissue laxity.

Methods.—Global wrist laxity in 60 healthy volunteers (30 men), aged 19–48 years, was determined during 2 hypermobility maneuvers of the thumb column and 2 passive extension and flexion movements of the wrist. Lunate motion was observed radiographically with the wrist in full radial deviation and in full ulnar deviation. Flexion-extension of the lunate was determined by measuring the change in length of the lunate bone, and the Lunate Flexion Index (LFI) was calculated (Fig 1). Hamate motion was determined by measuring the relative motion between ulnar and radial deviation (Fig 2). The relationship between the indices and wrist laxity was analyzed statistically.

Results.—The LFI, which ranged from 9.4% to 40%, and the LDI (Lunate Deviation Index), which ranged from 13% to 33%, were not correlated. However, the Scaphoid Flexion Index (SFI) and LFI and the Scaphoid Deviation Index (SDI) and LDI were significantly correlated. The SFI and SDI were significantly correlated with wrist laxity, but the LFI and LDI were not.

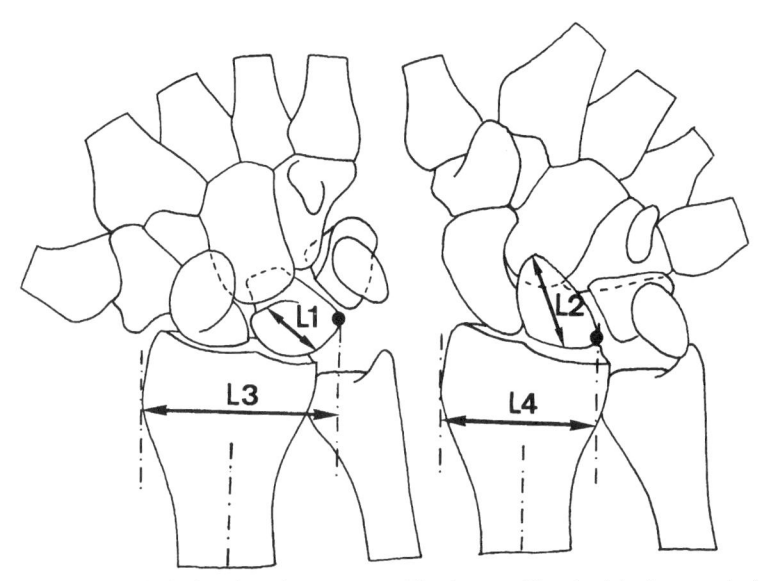

FIGURE 1.—Method of studying lunate motion. The changes of length of the lunate and of the distance between the ulnar edge of the lunate and a tangential line to the lateral border of the radius along the axis of the forearm are interpreted as representations of lunate flexion and deviation, respectively. The LFI is calculated using the formula:

$$LFI = \frac{(L2-L1)100}{L2}$$

The Lunate Deviation Index (LDI) is obtained by the formula:

$$LDI = \frac{(L3-L4)100}{L3}$$

(Courtesy of Freedman DM, Garcia-Elias M: The influence of joint laxity on periscaphoid carpal kinematics. *J Hand Surg [Br]* 22B:457–460, 1997.)

Conclusions.—Wrist laxity was related only to alterations in periscaphoid motion.

▶ What is the clinical significance of this study? It suggests that the clinical tests which are performed to diagnose scaphoid laxity be interpreted with caution, especially in the lax wrist. It also lends credence to the work of Craigen and Stanley,[1] which suggests that in the lax wrist, the scaphoid tends to show increased flexion/extension movement, and in the tight wrist, it tends to move more closely with the proximal row in radial/ulnar deviation. This also suggests that the scaphoid is the carpal bone which is most affected by generalized laxity.

L.K. Ruby, M.D.

Reference

1. Craigen MA, Stanley JK: Wrist kinematics: Row, column or both? *J Hand Surg [Br]* 20B:165–170, 1995.

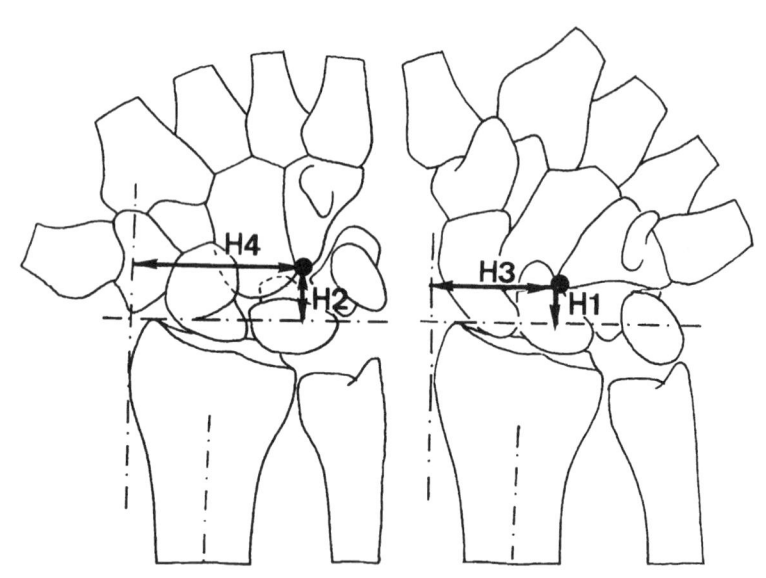

FIGURE 2.—Method of determining motion of the hamate. The changes in distance of the proximal tip of the hamate relative to 2 tangential lines to the lateral border and tip of the radial styloid indicate lateromedial and proximodistal motion of this reference point relative to the radius. The absolute value of displacement of this reference point (H) is calculated by the formula: $H = \sqrt{(H4-H3)^2 + (H2-H1)^2}$. (Courtesy of Freedman DM, Garcia-Elias M: The influence of joint laxity on periscaphoid carpal kinematics. *J Hand Surg [Br]* 22B:457–460, 1997.)

Reliability of Isometric Wrist Extension Torque Using the LIDO WorkSET for Late Follow-up of Postoperative Wrist Patients
Hudak P, Hannah S, Knapp M, et al (Univ of Toronto; Inst for Work & Health, Toronto)
J Hand Ther 10:290–296, 1997   8–4

Introduction.—For clients with upper extremity conditions, computerized work simulators have become integral components of rehabilitation. To quantify strength and endurance deficits, occupational and physical therapists can use the LIDO WorkSET, which assists therapists to implement appropriate rehabilitation programs. Little is known, however, about the reliability of the LIDO WorkSET. Using the LIDO WorkSET, the interobserver, intraobserver, and overall reliabilities of isometric wrist extension torque were determined. The minimal level of detectable change, using the standard error of measurement, was estimated.

Methods.—There were 18 postoperative patients who participated in the generalizability study. The mean torque of 3 trials was the primary outcome. To calculate generalizability coefficients for intraobserver, interobserver, and overall reliabilities variance components were used. Generalizability involved identifying and measuring sources of variance between repeated measurements.

Results.—To be 90% confident that true change has occurred, a change of more than 16 inch-lb is needed when the same therapist is evaluating a patient on different days. When different therapists evaluate a patient on different days, a greater value for change (23 inch-lb) is required. The LIDO WorkSET was successful in discriminating among patients who generated varying amounts of torque.

Conclusion.—In an applied setting, the LIDO WorkSET measures wrist torque in a reproducible manner. Among individuals, the testing protocol is sensitive to differences in wrist torque and is tolerated in the late postoperative period. Future studies should focus on determining the amount of change in torque that is clinically important, and should demonstrate the relationship between torque and more functional outcomes after surgery quantitatively.

▶ This article is a very insightful report of a research investigation into reliability of the LIDO WorkSET. Advanced computerized simulators provide evaluators with means to reproduce specific job and functional tasks. But we must question the reliability of the data being produced by these computerized simulators. The authors of this article questioned specifically the reliability of the wrist extension torque on the LIDO WorkSET, with late follow-up of post-operative wrist patients. Although we may have benefitted from a larger sample size, the study itself was very thorough and did prove the tool provided reliable testing. One issue we must look at, however, when using these tools, particularly for assessment or impairment ratings, is the degree of performance by the patient, because performance measures depend highly on the effort expended by the patient, and this challenges test reliability.

As a user of the LIDO WorkSET, I feel its capability of simulating numerous functional tasks is an asset to treatment, but I think it is important that we use supporting methodology to corroborate our data.

C. Gordon, O.T.R., C.H.T.

Customized Staple Fixation in Hand and Wrist Surgery
Looi KP, Chia J, Kour AK, et al (Natl Univ of Singapore)
J Hand Surg [Br] 22B:726–729, 1997   8–5

Introduction.—It is difficult to perform fixation in complex wrist conditions, in small bones, and for phalangeal epiphysiodeses in young children, with the wires, screws, plates, and pins that are commonly used. The smallness of the bone fragments and their ligament and muscle attachments make fixation a challenge. For many years, staples have been used for triple arthrodesis of the foot and high tibial osteotomy, but it is difficult to obtain control of the instrumentation during the procedure. The authors made customized staples intraoperatively from various diameters of K-wires (0.9–1.6 mm) and used them for definitive or supplementary bone fixation of the wrist and hand. A review of the technique is given.

Methods.—The purpose of the technique is to provide axial alignment and rotational stability for epiphysiodesis in phalanges and for carpal bone fixation. There were 14 patients, 3 children and 11 adults, who had this procedure performed. Follow-up ranged from 3 months to 3 years.

Results.—There was no occurrence of bone shattering, implant breakage, implant loosening, or infection. To give a more exact fixation, customsized and -shaped staples, which follow the bone contours, could be made, particularly since K-wires are quite malleable. One patient had removal of staples together with other larger implants in the forearm. Satisfactory outcomes were achieved in all patients, with preoperative objectives of bony fixation attained.

Conclusion.—The technique is versatile, precise, and reliable. Three-dimensional control of bone alignments is possible, as is adequate holding strength to the small bone fragments. The technique is also relatively cost-effective because it requires only simple, standard instruments. This method is advocated for limited and total arthrodesis of the wrist, nonunion of scaphoid fracture, interphalangeal arthrodeses, and epiphysiodesis in small phalanges.

▶ This article presents an interesting technique that may help in difficult technical situations requiring supplementary or definitive bone fixation. The authors advocate the use of customized staples made from 0.9 to 1.6 mm K-wire, which provide axial alignment and rotational stability for carpal bone fixation and for epiphysiodesis. Simple, standard instruments can be used to provide the fixation staples.

E. Akelman, M.D.

Carpus

Proximal Scaphoid Costo-Osteochondral Replacement Arthroplasty
Sandow MJ (Wakefield Orthopaedic Clinic, Adelaide, Australia)
J Hand Surg [Br] 23B:201–208, 1998   8–6

Background.—Compromise of the proximal pole of the scaphoid seriously destabilizes the wrist. Other surgeons have attempted to restore proximal scaphoid integrity by a medial column, scaphocapitate arthrodesis, proximal row carpectomy, complete wrist fusion, replacement of the proximal pole with a tendon anchovy, a piece of Silastic, or a scaphoid allograft. The results of using a rib bone/cartilage graft to replace the proximal pole of the scaphoid are discussed.

Methods.—Twenty-three patients without significant radioscaphoid arthritis were included in the study. Wrist function was assessed by a 100-point scoring system modified from Green and O'Brien. Pre- and postoperative radiographs were used to assess proximal pole union, with other imaging as needed. Twenty-two patients were available for follow-up. For the procedure, the patient was placed under general anesthesia and positive pressure ventilation was used during rib harvest. The harvested section was from the fifth or sixth rib and included bone, cartilage, and the

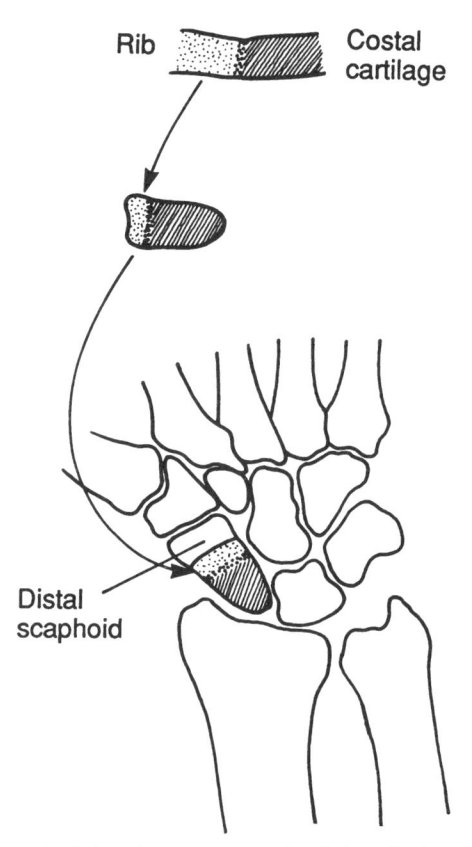

FIGURE 1.—Diagram of technique. Bone component of graft abuts distal scaphoid with the chondral portion of the graft articulating with the scaphoid facet of the distal radius. (Courtesy of Sandow MJ: Proximal scaphoid costo-osteochondral replacement arthroplasty. *J Hand Surg [Br]* 23B:201–208, 1998.)

perichondral sleeve. The proximal scaphoid pole was then excised, retaining the dorsal scapholunate ligament when possible. Intra-articular debris was removed, with limited removal of the radial styloid, if necessary. Then the surface of the distal scaphoid was prepared until it was smooth and cancellous. Next, based on the excised piece of the scaphoid or a bone cement mold, the osteochondral graft was carefully shaped to mimic the scaphoid defect. The graft usually contained 2–3 mm of bone and at least 5 mm of costal hyaline cartilage. The graft was placed into the scaphoid defect, with the bone touching the distal scaphoid and the chondral area articulating with the distal radius (Fig 1) and was stabilized with Kirschner wires.

Findings.—Wrist function scores and grip strength improved significantly after the procedure. Wrist function scores changed from an average of 53 before surgery to 75 at 6 months. Function continued to improve, and at the most recent review (from 12 to 72 months postoperative, median of 24 months), the scores averaged 80. Grip strength improved

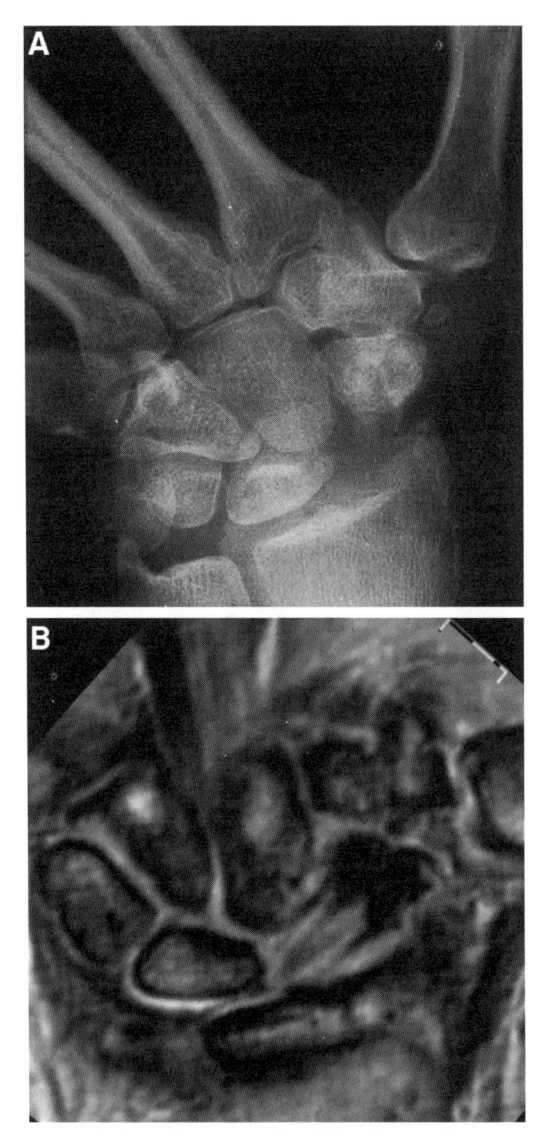

FIGURE 3.—Patient 12. **A,** x-ray of costo-osteochondral graft 6 months postoperatively. **B,** magnetic resonance scan 6 months postoperatively. Changes in the proximal pole of the capitate reflect pre-existing damage by a Herbert screw inserted for original unsuccessful treatment of scaphoid non-union. (Courtesy of Sandow MJ: Proximal scaphoid costo-osteochondral replacement arthroplasty. *J Hand Surg [Br]* 23B:201–208, 1998.)

from 59% before surgery to 80% at the most recent review. Integration of the bony component of the graft was satisfactory and occurred by 10 weeks (Fig 3). No evidence of nonunion was present, but 4 patients have undergone reoperation because of poor motion or suspected radial styloid impingement. Biopsy of the graft in these 4 patients confirmed the incorporation of the graft. Carpal alignment and degenerative changes could not be assessed by radiographs, because the costal cartilage of the proximal scaphoid pole is radiolucent.

Conclusions.—The use of a costo-osteochondral autograft to replace the proximal pole of the scaphoid has restored wrist stability for up to 6 years so far in these patients. This method avoids the risks of rejection, silicone synovitis, and infection transmission inherent in other techniques.

▶ The 12- to 72-month follow-up is not long enough for a definitive opinion. Carpal height is not reported, and the x-rays provided are not very impressive. It is well established that many patients with awful wrist x-rays have satisfactory wrist function, so the good functional scores reported need to be taken with a grain of salt. Nonetheless, for the small, proximal, unstable, symptomatic nonunion, rib osteochondral grafting may be an alternative to vascularized grafting.

P.C. Amadio, M.D.

Occult Fractures of the Scaphoid: The Diagnostic Usefulness and Indirect Economic Repercussions of Radiography Versus Magnetic Resonance Scanning
Kukla C, Gaebler C, Breitenseher MJ, et al (Vienna Univ)
J Hand Surg [Br] 22B:810–813, 1997
8–7

Introduction.—To be treated successfully, fractures of the scaphoid must be identified at an early stage. These fractures are difficult to diagnose, however, and a delay in detection may result in nonunion. Twenty-five patients with clinical signs and symptoms of scaphoid fracture but normal standard radiography findings at initial examination were studied with high-definition macroradiography (HDMR) and MRI to determine the value of these techniques in the early detection of scaphoid fractures.

Methods.—Patients were 16 men and 9 women with a mean age of 30.4 years. A common cause of injury (24% of cases) was a fall onto the hand. All patients had tenderness in the radial fossa and axial stress tenderness on thumb manipulation. Four-view plain radiography, performed at an average of 14 days after the injury, was compared with HDMR (an average of 2 days after injury) and MRI (an average of 3 days after injury).

Results.—Repeat scaphoid radiography showed bony abnormalities in 5 cases; 3 patients had a fracture of the scaphoid, 2 had an avulsion fracture, and 4 had other bony lesions. Using HDMR, fractures of the body of the scaphoid were identified in 2 patients, avulsion fractures of the scaphoid in 2 patients, and other bony lesions in 2 patients; no radiologic abnormalities were seen in the remaining 19 cases. Eight bony abnormalities of the scaphoid were identified with MRI, including 4 fractures of the body of the scaphoid and 4 avulsion fractures of the scaphoid.

Conclusion.—With plain radiography, the mean time to the detection of scaphoid fracture was 15 days. A repeat set of scaphoid views 2 weeks

TABLE 1.—Success Rates (Absolute Numbers) of the Different Techniques in the Detection of Ligamentous and Bony Lesions

	Scaphoid fracture	Bony lesions Avulsion from scaphoid	Others	Lig. lesions	Normal
MRI	4	4	5	3	9
R-SSV	3	2	4	—	16
HDMR	2	2	2	—	19
I-SSV	0	0	0	—	25

Abbreviations: Lig. lesions, ligamentous lesions; *R-SSV*, repeat set of scaphoid views; *HDMR*, high-definition macroradiography; *I-SSV*, initial set of scaphoid views.
(Courtesy of Kukla C, Gaebler C, Breitenseher MJ, et al: Occult fractures of the scaphoid: The diagnostic usefulness and indirect economic repercussions of radiography versus magnetic resonance scanning. *J Hand Surg [Br]* 22B:810–813, 1997.)

after injury was more successful, but not as accurate as initial MRI (Table 1). High-definition macroradiography proved unsuitable for screening for occult scaphoid fractures. Initial MRI, although an expensive test, can reduce the need for further imaging procedures and shorten time off work.

▶ MRI is an expensive examination. However, when used to detect non-displaced fractures such as a scaphoid fracture or other injuries at the patient's first visit, MRI can still be cost-effective as a result of savings in repeat radiographs, clinic visits, lost work time, etc. In Table 1, the number of lesions detected with use of early MRI vs. conventional radiography, magnification radiography, and repeat radiography after 14 days is shown.

G. Bergman, M.D.

Vascularized Bone Graft From the Palmar Carpal Artery for Treatment of Scaphoid Nonunion
Mathoulin C, Haerle M (Institut de la Main, Paris)
J Hand Surg [Br] 23B:318–323, 1998   8–8

Background.—Deciding how to treat scaphoid nonunion is difficult. The use of a bone graft obtained from the ulnar and palmar aspect of the distal radius and vascularized by the palmar carpal artery is described.

Methods and Outcomes.—Seventeen scaphoid nonunions were treated with this method between 1994 and 1996. Ten patients had previously undergone surgery with no success. The procedure was done on an outpatient basis, under pneumatic tourniquet control and regional anesthesia. In all patients, harvesting the vascularized bone graft was relatively difficult and delicate. In cutting the graft, about 1 cm³ was removed and pedicled on the palmar carpal artery (Fig 2). Mean follow-up was 16 months. As assessed by a normal appearance of the scaphoid on radiograph, union was achieved in all patients, occurring between 45 and 90 days.

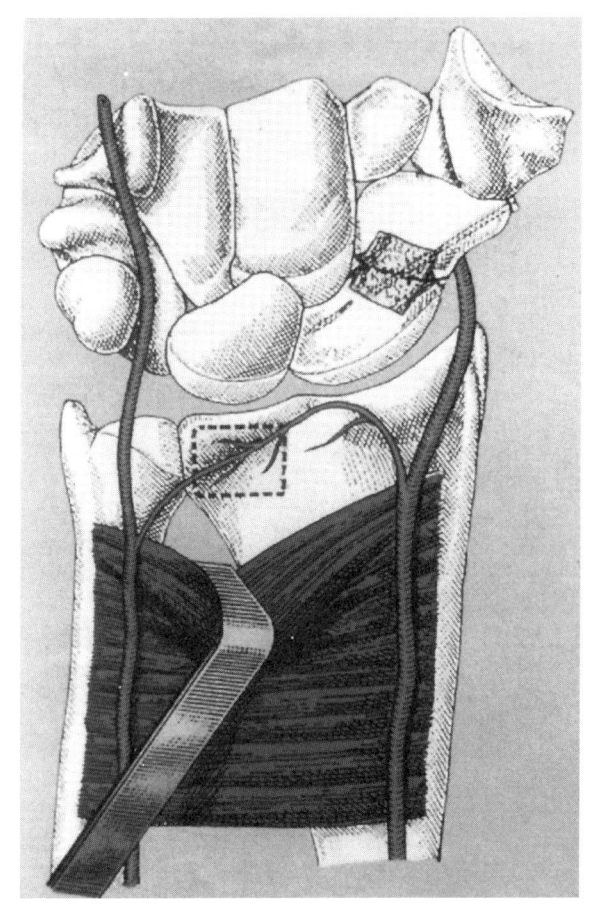

FIGURE 2.—Harvesting the bone graft pedicled on the palmar carpal artery. (Courtesy of Mathoulin C, Haerle M: Vascularized bone graft from the palmar carpal artery for treatment of scaphoid nonunion. *J Hand Surg [Br]* 23B:318–323, 1998.)

Conclusions.—The use of a bone graft harvested from the palmar and ulnar aspect of the distal radius and vascularized by the palmar carpal artery is recommended for scaphoid nonunion. The procedure can be done through a single approach and results in very rapid union with limited bone loss and no displacement of the bone fragments.

▶ It seems clear that the use of a vascularized bone graft increases the union rate in reoperation for scaphoid nonunion. Most commonly, a dorsal vascular pedicle is used; the approach has the advantage that the dissection is relatively straightforward. However, the dorsal approach requires either a second palmar incision for implant insertion, or fixation that pierces the articular cartilage of the scaphoid. For those who would prefer to do everything through a palmar approach, the technique described by Mathoulin and Haerle offers the same advantages of improved union rate, although at the price of a more difficult dissection. My personal preference remains the dorsal pedicle graft, because of its relative simplicity and reliability, but this palmar alternative is another option to keep in mind.

P.C. Amadio, M.D.

The Ulnocarpal Stress Test in the Diagnosis of Ulnar-sided Wrist Pain
Nakamura R, Horii E, Imaeda T, et al (Nagoya Univ, Japan)
J Hand Surg [Br] 22B:719–723, 1997   8–9

Introduction.—For ulnocarpal abutment syndrome, also referred to as ulnocarpal impingement syndrome or ulnar impaction syndrome, the ulnocarpal stress test is provocative, because it can differentiate ulnar-sided

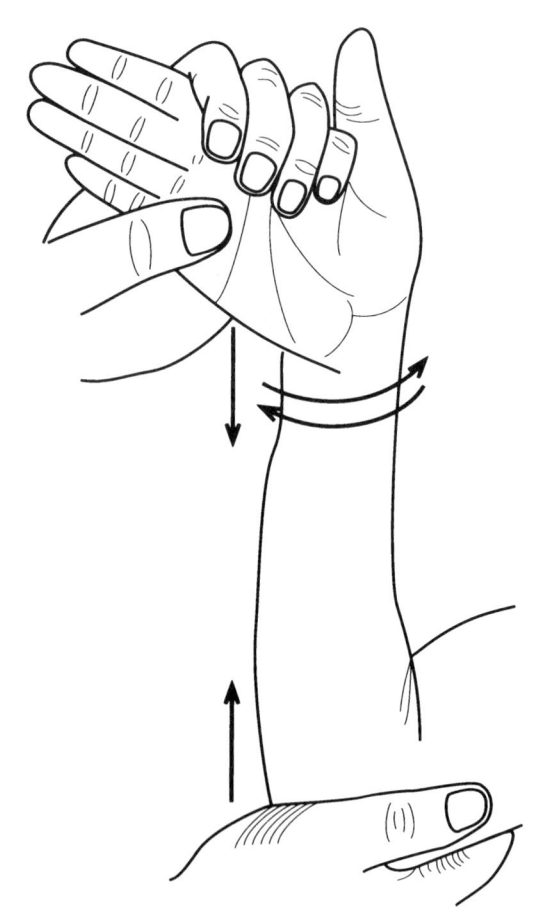

FIGURE 1.—Diagram demonstrating the performance of the ulnocarpal stress test. The test is positive when axial stress produces ulnar wrist pain during passive supination-pronation with the wrist in maximum ulnar deviation. (Courtesy of Nakamura R, Horii E, Imaeda T, et al: The ulnocarpal stress test in the diagnosis of ulnar-sided wrist pain. *J Hand Surg [Br]* 22B:719–723, 1997.)

wrist pain caused by ulnocarpal pathology from wrist pain of other etiologies. The test is positive when axial stress produces ulnar wrist pain during passive supination-pronation with the wrist in maximum ulnar deviation (Fig 1). In patients with positive ulnocarpal stress tests by radiograph, underlying wrist pathology was investigated.

Methods.—Radiocarpal arthrography, bone scanning, MRI, and arthroscopy were used to investigate 45 patients who complained of persistent ulnar wrist pain of more than 3 months duration and who had a positive ulnocarpal stress test. The patients ranged in age from 15 to 67 years and had a mean of 36 years. Tenderness was reported just distal to the ulnar head by all patients, with 5 also reporting tenderness over the distal radioulnar joint.

Results.—In 9 of 45 patients, ulnar wrist pathology was positively identified by radiograph. Arthrography identified ulnar wrist pathology in 18 of 37 patients; bone scan identified ulnar wrist pathology in 19 of 27 patients; and MRI identified pathology in 4 of 33. All 45 patients had wrist pathology identified by arthroscopy. The final diagnosis was ulnocarpal abutment syndrome in 28 patients, traumatic triangular fibrocartilage tear in 6, lunotriquetral ligament tear in 5, traumatic triangular fibrocartilage and lunotriquetral ligament tear in 1, wrist arthritis in 4, and cartilaginous free body in 1. Ulnar-sided wrist pathology is suggested by a positive test.

Conclusion.—The test is sufficiently sensitive to warrant further investigation and is useful for determining the etiology of ulnar-sided wrist pain. The presence of ulnocarpal abutment syndrome, triangular fibrocartilage injury, linotriquetral ligament tear, ulnocarpal arthritis, or free body is suggested by a positive test.

▶ The initial diagnosis and treatment of ulnar-sided wrist pain continue to be problematic. Nakamura and his colleagues provide data on the ulnocarpal stress test as initially described by Friedman and Palmer in 1991.[1] This current study analyzed 45 patients with ulnar-sided wrist pain and a positive ulnar carpal stress test. A positive test suggested the presence of either ulnar carpal abutment syndrome, a traumatic triangular fibrocartilage complex tear, a lunotriquetral ligament tear, a combination of triangular fibrocartilage complex and lunotriquetral ligament tears, wrist arthrosis and/or chondromalacia, or a cartilaginous free body. All patients had a positive finding. Of interest, radiographs confirmed diagnoses in 20% of patients and radiocarpal arthrography in 49%; a technetium bone scan was positive in 70% of patients, MRI in 12%, and wrist arthroscopy in 100%. This study suggests that the ulnar carpal stress test is sufficiently sensitive to warrant further investigation surgically by arthroscopy, if there is any question about a diagnosis in ulnar-sided wrist pain.

E. Akelman, M.D.

Reference

1. Friedman SL, Palmar AK: The ulnar impaction syndrome. *Hand Clin* 7:295–310, 1991.

Management of Trans-Scaphoid Perilunate Dislocations: Herbert Screw Fixation, Ligamentous Repair and Early Wrist Mobilization
Inoue G, Imaeda T (Nagoya Univ, Japan)
Arch Orthop Trauma Surg 116:338–340, 1997   8–10

Introduction.—Open reduction and internal fixation of the scaphoid is currently recommended for patients with transscaphoid perilunate dislocations. The optimal time of postoperative cast immobilization of the wrist has varied in published reports from 4 weeks or less to 7 weeks or more. A retrospective review of 29 cases evaluated the results of internal fixation by a Herbert screw and the effect of cast immobilization duration on outcome.

Methods.—Twenty-eight patients with 29 transscaphoid perilunate dislocations were treated at the study institution between 1985 and 1994. The average age of the patients was 26 years; 8 had associated injuries. Surgery was performed at an average of 15 days after the injury, using a palmar approach in 22 hands, a dorsal approach in 1, and a combined dorsal and palmar approach in 6. Treatment, in all cases, consisted of open reduction, internal scaphoid fixation using a Herbert screw, and repair of the torn palmar and/or dorsal carpal ligament. The average period of cast immobilization was 6.3 weeks.

Results.—Follow-up clinical examinations were conducted at an average of 24 months after treatment. Carpal instability patterns were evaluated by radiographic analysis of the radiolunate angle (greater than 10 degrees was considered abnormal). Results were excellent in 4 fractures, good in 15, fair in 8, and poor in 2. One of the patients with a poor outcome failed to achieve bony union because of a screw malposition and the other had a reflex sympathetic dystrophy. Both patients had the wrist immobilized for 8 to 10 weeks. The wrists were divided into 2 groups on the basis of cast immobilization time. Twelve wrists were immobilized for 4 weeks and 16 for more than 5 weeks. The average postoperative flexion-extension arc of the wrist was greater in the group with shorter immobilization time than in the other group (114 vs. 96 degrees). The 2 groups did not differ significantly in average grip strength or average wrist score.

Conclusion.—A lengthy cast immobilization makes stiffness of the wrist likely in patients with transscaphoid perilunate dislocation. The findings of this study support open reduction, internal scaphoid fixation using a Herbert screw, carpal ligament repair, and earlier removal of the cast.

▶ The authors report that 28/29 transscaphoid perilunate dislocations resulted in scaphoid healing after internal fixation with the Herbert screw. Palmar carpal ligaments were repaired and the carpus fixated with K-wires. Immobilization for 4 weeks resulted in a greater wrist motion when compared with immobilization extended beyond 5 weeks. The average radiographic follow-up was 24 months. The principles of scaphoid fixation and repair of the associated ligamentous injury remain the objective of care. If the wrist can be moved at 4 weeks without jeopardizing healing, a greater arc of motion will be achieved.

P.C. Dell, M.D.

Early Results of a Modified Brunelli Procedure for Scapholunate Instability
Van Den Abbeele KLS, Loh YC, Stanley JK, et al (Wrightington Hosp NHS Trust, Appley Bridge, UK)
J Hand Surg [Br] 23B:258–261, 1998   8–11

Introduction.—Scapholunate instability may be the most common form of carpal instability. Described is a modified Brunelli procedure in 22 patients with scapholunate instability.

Surgical Technique.—A palmar incision is made over the scaphoid tubercle, exposing the distal pole of the scaphoid and sheath of the flexor carpi radialis (FCR) tendon. The sheath is incised and a tendon-grasping forceps is passed about 10 cm proximally in the sheath along the FCR. Another proximal palmar incision is made over the grasping forceps and nearly one third of the FCR tendon is detached from the main body of the tendon on its anterior surface and stripped proximally to distally to deliver the tendon strip into the distal tubercle incision. A dorsal 5-cm transverse

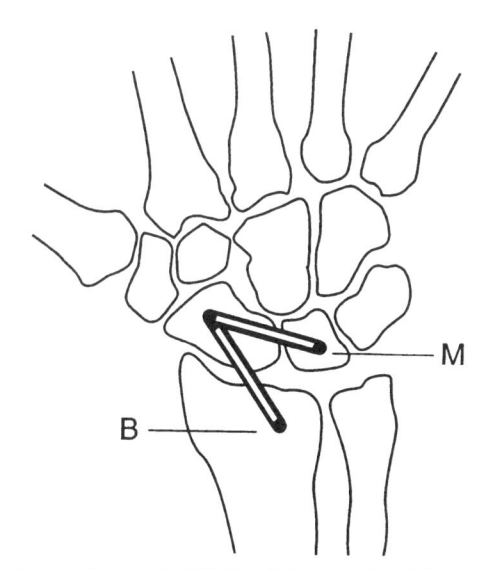

FIGURE 2.—Posterior view showing the FCR sling. *B*, fixation point of the original Brunelli technique. *M*, fixation point in the lunate with the modified technique. (Courtesy of Van Den Abbeele KLS, Loh YC, Stanley JK, et al: Early results of a modified Brunelli procedure for scapholunate instability. *J Hand Surg* [Br] 23B:258–261, 1998.)

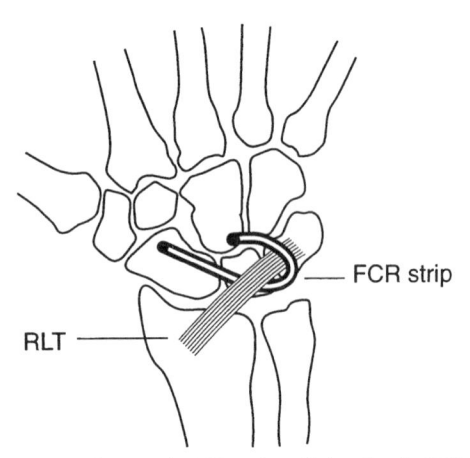

FIGURE 3.—Posterior view showing the FCR strip pulled under the RLT and fixed upon itself. *Abbreviation:* RLT, radiolunotriquetral ligament. (Courtesy of Van Den Abbeele KLS, Loh YC, Stanley JK, et al: Early results of a modified Brunelli procedure for scapholunate instability. *J Hand Surg [Br]* 23B:258–261, 1998.)

incision is created at the level of the scapholunate joint. This joint and the scapho-trapezio-trapezoidal joint are exposed. Scar tissue is removed from both joints. If needed, the rotary subluxation of the scaphoid is reduced by the "joy-sticking" technique. Temporary K-wires are placed in the scaphoid and lunate to manipulate the bones into a reduced position. A K-wire is drilled from the front of the scaphoid tubercle to the posterior bare area to determine the right direction of the tunnel through which the FCR tendon slip will run. A cannulated AO 3.5-mm drill is passed over the K-wire; radiographs may be taken to ensure accurate placement of the guide before the FCR-tendon slip is passed through the tunnel. The slip is tightened to assure scaphoid reduction. The tendon slip was attached to the lunate with an Acufex tag in 13 patients and passed under the dorsal radiolunotriquetral ligament (actually a capsular thickening) in 9 patients. The slip is pulled through the ligament close to the dorso-ulnar border of the radius and the tendon is sutured back on itself after sufficient tension is achieved (Figs 2 and 3). Care is taken to avoid damaging the posterior interosseous nerve.

Results.—Seventeen of 22 patients had relief of pain at short-term follow-up. Good recovery of grip strength was observed. Postoperative range of motion was diminished in extension and flexion, remained unchanged for radial deviation, and improved for ulnar deviation. Radiologic appearance of the dynamic or static scapholunate instability was unchanged after the procedure. Seventeen patients reported subjective improvement and would undergo the surgery again. Patients with unresolved medicolegal claims had significantly poorer results than those who were not undergoing litigation.

Conclusion.—Outcome was encouraging in some patients, particularly those not involved in medicolegal claims. Long-term evaluation is needed to determine advantages and disadvantages of a modified Brunelli procedure.

▶ The Brunelli procedure was originally aimed at supporting both the palmar aspect of the scapho-trapezio-trapezoidal joint and the dorsal aspect of the radioscaphoid joint to restrict rotatory subluxation ot the scaphoid. Along with other radioscaphoid tethering techniques, this fails to address ulnar translation of the lunate as part of the scapholunate dissociation problem. The authors' modification attempts to close the scapholunate gap by anchoring the slip of FCR to the lunate with sutures or passing it under and back around the dorsal radiotriquetral ligament. The latter is similar to a procedure we have used for some time with reasonable results. The drawbacks are as follows: (1) Tendon slips still have a propensity to stretch out with time and (2) closing the gap dorsally does not reinforce the palmar aspect of the scapholunate interosseous ligament, leaving a potential weakness for the intruding capitate head to exploit. Until a satisfactory scapholunate interosseous ligament replacement or repair has shown proven efficacy, their procedure offers a reasonable choice for repair.

R.L. Linscheid, M.D.

Isolated Scaphotrapeziotrapezoid Osteoarthritis: A Possible Radiographic Marker of Chronic Scapholunate Ligament Disruption
Wadhwani A, Carey J, Propeck T, et al (Boston Med Ctr)
Clin Radiol 53:376–378, 1998
8–12

Background.—Isolated osteoarthritis is rare. Cadaveric studies have shown isolated osteoarthritis of the scaphotrapeziotrapezoid (STT) in conjunction with scapholunate ligament disruption. This condition in patients is described, and the usefulness of STT osteoarthritis as a diagnostic marker of scapholunate ligament disruption is discussed.

Methods.—Six patients (3 men and 3 women, mean age 56 years) with chronic wrist pain and isolated STT osteoarthritis were included in the study. Radiographs were used to determine the scapholunate interspace distance, the scapholunate angle, the lunatocapitate angle, and the extent of any degeneration at the STT joint. Widening of the scapholunate interspace by more than 4 mm on neutral or stressed views was determined to represent scapholunate ligament disruption. Normal angles were determined as a lunato-capitate angle of 0 to −30 degrees and a scapholunate angle of 30 to 60 degrees.

Findings.—All patients had widening of the scapholunate interspace (from 4 to 10 mm), an abnormal scapholunate angle (from 65 to 90 degrees), and an abnormal lunato-capitate angle (from −45 to −60 degrees). None of the patients had volar angulation and flattening of the scaphoid (the Ring sign). Radiographs showed that the distal pole of the scaphoid appeared to impact the STT joint. The degenerative osteoarthritis present at the STT articulation was mild in 1 patient and severe in the other 5. Radiographs also suggested scapholunate ligament disruption in 3 patients; this was confirmed at arthroscopy.

Conclusions.—This study showed in 6 patients that isolated osteoarthritis of the STT occurs in the presence of scapholunate ligament disruption. A previous cadaveric study showed STT osteoarthritis in almost half of the wrists with a scapholunate ligament tear, but indicated the condition in only 14% of wrists that did not have such disruption. When osteoarthritis is isolated to the STT articulation, the practitioner should be alert to a possible scapholunate ligament disruption.

▶ This observation is interesting, but I remain to be convinced. STT arthritis occurs in older people, and older people often have degenerative perforations of the scapholunate and lumbrical tendon interosseous membranes. Such perforations are not the cause of instability, as the membranous portion of the scapholunate and lumbrical tendon ligaments has little mechanical holding power. Unfortunately, the diagnosis of scalpholunate pathology was made radiographically, and not clinically or surgically. Thus I believe this observation, though interesting, should remain in the category of "unproven."

P.C. Amadio, M.D.

Lunotriquetral Lesions and Their Sequelae in Perilunate Carpal Dislocations and Fracture-Dislocations [French]
Clément P, Laulan J, Sicre G (CHU Trousseau, Tours, France)
La Main 3:109–118, 1998   8–13

Objective.—Perilunate carpal dislocations (PLCD) and fracture-dislocations (PLCFD) are classically the result of a violent trauma in extension, ulnar inclination, and intercarpal supination with a sequence well defined by Mayfield. An analysis of triquetro-lunate lesions to isolate a reverse mechanism produced by intercarpal pronation has been attempted.

Method.—Sixteen patients were retrospectively reviewed: 9 were posterior trans-scaphoid PLCFD, 6 posterior PLCD and 1 anterior trans-scaphoid PLCFD. Primary X-rays were reviewed and patients were assessed clinically and radiologically after a mean follow-up of 52 months.

Results.—Luno-triquetral lesions were present in all cases radiologically and in 8 cases surgically assessed. A reverse mechanism beginning at the luno-triquetral space through pronation could be suspected in 12 (75%) patients and affirmed in 5 (42%) where the displacement was posteromedial with a scaphoid still in normal relationship with the radius. At follow-up clinical results were considered as good in 6 patients, fair in 7 and poor in 3. With good reduction and contention a good result was constant in all 5 patients. All patients without good reduction of lunotriquetral relationship had some pain, and all except 1 had some carpal collapse. Arthrosis was visible in 5 patients at mediocarpal level and in 3 patients at the radiocarpal joint.

Conclusion.—In PLCD and PLCFD, lesions can originate on the medial side and progress radially by intercarpal pronation.

▶ Mayfield, applying always the same type of deforming force with a component of intercarpal supination, demonstrated a sequence of lesions beginning at scaphoid level and progressing ulnarly. The authors have identified, in at least 5 of their 16 cases, a "reverse" sequence beginning at luno-triquetral level and progressing radially under a pronation of the second carpal row. Saffar[1] described such a mechanism as soon as 1983. Careful reduction of all lesions is mandatory, but it seems surprising that a correlation could exist between the clinical result and the quality of triquetro-lunate joint reduction. Usually isolated lesions at this level are not followed by arthrosis. A definite conclusion could not be drawn from this article because a precise assessment of cartilage lesion, under arthroscopy, was not attempted. These lesions are frequently observed in a violent trauma and could better explain mediocarpal and radiocarpal arthrosis.

G. Foucher, M.D.

Reference

1. Saffar PH: Les luxations rétro-lunaires du carpe, in Razemon JP, Fisk GR (ed): *Le Poignet*, Monographie du GEM Expansion Scientifique 12:120–128, 1983.

Ulnar Shortening Osteotomy for Ulnar Carpal Instability and Ulnar Carpal Impaction

Köppel M, Hargreaves IC, Herbert TJ (St Luke's Hosp, Sydney, Australia)
J Hand Surg [Br] 22B:451–456, 1997   8–14

Background.—Ulnar shortening osteotomy for disorders of the distal radioulnar joint is a common treatment for ulnar impaction syndrome. It is possible for ulnar impaction syndrome to result in secondary ulnar carpal instability, and vice versa. It is also possible for both conditions to coexist in 1 wrist. Ulnar shortening osteotomy is used to treat both disorders. The effectiveness of ulnar shortening osteotomy for ulnar impaction syndrome, ulnar carpal instability, and a combination of these conditions was evaluated. The effect of osteotomy type on functional outcome was also evaluated.

Methods.—The medical records of 47 patients who had ulnar shortening osteotomy for ulnar impaction syndrome and/or ulnar carpal instability were reviewed. A modified assessment system from Chun and Palmer was used to grade preoperative and postoperative wrist function. There were 19 men and 28 women; the mean patient age was 33 years. The mean follow-up was 18 months.

Results.—Distal ulnar shortening osteotomy reduced pain and improved wrist function in patients with ulnar impaction syndrome, as well

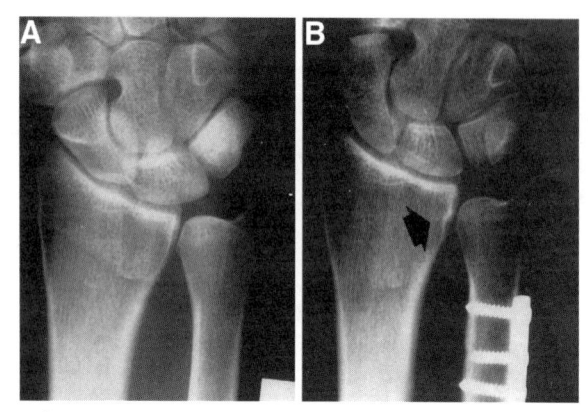

FIGURE 3.—Before (**A**) and after (**B**) osteotomy. Radiologic changes in the distal radioulnar joint were observed in 18 patients between 6 and 12 months after ulnar shortening osteotomy. The *arrow* indicates a focal osteolysis with sclerosis in the sigmoid fossa of the radius and a change in the slope of the ulnar head. These changes were considered as remodeling in response to the new load distribution in the joint, as they had no influence on the functional outcome. (Courtesy of Köppel M, Hargreaves IC, Herbert TJ: Ulnar shortening osteotomy for ulnar carpal instability and ulnar carpal impaction. *J Hand Surg [Br]* 22B:451–456, 1997.)

as in patients with ulnar carpal instability. The osteotomy was just as effective in patients with combined ulnar impaction syndrome and ulnar carpal instability. The procedure significantly improved grip strength and wrist stability but had little effect on range of wrist and forearm motion. Oblique osteotomies healed faster and had a lower nonunion rate compared with transverse osteotomies. At 6 and 12 months, radiologic changes in the distal radioulnar joint were seen in 18 patients (Fig 3).

Discussion.—Although adaptive changes in the distal radioulnar joint were seen on the radiographs of a significant number of patients in this study, there is no evidence to date that this causes secondary osteoarthritis. The authors recommend oblique osteotomy because it provides a larger surface area for healing and allows direct compression at the osteotomy site, even though it is technically more difficult.

▶ The authors reconfirm previous reports that ulnar shortening osteotomy is an effective method for reliably decreasing ulnar-sided wrist pain secondary to ulnocarpal impaction. Additionally, they have extended the procedure to distal ulnar dorsal instability of varying severity. Presumably, any improvement in the latter condition may be secondary to resultant tightening of the soft tissue sleeve around the distal ulna. A nonunion rate can always be anticipated but may be decreased by proper technique. Cooling during the osteotomy may decrease osteonecrosis, which is manifest later on x-ray film by a zone of bone resorption suggestive of inadequate compression through the plate.

Generally, 3.5 plates are recommended instead of the smaller 2.7 system. An oblique osteotomy will heal faster than a transverse, particularly when there is a well-placed lag screw across the osteotomy, either through the plate or at 90 degrees to the plate. The authors do not document dorsal ulnar subluxation by any studies but rely on clinical evaluation.

P.C. Dell, M.D.

Biomechanical Analysis of Limited Intercarpal Fusion for the Treatment of Kienböck's Disease: A Three-dimensional Theoretical Study
Iwasaki N, Genda E, Barrance PJ, et al (Johns Hopkins Univ, Baltimore, Md; Hokkaido Univ, Sapporo, Japan)
J Orthop Res 16:256–263, 1998   8–15

Introduction.—Avascular necrosis of the lunate from repetitive compressive minor trauma may be a key factor in the etiology of Kienböck's disease. Several fusion procedures performed to decrease the load on the lunate have yielded variable clinical outcomes. Effects of each type of carpal fusion on healing of the lunate, osteoarthritic changes, and ligament insufficiency throughout the entire wrist joint are not clear. Joint load and ligament tension were measured in a 3-dimensional model of joint geometry to determine which intercarpal fusion procedures unload the lunate and whether they change the force transmission through the entire wrist joint.

Methods.—Ten theoretical models of wrists were used to simulate 3 separate surgical procedures: capitate-hamate fusion, scapho-trapezial-trapezoidal fusion, and scaphocapitate fusion. A discrete element analysis technique was used in these experiments. Joint force and ligament tension of normal wrists and of simulated surgical procedures were calculated according to the deformation of each spring element to simulate the articular cartilage and carpal ligaments.

Results.—There was a significant reduction in joint force at the radiolunate joint and the lunocapitate joint and a significant increase in joint force at the radioscaphoid joint, compared with the intact wrist in scaphocapitate and scapho-trapezial-trapezoidal fusions. Joint force was increased by scaphocapitate fusion at the scapho-trapezial-trapezoidal joints and the triquetral-hamate joint. Scapho-trapezial-trapezoidal fusion increased joint force at the scaphocapitate joint. No significant changes in joint forces through the entire wrist joint were detected with capitate-hamate fusion (Fig 4). In an analysis of ligament tension, scaphocapitate and scapho-trapezial-trapezoidal fusions significantly diminished the tension only in the dorsal scapholunate ligament.

Conclusion.—Scaphocapitate and scapho-trapezial-trapezoidal fusions were effective in decompressing the lunate in a 3-dimensional wrist model. The capitate-hamate fusion was not effective in decreasing lunate compression. Scaphocapitate and scapho-trapezial-trapezoidal fusions are recommended for treatment of Kienböck's disease yet clinicians need to be aware that the increase of force transmission through the radioscaphoid and midcarpal joints may cause early degenerative changes.

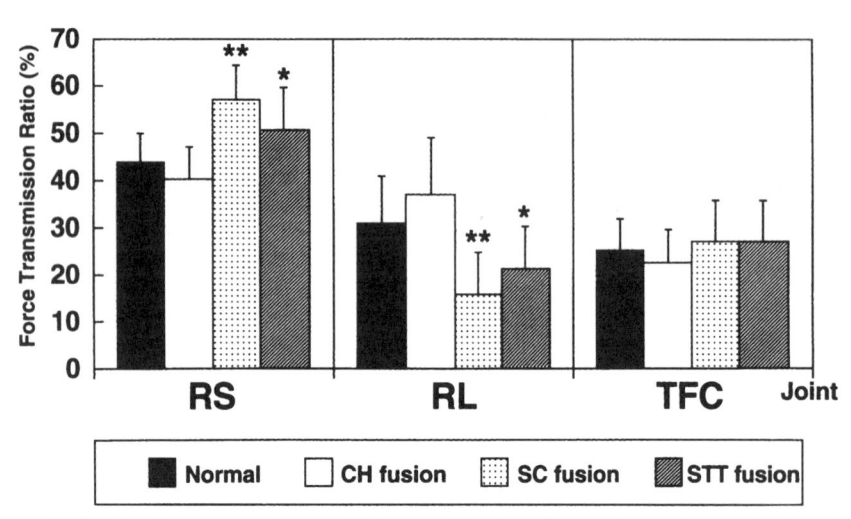

FIGURE 4.—Force transmission ratio (%) (mean ± SD) at the radiolunate joint in the normal wrist and that with simulated intercarpal fusion. Scapho-trapezial-trapezoidal (*SST*) fusion results are illustrated by bars with hash marks. *$P < 0.05$ †$P < 0.005$ in comparison with normal. *Abbreviations*: RS, radioscaphoid joint; RL, radiolunate joint; and TFC, triangular fibrocartilage. (Courtesy of Iwasaki N, Genda E, Barrance PJ, et al: Biomechanical analysis of limited intercarpal fusion for the treatment of Kienböck's disease: A three-dimensional theoretical study. *J Orthop Res* 16:256–263, 1998.)

▶ This is a good illustration of the power of computer analysis available for complex musculoskeletal problems. The 3-dimensional capabilities of the discrete element analysis technique increases the validity over previous 2-dimensional programs. The results are not unexpected and correlate well with previous computer simulations and stress measurements in the cadaver model. The drawbacks to this technique include the difficulty in addressing the amount of joint resection, the quantity of bone graft inserted, and angulations and translations that may take place between the carpal bones during surgery. It is also a static study, which doesn't address the effects of motion of the wrist on the intracarpal stress distribution. Nevertheless, it is impoertant to realize that the time is drawing near when computer simulation will allow a reasonable projection of the efficacy of a procedure before it is ever tried in the patient.

R.L. Linscheid, M.D.

Kienböck Disease Treated by Skeletal Traction
Kozuki K, Shakya IM, Tanaka H, et al (Sogo Aizu Chiuo Hosp, Fukushima, Japan)
J Jpn Soc Surg Hand 14:788–793, 1997   8–16

Objective.—Many different methods of treatment for Kienböck's disease have been proposed. One approach is to remove axial loading from the lunate, which can be achieved through a number of surgical procedures. The use of skeletal traction with an external fixation device for the treatment of Kienböck's disease is discussed.

Patients.—The study included 6 patients with Kienböck's disease: 3 with stage 1 and 3 with stage 2 disease. Two of the patients with stage 1 disease received conservative treatment, to no avail. In all the stage 1 patients, lunate findings on radiographs were negative; the diagnoses were finally confirmed by low MRI signal intensity on T1-weighted scans. The 3 patients with stage 2 disease did not receive conservative treatment.

> *Technique.*—All patients were treated with skeletal traction, produced by an external fixation device applied to the radius and metacarpal. Fixation was achieved with 2 pins in the distal radius and 2 in the second or third metacarpal. Distraction was gently applied to increase the width of the radiolunate joint by 3–4 mm. Initial problems with pain, tenderness, and swelling resolved after 3–11 days. The external fixators were left in place for 3–6 weeks.

Results.—Average follow-up in the stage 1 patients was 2 years, 4 months. All 3 patients had significant improvement in pain, tenderness, and swelling, although 1 patient reported dull pain after heavy work. Compared with preoperative measurements, wrist extension improved from 47.5 to 85.0 degrees and wrist flexion from 57.5 to 73 degrees. Grip strength returned from 51% to 93% of strength on the unaffected side, and all 3 patients returned to their original jobs within 6 weeks after removal from traction. Follow-up MRI scans showed dramatic improvement.

In the stage 2 cases, all symptoms had completely resolved by the time the external fixators were removed. However, symptoms returned within 6 weeks, followed in 3–5 months by radiographic progression. All 3 patients in this group eventually required radial-shortening osteotomy.

Conclusions.—Skeletal traction with an external fixator is apparently an effective treatment for stage 1 Kienböck's disease. However, for patients with stage 2 or more advanced disease, more sustained decompression, such as that provided by radial shortening osteotomy, is required. More research is needed to define the optimal strength and duration of traction for use in Kienböck's disease.

▶ This article proposes a new treatment for early Kienböck's disease. Three patients were diagnosed to have Kienböck's disease in stage 1 by clinical symptoms, x-ray, and MRI. Distraction and immobilization of the wrist was continued for 3 weeks, using an external fixator. Pain, swelling, and tenderness at the wrist disappeared during the period. At the time of follow up 1 to 5 years after the treatment, those patients were free from pain, swelling, and tenderness of the wrist. Only 1 patient complained of dull ache after heavy manual work. The range of motion in both extension and flexion were remarkably improved by the treatment. Grip power increased to 93% of the opposite hand. The rationale of this treatment is that distraction and immobilization for 3 weeks not only sedate the inflammation, but also promote revascularization and mechanical strength of the lunate in the very early stage of Kienböck's disease. As reported here, this treatment was ineffective for the disease in stage 2. I think this relatively simple treatment with an external fixator would be a treatment of choice for very early Kienböck's disease after making the correct diagnosis.

Y. Ueba, M.D., D.M.Sc.

Osteotomy of the Radial Styloid in the Treatment of Scapho-Lunate Collapse and Radio-Styloid Pain Syndrome [Spanish]
Galán V, Izquierdo de la T J, Cruchaga C A, et al (Hosp de Galdácano)
Rev Esp Cir Mano 24:15–19, 1997   8–17

Introduction.—Degenerative arthritis of the radioscaphoid joint is a frequent cause of pain and the most common presentation in wrist degenerative arthritis. A procedure for managing this condition is discussed.

Methods.—Sixteen patients underwent a closing wedge osteotomy of the radial styloid. In 8 patients, radioscaphoid arthritis was secondary to pseudoarthritis of the scaphoid; in 6 patients, the condition occurred after an intrarticular fracture of the distal radius; and in the remaining 2 patients, it was secondary to a scapho–trapezium-trapezoid arthrodesis. The osteotomy line went from the lateral aspect of the radial metaphysis to the crest between the lunate and scaphoid fossa. The average correction of radial angulation was 7.6%. Internal fixation was provided by 1 or 2 Herbert screws, plus 1 or 2 K-wires.

Results.—Eight patients were completely relieved from pain, 5 complained of occasional pain, and 3 of pain only after vigorous exercises.

Conclusion.—This procedure can be effective for the relief of pain caused by degenerative arthritis of the radioscaphoid joint.

▶ It is difficult to evaluate the outcome of this procedure in these types of painful wrists, as there is an underlying pathologic condition that is not solved by the surgical technique, such as a scaphoid pseudoarthrosis. This procedure was proposed by Giannikas and Papachritov[1] and seems to be a valid alternative to a radial styloidectomy.[2] The closing wedge osteotomy of the radial styloid will also decompress the radioscaphoid joint with the advantage of preserving the radiocarpal ligaments. Bone healing should not be a problem, and the only drawback would be that a very precise surgical technique is required to avoid complications.

A. Luch, M.D., Ph.D.

References

1. Giannikas A, Papachritov G: Wedge osteotomy of the lower end of the radius in the treatment of painful pseudoarthrosis of the carpal scaphoid bone. *Clin Orthop* 246:16, 1989.

2. Siegel DB, Gelberman RH: Radial styloidectomy: An anatomical study with special reference to radiocarpal intracapsular ligamentous morphology. *J Hand Surg [Am]* 16A:40–44, 1991.

Resection of the Proximal Row of the Carpus: A Review of 45 Cases
Alnot JY, Apredoaei C, Frot B (Hôpital Bichat, Paris)
Int Orthop 21:145–150, 1997   8–18

Background.—Removal of the scaphoid, lunate, and triquetrum is often used to reconstruct the wrist with scapholunate advanced collapse (SLAC). This article studies proximal row carpectomy in patients with varying degrees of SLAC.

Methods.—There were 45 patients in total, 33 men and 11 women, 23 to 71 years old. All patients underwent a proximal row carpectomy for pain due to ligamentous instability (n = 23) or due to an osseus origin (n = 22; Kienbock's disease, Preiser's disease, and pseudoarthrosis). Imaging studies were performed for each patient to determine the extent of degeneration. Before surgery, the average extension was 31 degrees and average flexion was 37 degrees (arc of 68 degrees). Average radial deviation was 15 degrees and average ulnar deviation was 25 degrees. Grip strength averaged 40% lower with the affected hand than with the unaffected hand.

Findings.—Follow-up ranged from 1 to 7 years (average, 30 months). Surgery failed to relieve pain permanently in 3 patients; all 3 previously had hand surgery, and all 3 ultimately required fusion. Of the remaining 42 patients, 34 (81%) experienced a 90% improvement in pain. Most patients maintained good range of movement, with an average extension of 30 degrees, average flexion of 31 (arc of 61 degrees), average radial deviation of 10 degrees, and average ulnar deviation of 20 degrees. Grip strength improved, to average only 20% lower with the affected hand than the unaffected hand. As seen on radiographic studies, 9 patients experienced a 50% decrease in joint space, and 1 patient with severe SLAC developed painful osteoarthritis because of scapholunate instability. Pain relief was less in the 6 patients in whom lesions were noted on the radial side of the radiolunate joint.

Conclusions.—Resection of the proximal row of the carpus improved grip strength and relieved pain in these patients with SLAC. Although range of motion after surgery was less than that before surgery, surgery nonetheless provided adequate range of motion, with the added benefit of pain relief. Proximal row carpectomy remains a useful approach to pain relief in the wrist with SLAC.

▶ Articles reporting good results using proximal row carpectomy for various degenerative conditions of the carpus are becoming more frequent. This article reports a "medium term" follow-up (average, 30 months) in a mixed group of conditions. Approximately half were perilunate injuries with the remaining being Kienböck's disease and scaphoid nonunions. Their results are similar to most reported series, with over 90% obtaining relief of pain and a less than 10% failure rate. The average flexion-extension arc of motion was 60% and average grip strength was 80% of opposite wrist. Follow-up x-rays showed some loss of joint space in 10 of 42 cases which was attributed to remodeling. It is interesting to note that of the 3 patients who were ultimately fused, 2 had undergone operations prior to the proximal row carpectomy.

W.D. Engber, M.D.

Proximal Row Carpectomy Through a Palmar Approach
Luchetti R, Soragni O, Fairplay T (State Hosp, San Marino, Republic of San Marino)
J Hand Surg [Br] 23B:406–409, 1998   8–19

Introduction.—Though usually performed through a dorsal approach, proximal row carpectomy (PRC) can also be performed through a palmar approach. Some reports have expressed concern that the palmar approach might lead to instability resulting from the excision arthroplasty. The results of PRC performed through a palmar approach are reported.

Methods.—The experience included 7 men and 2 women, average age 34. Severe wrist pain was caused by scaphoid pseudoarthritis in 5 patients, Kienböck's disease in 5, and scapholunate advanced collapse-type osteoarthritis in 1. The procedure was performed through a curved palm-wrist incision. After opening of the capsule, the bones were sectioned with an osteotome and removed with rongeurs: the lunate first, then the triquetrum. No Kirschner wire stabilization was used. After the palmar capsule and skin were sutured, the wrist was placed in a palmar trough splint in 25–35 degrees of extension.

Results.—Seven patients reported no pain at an average follow-up of 20 months. There was no change in average range of wrist flexion/extension, though average radial/ulnar deviation increased from 25 to 46 degrees. Grip strength was increased in all patients. In 4 cases, the articular space was slightly reduced and there was subchondral sclerosis in the radiocapitate joint. However, function was good. There was no evidence of radiocarpal instability on dynamic joint studies. Patient satisfaction was high, with return to work after an average of 2 months.

Conclusions.—The authors report good results with PRC performed through a palmar approach. This procedure eliminates wrist pain, provides good functional mobility of the wrist, and increases grip strength. Patients are able to return to work in a very short time, and express a high level of satisfaction.

▶ Although this article shows that PRC can be done, with reasonable results, through a palmar approach, it is hard to imagine that the technique is any easier than carpectomy done through a dorsal approach. The authors never give their rationale for using a palmar approach, and it would be useful to know if there are any actual or theoretical advantages to a palmar PRC. If not, the dorsal approach, being simpler, would remain my method of choice.

P.C. Amadio, M.D.

Denervation of the Radiocarpal Joint: A Follow-up Study in 22 Patients
Grechenig W, Mähring M, Clement HG (Univ Clinic for Traumatology, Graz, Austria)
J Bone Joint Surg Br 80B:504–507, 1998

Background.—Selective denervation of the wrist can be performed to relieve chronic wrist pain, while preserving some sensation and mobility. Denervation is preferred over arthrodesis for patients with useful movement at the wrist. Results of wrist denervation surgery are reviewed.

Methods.—The experience included 22 patients who had undergone selective denervation a mean of 50 months previously. The most frequent indications were fracture of the radius and scaphoid, usually with secondary arthritis. All patients had failed to respond to conservative therapy, and showed considerable pain relief on preoperative nerve blockade. Sixteen patients were treated with surgery only, consisting of division of the posterior interosseous nerve, the articular branch of the superficial radial nerve to the first intermetacarpal space, the articular branches of the lateral cutaneous nerve of the forearm, the articular branch of the superficial radial nerve, the anterior interosseous nerve, and the dorsal articular branch of the ulnar nerve. Six patients underwent other procedures, such as synovectomy or carpal tunnel release, as well.

Results.—Seventeen patients said they were very satisfied with their results, and 3 said they were satisfied. Two patients reported dissatisfaction, but none was made worse. Fifteen of the 22 patients reported no adverse symptoms or only minor pain on stressing the wrist joint, 6 reported pain on normal use of the joint, and 2 reported no improvement. No patient had postoperative complications. No patient desired supplementary arthrodesis.

Conclusions.—Selective denervation surgery is a useful procedure for patients with chronic wrist pain. Preoperative nerve blockade tests are essential. The surgeon must have detailed knowledge of the nerves supplying sensation to the radiocarpal joint.

▶ Denervating a painful joint, such as the wrist, is certainly attractive in the face of the substantial morbidity from alternative procedures. The concept of wrist denervation has been applied, largely in Europe, from as early as 1966 (by Wilhelm), and was reintroduced by Buck-Gramcko in 1977. There have been no reports of Charcot joints, and the perioperative morbidity is very limited. Many patients with intractable wrist pain experience substantial relief with a partial denervation, focusing on the anterior and posterior interosseous nerves. The advantage of this particular procedure is its ability to block the nerves with a local anesthetic preoperatively to predict the efficacy of the procedure, described in the article noted below.[1]

R.A. Berger, M.D., Ph.D.

Reference

1. Berger RA: Partial denervation of the wrist: A new approach. *Techniques in Hand and Upper Extremity Surg* 2:25–35, 1998.

Limited Wrist Arthrodesis for the Salvage of SLAC Wrist
Gill DRJ, Ireland DCR (Cliveden Hill Private Hosp, East Melbourne, Australia)
J Hand Surg [Br] 22B:461–465, 1997
8–21

Background.—Wrists with scapholunate advanced collapse (SLAC) are often salvaged by a 4-corner fusion of the wrist joint articulations into 1 articulation of the radiolunate joint and stabilization of the midcarpal joint. This article reports the results of an approach that avoids lunotriquetral joint fusion, instead using the capitate as the apex for the fusion (limited wrist arthrodesis).

Methods.—A total of 24 wrists in 22 patients (21 men and 1 woman, 26–69 years old) were treated by limited wrist arthrodesis. A midline dorsal skin incision was made and the carpal bones were exposed. The scaphoid was removed and a radial styloidectomy was performed to keep the midcarpal joint from impinging on the trapezium. The midcarpal joint was then reduced to maintain its original contour. The lunate was flexed outward and attached to the capitate with cancellous screws (early in the series, K wires were also used). This approach avoided involvement of the normal lunotriquetral and capitatohamate joints. After surgery, compression dressing and splints were used for 2 weeks, then a below-elbow cast was used for 6 weeks.

Findings.—After 6–81 months (mean, 23 months), 17 patients (19 [79%]) of 24 wrists had no or only mild pain, 1 with moderate pain was diagnosed as having osteoarthritis of the distal radioulnar joint, and 4 had severe pain that required further surgery. After surgery, range of motion decreased to a mean flexion/extension arc of 48 degrees and a mean radial/ulnar deviation arc of 19 degrees. Nonetheless, after surgery 6 patients still had functional range of motion in all planes, and 9 had functional range of motion in flexion and extension. Grip strength in the operated hand averaged 70% that of the unoperated side. All 4 of the patients in whom the procedure failed had nonunions of the lunocapitate joint. Two underwent a second limited wrist arthrodesis with cancellous bone graft and 2 underwent pan arthrodesis; revision surgery was successful in all 4 patients. Other adverse effects included pisotriquetral impingement because of the second screw (Removal of the screw relieved symptoms in 2 patients), continued pain after a successful limited wrist arthrodesis (2 patients required pan arthrodesis), and extensor tendon rupture due to a retained K-wire (reconstruction of the tendon and removal of the wire was successful in 1 patient). Ten patients elected to have the screws removed because the heads were prominent and were becoming loose at the base of the third metacarpal.

Conclusions.—Pain relief, range of motion, and grip strength with this limited wrist arthrodesis are similar to results after 4-corner fusion. Yet the limited wrist arthrodesis requires fewer steps, provides a greater contact area for the fusion mass, and avoids disturbing normal lunotriquetral and capitatohamate joints. Limited wrist arthrodesis is a good alternative to other approaches for SLAC salvage, particularly in patients who have severe wrist pain or stiffness or a weak grip.

▶ The authors describe their modification of Watson's SLAC wrist reconstructions (scaphoid excision and 4-corner arthrodesis). In their technique, a scaphoid excision was combined with a capito-lunate and a triquetrial-hamate fusion using cancellous lag screws. Their short term results (average 23 months) show approximately 75% of patients had minimal or no pain and a flexion-extension arc of motion of 48 degrees. Over 50% of patients required reoperation—most for hardware problems. Nonunion occurred in about 20% and four out of 24 wrists required pan carpal arthrodesis.

This technique has a higher incidence of reoperation and a smaller flexion-extension arc than most published series of proximal row carpectomy—an alternative surgical procedure.

W.D. Engber, M.D.

A Comparison of Fixation Screws for the Scaphoid During Application of Cyclical Bending Loads
Toby EB, Butler TE, McCormack TJ, et al (Univ of Kansas, Kansas City)
J Bone Joint Surg Am 79-A:1190–1197, 1997   8–22

Background.—Scaphoid fractures pose significant treatment challenges related to persistent bending forces applied to this bone. The Herbert screw is a popular choice for the fixation of scaphoid fractures and nonunions, and has given good clinical results, although biomechanical studies suggest that it provides less pull-out strength and generates less compressive force than standard screws. Various scaphoid fixation devices were tested using a cyclical bending test to simulate a more physiologic pattern of loading.

Methods.—Thirty-five matched pairs of human cadaver scaphoids were used. After osteotomy, 1 scaphoid of each pair was fixed with a Herbert screw and the other with an AO 3.5-mm cannulated screw, a Herbert-Whipple screw, an Acutrak cannulated screw, or a Universal Compression screw (Fig 1). Each specimen was stressed with ramped-intensity cyclical bending loads to simulate the bending forces applied to the scaphoid, which tends to subside into a palmar-flexed position in cases of nonunion. In a further experiment, the AO and Herbert screws were compared in

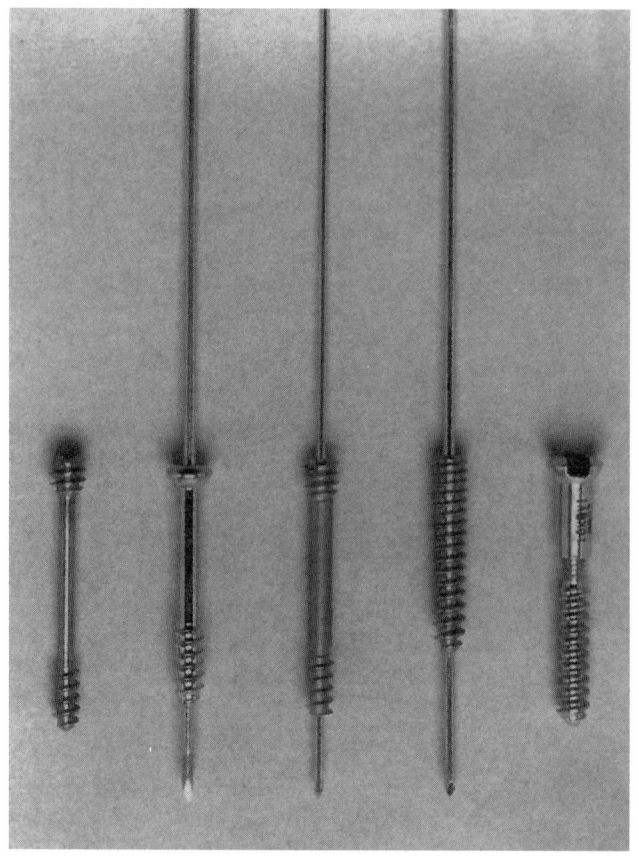

FIGURE 1.—Photograph of the fixation devices for the scaphoid used in the present study: *from left,* Herbert screw, AO 3.5-millimeter cannulated screw, Herbert-Whipple screw, Acutrak cannulated screw, and Universal Compression screw. (Courtesy of Toby EB, Butler TE, McCormack TJ, et al: A comparison of fixation screws for the scaphoid during application of cyclical bending loads. *J Bone Joint Surg Am* 79-A:1190–1197, 1997.)

scaphoids from which a piece of volar segment had been removed, in addition to osteotomy.

Results.—Resistance to cyclical bending loads was greater with the AO, Acutrak, and Herbert-Whipple screws than with the Herbert screw. The Universal Compression screw was associated with a tendency for fractures to occur at the time of insertion. In the additional experiment, removal of a portion of the volar cortex greatly reduced the fixation provided by both the AO and Herbert screws.

Conclusions.—The various screws available for fixation of scaphoid fractures vary considerably in their resistance to cyclical bending loads. Fixation appears to be superior with the Herbert-Whipple screw than with the standard Herbert screw, mainly because of the larger size of the former screw. The same factor may make it more difficult to place the Herbert-

Whipple screw. This is among the many factors that should be considered when selecting a fixation device for scaphoid fracture or nonunion.

▶ This is a clinically useful and well-designed follow-up study to the original performed by Shaw.[1] Cyclical bending was performed on cadaveric scaphoids. This model was chosen, rather than load to failure, to imitate the effect of repetitive use, an important consideration for a fracture prone to nonunion. This study underscores the previous compressive tests,[1] that screws with a wider diameter provide better fixation, even with the new, biomechanically weaker, cannulated screws. The variables of pitch and thread are important as well. This study reminds us to use the strongest device to get the job done, within the technical limits of an often difficult fracture.

A.L. Ladd, M.D.

Reference

1. Shaw JA: A biomechanical comparison of scaphoid screws. *J Hand Surg [Am]* 12A:347–353, 1987.

Suggested Reading

Kobayashi M, Berger RA, Nagy L, et al: Normal kinematics of carpal bones: A three-dimensional analysis of carpal bone motion relative to the radius. *J Biomech* 30:787–793, 1997.
▶ The authors describe an elegant study in which they try to describe the 3-dimensional kinematics of carpal bones relative to the radius. To date, their study includes the largest number of specimens reported in the literature. The authors are truly to be commended on this excellent piece of work, and there is much information that can be gathered from the data listed in this paper.

It is interesting and, I believe, important to note that in the authors' discussion, they acknowledge a number of reports in the literature trying to detail kinematics of the wrist with findings that differ from one to another. I believe this is a reflection of the type of motion and methods used to try to measure kinematics of the carpal bones, as well as the anatomy and variability of physiologic laxity from one specimen to another. Previous studies we have carried out have, in fact, found a quantifiable difference between carpal bone motion resulting from passive movement of the wrist, static analysis in comparison of different postures of wrist position, and dynamic motion analysis. The experimental model that was used in this study transfixed the radius and ulna with a pin and constrained the wrist to planar motion, as directed by a Steinmann pin placed in the third metacarpal, and analyzed the position of the carpal bones in different wrist positions. The actual difference in the measured motion that this would result in, compared with unconstrained dynamic kinematics, is not fully known. However, the wrist and digital flexor and extensor tendons are believed to stabilize the carpal bones and may contribute to the dynamic kinematics of the carpal bones. In addition, translational motion has been shown to be a real component of carpal bone motion but cannot be measured when simply analyzing different static positions of the wrist.

In our studies, we have found that in flexion, the radiolunate joint contributes more in extremes of flexion to overall wrist motion than the lunocapitate joint.

However, in extension—particularly the extremes of extension—the lunocapitate joint contributes more for overall wrist motion than the radiolunate joint. The authors in this study found a more equal sharing of the contribution to overall wrist motion between the radiocarpal and midcarpal joints.

I believe it is helpful and important to consider the experimental techniques that are used in measuring carpal bone motion so that we may better understand and compare the different reports in the literature. Since the literature reports what has actually been measured, it is not a question of what is right or wrong, but more a measurement of how the particular anatomy responds to a particular combination of forces. All of the data are pieces of a puzzle that, when placed together, should offer us a better picture of the kinematics of the carpal bones.

S.F. Viegas, M.D.

Kobayashi M, Garcia-Elias M, Nagy L, et al: Axial loading induces rotation of the proximal carpal row bone around unique screw-displacement axes. *J Biomech* 30:1165–1167, 1997.
▶ This study evaluated the displacement of the normal carpus under load in a cadaver model. Under compressive loading, all 3 proximal row bones moved in the general directions of flexion, radial deviation, and supination, although each had its own axis of displacement/rotation. The authors concluded that, in the normal carpus, the oblique alignment of the scaphoid predominates, and it induces the flexion/radial deviation/supination movement of the lunate and triquetrum.

P.C. Amadio, M.D.

Sie TH, Abdel-Kader KFM, Allcock S: A useful technique for removal of Herbert screws from the scaphoid. *J Hand Surg [Br]* 23B:332–333, 1998.
▶ A 3.5-mm drill guide just fits over the head of a Herbert screw. These authors describe the use of the serrated end of the guide as a trephine to expose the buried head of a Herbert screw. A nice trick!

P.C. Amadio, M.D.

Wulff RN, Schmidt TL: Carpal fractures in children. *J Pediatr Orthop* 18:462–465, 1998.
▶ This report confirms the rarity of carpal fractures in children, especially in those under the age of 12.

P.C. Amadio, M.D.

Yuceturk A, Isiklar ZU, Tuncay C, et al: Treatment of scaphoid nonunions with vascularized bone graft. *J Hand Surg [Br]* 22B:425–427, 1997.
▶ This is a small but interesting study of 4 patients with chronic nonunion of the scaphoid who are treated with vascularized bone graft from the first metacarpal. In view of the paper published by Zaidemberg et al.[1] using the distal radius as a vascularized bone graft site for the same problem, this seems a more technically demanding and possibly riskier technique that may be considered as a secondary option.

L.K. Ruby, M.D.

Reference

1. Zaidemberg C, Siebert JW, Angrigiani C: A new vascularized bone graft for scaphoid nonunion. *J Hand Surg [Am]* 16:474–478, 1991.

Distal Radius

Evaluation of Simplified Frykman and AO Classifications of Fractures of the Distal Radius: Assessment of Interobserver and Intraobserver Agreement
Illarramendi A, González Della Valle A, Segal E, et al (Italian Hosp, Buenos Aires, Argentina)
Int Orthop 22:111–115, 1998   8-23

Background.—Many classification systems have been used for distal fractures of the radius, preventing meaningful comparisons of treatments and outcomes from different studies. The interobserver and intraobserver agreement of the Frykman and AO classifications and their variations among evaluators with different levels of experience were determined.

Methods.—Three hand specialists, a fellow and 2 senior residents, were asked to classify the radiographs of 200 fractures of the distal radius in anteroposterior and lateral views. Reproducibility was determined using the proportion of agreement and kappa coefficient between observer pairs.

Findings.—For the Frykman classification system, interobserver reproducibility was moderate, with a kappa value of 0.43, and intraobserver reproducibility was good, with a kappa of 0.61. For the AO system, the kappa values were 0.37 and 0.57 for interobserver and intraobserver reproducibility, respectively. Intraobserver agreement was higher for the residents than for the fellow. Evaluator experience did not significantly influence either variable.

Conclusions.—The interobserver and intraobserver reproducibilies of both the Frykman and AO classification systems for distal fractures of the radius are questionable. Thus, neither system is recommended for clinical use.

▶ This article once again suggests that our ability to classify distal radius fractures is limited not only by the internal logic or theoretical completeness of the various classification schemes, but also by the reliability of the classification process itself. The reader should note that the authors here did not use the AO classification as recommended by the AO group, but instead used a 5-type modification of it suggested by Saffar. This may explain the difference in results between this study, which found little reliability of the AO classification, and that of Kreder et al.,[1] which did find that the A,B,C, 1,2,3 3-part, 2-level classification was reasonably reliable. The fact that Saffar's modification was not shown to be reproducible among examiners may be more a criticism of that particular grouping and not of the AO system itself.

As for the Frykman classification, as it appears here to be poorly reproducible, and because it has never been shown to have any prognostic import, perhaps it is time to consider whether we should continue to use it. At least in the United States, it remains extremely popular; the data would suggest inappropriately so.

P.C. Amadio, M.D.

Reference

1. Kreder H, Hanel D, McKee M, et al: Consistency of AO fracture classification for the distal radius. *J Bone Joint Surg Br* 78:726–731, 1996.

AO and Frykman's Classifications of Colles' Fracture: No Prognostic Value in 652 Patients Evaluated After 5 Years

Flinkkilä T, Raatikainen T, Hämäläinen M (Oulu Univ Hosp, Finland)
Acta Orthop Scand 69:77–81, 1998   8–24

Background.—Two common methods to classify fractures are the AO method and Frykman's method. However, whether these classification methods have any prognostic value is a matter of debate. These authors studied long-term outcomes after Colles' fracture to see if either classification method had significant prognostic value.

Methods.—During 6 years, 652 patients with Colles' fracture and a healthy contralateral arm were studied. About 80% of the patients were women and the mean patient age was 56 years. Each fracture was radiographed and films were assessed by 1 author. Each fracture was classified according to the AO system (only main groups A2, A3, C1, C2, and C3) and the Frykman class (classes 1 through 8). After a mean of 5 years of follow-up, patients were sent questionnaires to assess forearm and hand symptoms of pain (at rest, during exercise, after exercise), stiffness, restricted range of motion, finger numbness, reduced grip strength, and wrist deformity in both arms.

Findings.—At follow up, the arm with the fracture had significantly more symptoms than the contralateral arm. For example, 28% of cases reported no symptoms in the fractured arm, compared with a majority (81%) reporting no symptoms in the control arm. Similarly, severe or very severe symptoms were present in 6.4% of fractured arms but in only 0.5% of control arms. Almost half the patients (46%) had impaired function, and 8% of these patients had to modify their leisure activities or make special work arrangements. No associations with symptoms or impairment were seen for age, sex, duration of follow-up, side of the fracture, hand dominance, cause of injury, any associated injuries, the number of repositions, the type of treatment, or whether the patient had retired. Also, symptom severity scores did not differ significantly whether measured by the AO method or Frykman's classification.

Conclusions.—The system of classification (AO or Frykman's) had no predictive value for clinical outcome after Colles' fracture. Shortcomings of these methods to predict outcome may be that the AO classification does not factor in the degree of dislocation (which may indicate the severity of trauma) and that interobserver reliability and intraobserver reproducibility are poor.

▶ This paper looked at symptoms in patients with Colles' fracture at a minimum 2.5 years post fracture, and found no correlation of symptoms at follow-up with fracture classification by either the Frykman or AO methods, or by treatment method or age. At first blush, this finding may seem counterintuitive; shouldn't more comminuted fractures do worse? Don't the Frykman and AO methods assess comminution? Are these methods of no use? Sometimes, yes, and it depends.

Comminuted fractures will do worse only if they lead to poorer anatomic results, with articular incongruity, shortening and angulation. If these are treated, the results are not necessarily worse than those of less severe fracture types. Thus, it is the classification of final anatomy, not initial, which should be correlated with outcome.

The Frykman and AO methods do, indeed, measure comminution, although there is some evidence to suggest that the AO method does a better job of it. Again, these methods are helpful in guiding treatment; I would not expect them to predict results unless the fractures were left untreated.

As to whether fracture classification is of any use, I would reply yes, as a shortterm means of communication between treating orthopedists, and perhaps as a guide to treatment. To me, the main issues are displacement, especially articular displacement, angulation, shortening, comminution, and bone stock. These 5 factors need to be assessed and addressed in every case, tailoring of course to the patient's needs and functional status. When I am considering how to treat the fracture, none of the existing classification schemes serve me as well as an individual assessment of each of these 5 factors in each case. When I am concerned primarily with clustering anatomically similar fractures for purposes of discussion, I find that the AO method produces more biologically similar clusters than the Frykman method, and possesses more flexibility than any of the other commonly used schemes.

P.C. Amadio, M.D.

Wrist Arthrography After Acute Trauma to the Distal Radius: Diagnostic Accuracy, Technique, and Sources of Diagnostic Errors
Grechenig W, Peicha G, Fellinger M, et al (Karl Franzens Univ of Graz, Austria)
Invest Radiol 33:273–278, 1998

8–25

Background.—Injuries to the carpal region and triangular fibrocartilage complex (TFCC) accompanying fractures of the distal radius seem to markedly influence functional results. The diagnostic accuracy of wrist arthrography in detecting interosseous ligament and TFCC abnormalities in patients after acute injuries to the carpal region was assessed prospectively.

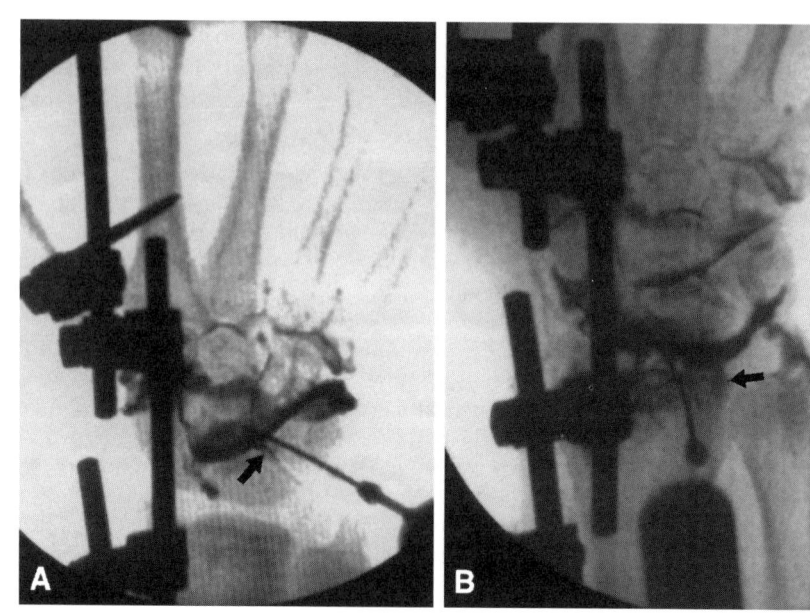

FIGURE 1.—Eighteen-year-old polytraumatized woman with an intra-articular fracture of the distal radius and initially far dislocation. After closed reduction and stabilization by an external fixator, a 2-compartment arthrography was performed. A, Injection of the midcarpal joint at the level of the lunate/hamate/triquetrum/capitate. There is a threadlike contrast fluid into the joint space between scaphoid and triquetrum (*arrow*) without penetration into the radiocarpal joint. This is the normal appearance of contrast medium filling in between the lunate and scaphoid representing the normal proximal attachment of the scapholunate ligament. B, Radiocarpal arthrography after injecting the joint between the third and fourth compartment of the tendon. There is no leakage of contrast dye into the scapholunate joint space or the distal radioulnar joint. Contrast material in the intra-articular fracture of the radius (*arrow*). (Courtesy of Grechenig W, Peicha G, Fellinger M, et al: Wrist arthrography after acute trauma to the distal radius: Diagnostic accuracy, technique, and sources of diagnostic errors. *Invest Radiol* 33:273–278, 1998.)

Methods.—Twenty-two patients with radial fractures after acute wrist trauma undergoing arthrography and arthroscopy of the wrist were included. Arthrography was done using standard techniques, by 2- to 3-compartment injection. Wrist arthroscopy was performed in the same session. Image analysis included the assessment of interosseous carpal ligaments, the TFCC, and osseous structures.

Findings.—Eleven injuries of the intrinsic ligaments and the TFCC were diagnosed by arthroscopy. Nine of these injuries were diagnosed correctly with arthrography preoperatively. A scaphoid fracture missed previously on conventional radiographs was also diagnosed by arthrography (Fig 1).

Conclusions.—Wrist arthrography is apparently a valuable tool in the diagnosis of acute wrist trauma. This technique seems to be very sensitive for detecting interosseous ligament disruptions and lesions in the TFCC, especially if the dual or triple compartment injection method is used.

▶ Ligament and TFCC lesions are easily overlooked and frequently not considered when interpreting radiographs in patients with wrist fractures. Subtle changes in the scapholunate distance or the distal radioulnar joint may be more obvious when traction is used for reduction or when evaluating fractures treated with external fixation frames.

Imaging of ligament and TFCC injuries can be accomplished with arthrography, ultrasound, or MRI. Ultrasound is suboptimal and MRI may be difficult to perform, particularly in the presence of fixation devices. This leaves arthrography as the most accurate and obvious choice. However, arthrography may be difficult to perform as well. The authors summarize certain pitfalls that may create errors in interpretation. Bottom line—arthrography should be reserved for patients with suggestive changes on radiographs and patients that would be surgically treated for their ligament or TFCC lesions. Delay in performing arthrograms could also be considered to avoid problems performing the technique associated with the acute injury.

T.H. Berquist, M.D.

Fracture of the Distal Forearm: Epidemiological Developments in the Period 1971–1995
Oskam J, Kingma J, Klasen HJ (Univ Hosp Groningen, The Netherlands)
Injury 29:353–355, 98
8–26

Background.—From 1960 to 1996 there were only 2 studies of the epidemiology of distal forearm fractures. One study, from Sweden, compared historical data from 1953 to 1957 and 1981 to 1982 and indicated a significant increase in the incidence of these fractures, particularly in people more than 60 years old. It also predicted the incidence to increase further. Another study from Norway assessed age and gender specific incidence rates for people aged more than 20 years. The current study evaluated the incidence rates of distal forearm fracture from 1971 through 1995 at a Dutch university hospital.

Methods.—The trauma registry for the largest trauma center in the northern region of the Netherlands was analyzed for cases of fracture of the distal forearm. The cause of the fracture was noted, as were patient demographics and admission information.

Findings.—During the 25 years reviewed, from a total of 256,431 trauma cases, there were 8,567 (3%) fractures of the distal forearm. From 1971 to 1981 the incidence rate across the entire population increased, but incidence rates gradually decreased after 1981. The age groups at greatest risk were people older than 79 years (90 fractures per 10,000 patients) and those aged 9 years or less (80 per 10,000 patients). Incidence rates remained stable for patients aged 20–49 years while rates for patients aged 50 to 79 years actually decreased. Before the age of 40, no difference in incidence rates between men and women were noted; after age 40, more women than men experienced fractures (odds ratios at least 1:4 for age groups more than 50 years). Across the lifespan, falls were responsible for more fractures (62%) than sports and leisure activities (19%) or traffic accidents (14%). However, accidental fall incidence rates decreased gradually from 1971 (32 per 10,000 patients) to 1995 (22 per 10,000 patients). Sport and leisure activities accounted for many injuries in patients aged 0–9 and 10–19 years. Hospitalization rates over the period doubled, from 6% in 1971 to 14% in 1995; most of these hospitalizations occurred in patients aged less than 50 years.

Conclusions.—This report is in agreement with a previous report that elderly people are at the greatest risk of distal forearm fracture. However, unlike the previous report, the current study indicates that incidence rates have decreased in recent years. Significant numbers of pediatric patients with distal forearm fracture were also seen. Thus the clinician must be aware of the special needs of geriatric and pediatric patients. A possible explanation for the greater number of hospital admissions is that beginning in the 1980s, displaced fractures in children were treated with the patient under general rather than local anesthesia. Furthermore, since the 1980s, there has been a push to ensure optimal anatomical results, and thus more patients have undergone surgery.

▶ This report from a trauma center presumably includes the vast majority of distal radius fractures from its catchment area, but as a comprehensive survey was not done, we cannot be sure. The data suggests, in contrast to an earlier study from Sweden, that the rate of distal radius fractures has slightly decreased over time, when one factors in the aging of the population that has occurred. The reason is mostly a lower accident rate. Previous studies, which had shown an increased rate over time, may have in retrospect simply recorded changes in detection rate, associated with the development of trauma registries in the late 1970s.

P.C. Amadio, M.D.

External Fixation Versus Percutaneous Pinning for Unstable Colles' Fracture: Equal Outcome in a Randomized Study of 60 Patients
Ludvigsen TC, Johansen S, Svenningsen S, et al (Aust-Agder Central Hosp, Arendal, Norway; Vest-Agder Central Hosp, Kristiansand, Norway)
Acta Orthop Scand 68:255–258, 1997   8–27

Background.—Although distal radius fracture is the most common type of fracture, classification, treatment, and correlation between radiographic and functional outcome have been controversial. The most common forms of treatment are K-wires and a plaster cast or external fixation. The radiographic and clinical outcomes of this type of fracture treated by external fixation or percutaneous pinning with K-wires were compared.

Methods.—There were 60 patients with Colles' fracture type Older 3 or 4 who were randomly assigned to external fixation or wire pinning. All patients were immobilized for 6 weeks in a plaster cast. Treatment was given within 5 days of injury and outcome was evaluated at 6 months. All patients were older than 20 years.

Results.—The treatment groups were similar in age, gender distribution, fracture type, and dislocation. Radiographic and functional outcomes were similar in both groups. All fractures healed. The complication rate was similar for both groups.

Discussion.—These results suggest that most unstable distal radial fractures can be successfully treated with percutaneous pinning and immobilization in a plaster cast. The authors recommend the use of 3 pins converging in both planes to prevent radial shortening, which is reported to be a potential problem. This percutaneous pinning technique is simpler and less expensive than external fixation.

▶ Sixty patients with more severe distal radial fractures were treated by either application of an external fixator, or percutaneous pinning. No open reductions or bone grafting was included. Both groups experienced ulnar shortening and dorsal collapse that did not differ statistically. This study points out that the most predictable results are derived from an algorithm that includes all facets of internal and external fixation, combined with appropriate bone grafting when indicated. As has been reported, the most reliable clinical outcome follows anatomical reduction and maintenance.

P.C. Dell, M.D.

Intraarticular Fractures of the Distal Radius Treated With Metaphyseal External Fixation
Krishnan J, Chipchase LS, Slavotinek J (Flinders Univ, Bedford Park, Australia)
J Hand Surg [Br] 23B:396–399, 1998
8-28

Objective.—There are many competing options for management of unstable intra-articular fractures of the distal radius. External fixation at the wrist, which immobilizes the wrist joint as well as the fractures, carries a risk of complications. Promising results of dynamic external fixation with the distal pins inserted into the fracture fragments, which avoids immobilization of the wrist, have been reported. The results of a new metaphyseal external fixation approach to intra-articular fractures of the distal radius are described.

Methods.—The experience included 22 patients with unstable Frykman grade 7 or 8 intra-articular fractures of the distal radius. There were 11 men and 11 women, mean age 50. All were treated with a new configuration using an AO interfragmentary external fixator, the "delta frame." The triangular frame did not extend across the joint, the distal pins were inserted into the distal radial fracture fragments, and thus the wrist and hand were not immobilized. A total of 4 2.5-mm self-tapping threaded pins were inserted into the distal radius in 2 horizontal planes. In addition, a 4-mm threaded pin was inserted into the proximal radial shaft.

Results.—The patients were studied for an average of 12 months. At follow-up, all patients had full functional ability and good range-of-motion. Scores indicated acceptable levels of function, pain, and range-of-motion within 4 weeks after removal of the external fixation device. Postoperative radiographs showed good maintenance of wrist position after reduction.

Conclusions.—External fixation using the delta frame provides good results in patients with unstable Frykman grade 7 or 8 intra-articular fractures of the distal radius. This technique achieved reliable maintenance of fracture fixation, and allowed early motion and exercise. Strength and range-of-motion were restored more quickly than possible with static external fixation.

▶ I agree that external fixation bridging the fracture alone is preferable to that bridging adjacent joints as well. The difficulty for me is finding fractures comminuted enough to require external fixation yet having solid enough distal fragments to hold fixator pins. When I find such fractures, I usually use some sort of interfragmentary or Kapandji-style pinning. Metaphyseal external fixation is clearly an alternative. It would have been nice if this article had included some radiographs, so the reader could see precisely what sort of fractures these authors select for this treatment option. Simply noting that the fractures were Frykman grade 7 or 8 provides little data, because the classification says nothing about comminution or displacement, and also because we have learned that the Frykman classification has relatively low interexaminer reliability.

P.C. Amadio, M.D.

Distal Radial Fractures: Kapandji's or Py's Pinning? [French]
Fikry T, Fadili M, Harfaoui A, et al (CHU Ibnou Rochd, Casablanca, Morocco)
Ann Chir Main 17:31–40, 1998   8–29

Background.—Distal radius fractures are typically treated by pinning. Numerous pinning techniques have been used, including the intrafocal pinning technique of Kapandji and the isoelastic pinning technique of Py. In this randomized, prospective study the efficacy of these 2 pinning methods in patients with distal radius fractures were compared.

Methods.—The subjects were 88 patients who had posterior displacement of a distal radius fracture. None had a comminuted fracture, radiocarpal subluxation, any associated carpal or same-limb lesions, or a major skin wound. Group 1 consisted of 42 patients (30 men and 12 women; mean age, 33 years) who underwent Kapandji's pinning technique, and group 2 consisted of 46 patients (38 men and 10 women, mean age, 35 years) who underwent Py's pinning technique. For the Kapandji procedure, 3 Kirschner wires (2 posterior and 1 external) were introduced into the fracture, advanced toward the top at a 45-degree angle, and fixed to the opposite side (Fig 1, B and C). For the Py procedure, 2 Kirschner wires

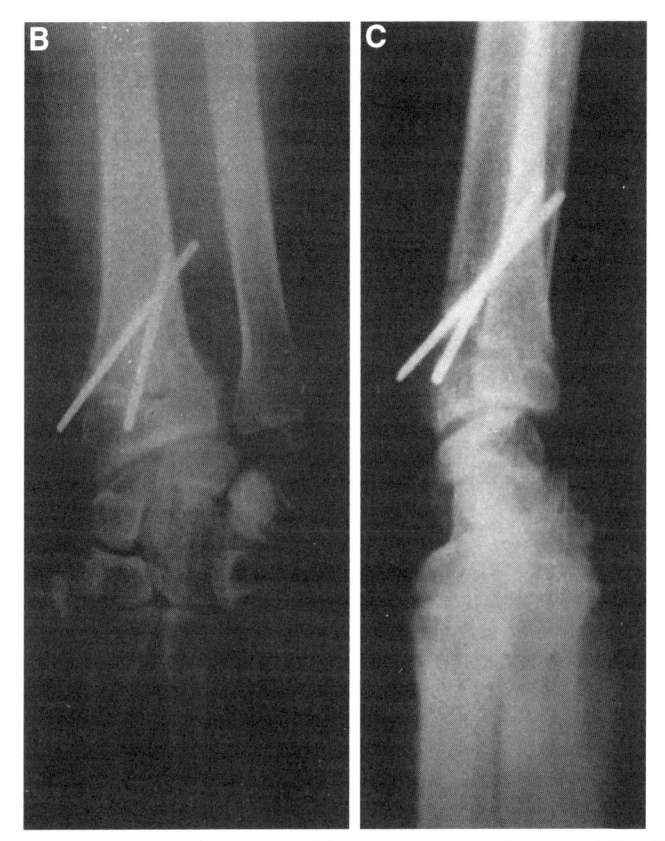

FIGURE 1, B and C.—Colle's fracture treated by Kapandji pinning. (Courtesy of Fikry T, Fadili M, Harfaoui A, et al: Distal radial fractures: Kapandji's or Py's pinning? [French] *Ann Chir Main* 17:31–40, 1998.)

(1 posterior and 1 external) were introduced into the radial epiphysis and pushed through the canal until reaching the level of the radial head. Careful wire placement and the use of fluoroscopy ensured good contact between the wire and the cortical bone (Fig 2, B). In all patients, the wires were cut at the skin and covered. The limb was immobilized for 4 weeks, and the wires were removed at 8 weeks. Mean follow-up was 27 months (range, 20–52 months).

Findings.—Seven patients (17%) in group 1 and 2 patients (4%) in group 2 had secondary displacement. By the fifth week, 6 patients (14%) in group 1 had displaced Kirschner wires; no patients in group 2 had this complication. There were 3 cases (7%) of superficial infection, all in group 1. There were 3 tendinous ruptures (7%) in group 1 and 1 (2%) in group 2. The scoring system of Jakim et al was used to rate the functional results. Patients in group 2 had significantly better global, objective, and radiologic scores than those in group 1.

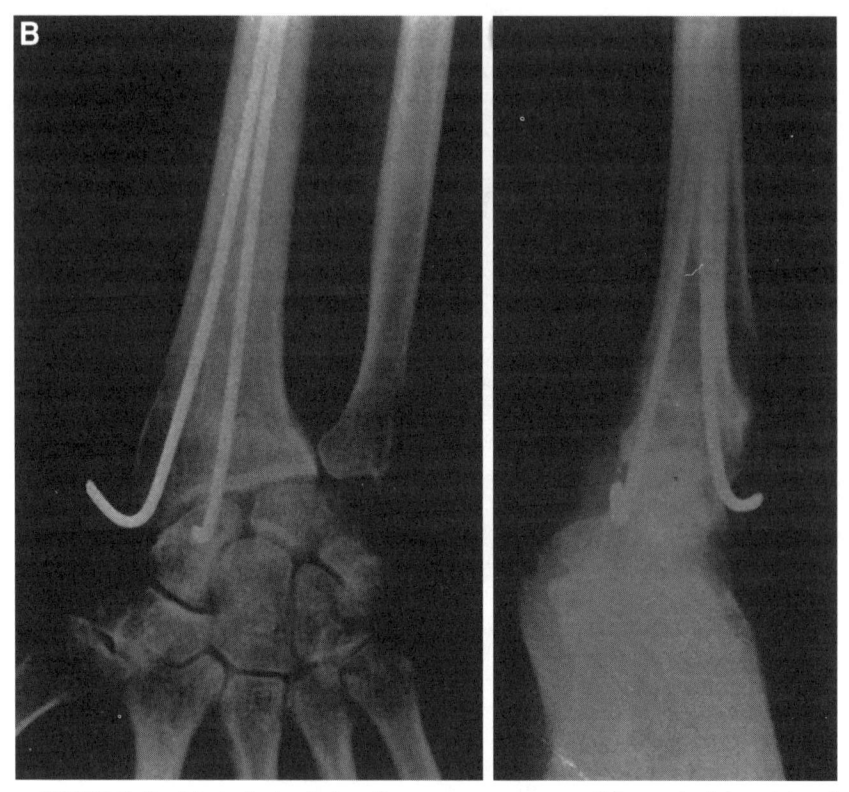

FIGURE 2, B.—Py's isoelastic pinning allows permanent anteromedial control of the epiphyseal fragment. Fluoroscopic control is optional. (Courtesy of Fikry T, Fadili M, Harfaoui A, et al: Distal radial fractures: Kapandji's or Py's pinning? [French] *Ann Chir Main* 17:31–40, 1998.)

Conclusions.—Py's pinning technique was superior to the technique of Kapandji in repairing distal metaphyseal fractures. Py's technique gave more stability because the isoelastic wires prevented posterior comminution. Furthermore, the wires can be inserted with or without fluoroscopy. Kapandji's technique might be more useful in cases in which focal comminution is absent, in teenagers with lower and unstable fractures, or in T fractures. Otherwise, Py's technique is preferred in the treatment of metaphyseal fractures with posterior displacement.

▶ Py pinning seems to be the winner in this contest, but both techniques seem to be most effective where they are needed least, that is, in minimally comminuted extraarticular fractures.

P.C. Amadio, M.D.

Displaced Intra-articular Fractures of the Distal Aspect of the Radius: Long-term Results in Young Adults After Open Reduction and Internal Fixation

Catalano LW III, Cole RJ, Gelberman RH, et al (Washington Univ, St Louis; Orthopaedic Clinic, Memphis, Tenn)

J Bone Joint Surg Am 79-A:1290–1302, 1997

8–30

Introduction.—Residual articular displacement of fractures of the distal aspect of the radius has been correlated to the prevalence of posttraumatic osteoarthrosis. Some experts have recommended that distal radial fracture fragments be reduced operatively to improve clinical outcomes after intra-articular fractures when articular incongruities exceed 1 or 2 mm. No long-term follow-up study has examined the relationship between the radiographic and functional outcomes after displaced intra-articular fractures of the distal aspect of the radius.

Methods.—There were 26 patients who had an acute displaced intra-articular fracture of the distal aspect of the radius, treated with operative reduction and stabilization, who were retrospectively reviewed to determine the long-term functional and radiographic outcomes. Follow-up included a physical examination, imaging with plain radiographs and computerized tomography, and completion of a validated musculoskeletal function assessment questionnaire at a minimum of 5.5 years.

Results.—On the plain radiographs and computerized tomograph scans of 16 (76%) of the 21 wrists, osteoarthrosis of the radiocarpal joint was evident at an average of 7.1 years. Residual displacement of articular fragments at the time of osseous union was strongly associated with the development of osteoarthrosis of the radiocarpal joint. The magnitude of the residual step and gap displacement at the time of fracture-healing did not correlate with the functional status as determined by physical examination and the responses to the questionnaire at the time of the most recent follow-up. Irrespective of radiographic evidence of osteoarthrosis of the radiocarpal or the distal radio-ulnar joint, or of non-union of the ulnar styloid process, all patients had a good or excellent functional outcome.

Conclusion.—Rather than radiographic evidence of osteoarthrosis of the radiocarpal joint, the presence of severe symptoms or a loss of function should be the indication for salvage operative procedures.

▶ This article reports functional and radiographic results after open reduction of intra-articular fractures of the distal radius. It confirms previous studies that have shown an inverse correlation of anatomic results with posttraumatic arthritis. The rate of arthritis here is highter, but this study uses tomography, whereas previous studies reported on plain radiographs. As in other articles reporting on many other wrist conditions, functional results were better than radiographic results. The authors should be commended for using a validated outcome questionnaire to assess functional results. However, the questionnaire chosen, the musculoskeletal functional assessment (MFA), is not specific for the upper limb, and the reported sensitivities and responsiveness suggest it may perform less well than other, more specific questionnaires like an upper extremity-specific questionnaire, or a wrist-specific instrument. Despite a significant wrist injury, half these patients received a perfect MFA score. This is an indication of a ceiling effect; the MFA is able to detect only fairly large differences in hand function, such as occur, for example, in advanced rheumatoid arthritis. Such an instrument may not be ideal to detect differences in outcome in patients with less severe impairments. Thus, the lack of correlation of function with anatomy in this study may be more a reflection of a lack of statistical power, resulting from both the small sample size of 26 and the relative insensitivity of the MFA, than of an actual lack of clinically significant correlation. Future studies in this area should address both the issue of statistical power (how many patients are needed to be 80% or 90% sure of detecting a clinically significant difference), and proper outcome instrument selection.

P.C. Amadio, M.D.

Arthroscopically-assisted Reduction of Intra-articular Fractures of the Distal Radius
Adolfsson L, Jörgsholm P (Univ Hosp, Linköping, Sweden; Univ Hosp, Odense, Denmark)
J Hand Surg [Br] 23B:391–395, 1998

Background.—In displaced intra-articular fractures of the distal radius, a residual incongruity as small as 2 mm between the surfaces can rapidly lead to the development of osteoarthritis. Thus anatomical reduction of the residual incongruity is required, typically by open reduction and internal fixation. However, with this method, the entire joint surface may not be visible. The efficacy of arthroscopy to perform reduction and percutaneous fixation in patients who had a displaced intraarticular fracture of the distal radius was assessed.

Methods.—During a 5-year period, 27 patients (16 men and 11 women; mean age, 44 years) who had displaced intra-articular distal radial fractures underwent reduction via arthroscopic guidance. All fractures had been previously treated at least once, but a step of more than 1 mm remained. The study excluded patients who had a fracture in osteoporotic bone, who required bone transplantation or fixation with screws or a plate, who had fractures in which closed reduction could not restore length, or who had an associated soft-tissue lesion requiring open repair. Under arthroscopic guidance, attempts were first made to reduce the displaced fracture fragments with percutaneous Kirschner wires. For fragments that could not be reduced from inside the joint, a skin incision was used to accomplish reduction. Percutaneously introduced Kirschner wires were used to stabilize the fragments in the reduced position in 26 patients. A fluoroscope was used to check the positioning of the wires and the alignment of the distal fragments with the long axis of the radius. For 4–6 weeks postoperatively, 22 patients received a dorsal plaster splint and 5 underwent external fixation. After about 8 weeks, patients resumed all activities. Follow-up ranged from 3 to 38 months (mean, 16 months).

Findings.—There was no measurable incongruence of the joint surface in any patient. Minor (5–10 degrees) dorsal angulation or compression occurred in 4 (14.8%) patients. Wrist function was evaluated by the Mayo Modified Wrist Score; results were excellent in 19 (70.3%) patients and good in 8 (29.6%). Sixteen patients (59%) had associated lesions. Only 3 (11.1%) patients experienced complications, consisting of superficial infections of the Kirschner wires in 2 patients and carpal tunnel syndrome in 1 patient who underwent reduction on the same day as the injury. Also, 5 (18.5%) patients had to undergo a second procedure to remove wires that had been cut too short and were left under the skin.

Conclusions.—Arthroscopically controlled restoration of joint congruity after intra-articular distal radius fractures is effective and safe. This method, however, is best reserved for situations in which closed reduction could restore the length and angulation.

▶ Arthroscopic-assisted reduction of intra-articular distal radius fractures has been getting increasing attention at meetings, and small numbers of cases have been reported,[1] but this is the first series to my knowledge to appear in print. The results are good in selected cases, and I agree with the indications noted by these authors: cases where length and overall alignment can be reduced by traction, where bone grafting is not needed, and where articular stepoff is significant. Several of my colleagues are pushing the envelope even further, using small incisions to add cancellous grafting in cases with significant subchondral comminution. This technique appears here to stay. Not only are the anatomical and long-term functional results good, but our results at Mayo Clinic suggest that the time to achieve these results can also be significantly reduced.[2]

P.C. Amadio, M.D.

References

1. Rettig M, Amadio PC: Wrist arthroscopy: Indications and clinical application. *J Hand Surg [Br]* 19B:774–777, 1994.
2. Berger RA, Stewart NJ, Bishop AT, et al: A retrospective analysis of matched cohorts of distal radius fractures treated by arthroscopic reduction versus open reduction. Presented at the International Federation of Societies for Surgery of the Hand, Vancouver, BC, May 25, 1998.

Intraarticular Lesions in Distal Fractures of the Radius in Young Adults: A Descriptive Arthroscopic Study in 50 Patients
Lindau T, Arner M, Hagberg L (Lund Univ, Sweden; Malmö Univ, Sweden)
J Hand Surg [Br] 22B:638–643, 1997   8–32

Objective.—Ligament injuries are found in the majority of distal fractures of the radius. The frequency and distribution of chondral and liga-

TABLE 5.—Isolated or Combined, Partial or Total Tears of the Major Intrinsic Ligaments and the Triangular Fibrocartilage Complex in Relation to Fracture

	Extraarticular fractures	Intraarticular fractures
Isolated tears (n = 18)		
TFCC	6	7
SL	1	3
LT	0	1
Combined injuries (n = 27)		
SL + TFCC	5	15
LT + TFCC	1	3
SL + LT	1	0
SL + LT + TFCC	1	1
Total	15	30

Abbreviations: SL, scapholunate ligament; LT, lunotriquetral ligament.
(Courtesy of Lindau T, Arner M, Hagberg L: Intraarticular lesions in distal fractures of the radius in young adults: A descriptive arthroscopic study in 50 patients. J Hand Surg [Br] 22B:638–643, 1997.)

ment injuries, the degree of instability in the interosseous ligaments, and correlations with specific fracture types in initial displaced distal fractures of the radius were investigated in young adults.

Methods.—Arthroscopy was performed 1–17 days after injury in 50 patients (24 men), aged 20–60 years, with displaced fractures. The radiocarpal, midcarpal, and radioulnar joints and the scapholunate ligament were examined. All patients had radiographic examinations.

Results.—There were 35 intra-articular and 15 extra-articular fractures. Arthroscopy showed 36 intra-articular fracture lines, 35 subchondral hematomas, 10 localized areas of osteoarthritis, and a scapholunate advanced collapse (wrist). There were 96 injuries to 37 palmar extrinsic or ulnocarpal ligaments. Triangular fibrocartilage complex tears arose most frequently, occurring in 39 patients (78%). Partial or complete tears in the scapholunate ligament occurred in 27 patients (54%). Only 1 patient had no ligament injury. No patient had major instability. Sixteen patients (32%) had chondral lesions. Triangular fibrocartilage complex (TFCC) injuries, including 39 tears, occurred in 41 patients. There were 13 Palmer classification type 1A tears, 17 type 1B, 5 type 1C, and 17 type 1D. Fracture of the ulnar styloid occurred in 24 patients with a TFCC tear and in 15 patients without a tear. The presence of a styloid fracture increased the risk of a TFCC tear (odds ratio, 5.1). There was no correlation between fracture type and ligament tear (Table 5). There were no arthroscopic complications.

Conclusion.—The frequency of chondral and ligamentous lesions may explain why many patients have a mediocre long-term outcome.

▶ With the advent of arthroscopically aided reduction of intra-articular fractures of the distal radius came the heightened awareness that many of these fractures had associated ligamentous and chondral injuries that were previ-

Reservation Card for the Year Book

Yes! I would like my own copy of *Year Book of Hand Surgery*® at the price of **$83.00** (**$92.00** outside the U.S.) plus sales tax, postage, and handling. Please begin my subscription with the current edition according to the terms described below.* I understand that I will have 30 days to examine each annual edition.

Name _____

Address _____

City _____ State _____ ZIP _____

Method of Payment

Check (in U.S. dollars, drawn on a U.S. bank, payable to *Year Book of Hand Surgery*®)

❏ VISA   ❏ MasterCard   ❏ Discover   ❏ AmEx   ❏ Bill me

Card number _____ Exp. date: _____

Signature _____

Prices are subject to change without notice.   PMC-348

Subscribe to the related journal in your field!

Yes! Begin my one-year subscription to *Journal of Shoulder and Elbow Surgery* (6 issues).

Name _____

Institution _____

Address _____

City _____ State _____

ZIP/PC _____ Country _____

Specialty _____
(Students/residents, please list Institution)

Subscription prices (through 9/30/99)

		USA	Canada*	Int'l
Individuals	❏	$116.00	$154.08	$144.00
Institutions	❏	143.00	182.97	171.00
Students, residents	❏	60.00	94.16	88.00

Method of payment

Enclose payment (check or credit card number) and we'll send an extra issue FREE!

❏ Check (in U.S. dollars, drawn on a U.S. bank, and payable to *Journal of Shoulder and Elbow Surgery*)

❏ VISA   ❏ MasterCard   ❏ Discover
❏ AmEx   ❏ Bill me   Exp. date_____

Card # _____

Signature _____

*Includes Canadian GST

Individual/student subscriptions must be in the name of, billed to, and paid for by the individual.

Canada/Int'l prices include airmail postage.
Prices subject to change without notice.

J032991YA

---

*Your Year Book service guarantee:

When you subscribe to the *Year Book*, you will receive advance notice of future annual volumes about two months before publication. To receive the new edition, you need do nothing—we'll send you the new volume as soon as it is available. If you want to discontinue, the advance notice allows you time to notify us of your decision. If you are not completely satisfied, you have 30 days to return any *Year Book*.

BUSINESS REPLY MAIL
FIRST-CLASS MAIL   PERMIT NO 135   ST LOUIS MO

POSTAGE WILL BE PAID BY ADDRESSEE

SUBSCRIPTION SERVICES
MOSBY, INC.
11830 WESTLINE INDUSTRIAL DRIVE
ST. LOUIS   MO 63146-9988

NO POSTAGE NECESSARY IF MAILED IN THE UNITED STATES

BUSINESS REPLY MAIL
FIRST-CLASS MAIL   PERMIT NO 135   ST LOUIS MO

POSTAGE WILL BE PAID BY ADDRESSEE

SUBSCRIPTION SERVICES
MOSBY, INC.
11830 WESTLINE INDUSTRIAL DRIVE
ST. LOUIS   MO 63146-9988

NO POSTAGE NECESSARY IF MAILED IN THE UNITED STATES

Want to speed up the process?

To order a *Year Book* or *Advances*, you also may call 1-800-426-4545

To subscribe to a journal today, call toll-free in the U.S.:
1-800-453-4351
or fax 314-432-1158
Outside the U.S., call: 314-453-4351

Visit us at: *www.mosby.com/periodicals*

Mosby, Inc.
Subscription Services
11830 Westline Industrial Drive
St. Louis, MO   63146   U.S.A.

M Mosby

ously unappreciated or underappreciated. This study confirms the findings of other authors: These lesions are common. What this study also says is that, even though some degree of ligament tear or chondral injury is common—e.g., 78% of TFCC tears and 54% of scapholunate ligament injuries—*complete* disruption of these ligaments, especially destabilizing injuries, is *not* common.

The authors hypothesize that the high percentage of cases with a ligament injury might help explain why many patients have mediocre long-term results, because of gradual attenuation of ligaments resulting in late destabilization. The authors do not provide definitive treatment recommendations, other than that surgeons should be cognizant of the high probability of a lesion in a patient with an intra-articular fracture.

One can argue, as the authors do, that the pros and cons of open reduction with internal fixation, open reduction and external fixation, different treatment methods of intra-articular fractures (arthroscopic reduction, external fixation, pinning, etc.), given the information learned from this study, are now even more uncertain than they were! This paper is chock full of data, including an excellent bibliography, which could be of value to anyone who wants to learn more about the complexities of this injury.

L.B. Lane, M.D.

A Comparison of 3 and 5 Weeks Immobilization for Older Type 1 and 2 Colles' Fractures
Vang Hansen F, Staunstrup H, Mikkelsen S (Silkeborg Centralsygehus, Denmark)
J Hand Surg [Br] 23B:400–401, 1998   8–33

Background.—Colles' fracture, one of the most common fractures, is usually treated by immobilization for 2–6 weeks, depending on the degree of displacement. Outcomes associated with 3 and with 5 weeks of immobilization were compared in the treatment of Older type 1 and type 2 Colles' fractures.

Methods and Findings.—One hundred patients were included in the prospective study. By random assignment, patients were treated with either 3 or 5 weeks of immobilization. All patients were immobilized with a below-elbow plaster splint. Seventy-three patients with 74 fractures were available for the 1-year follow-up. Assessment included measurements of dorsal angulation, radial length, wrist motion, grip strength, and pain. These parameters did not differ significantly between groups.

Conclusions.—Three weeks of immobilization is satisfactory in the treatment of type 1 or 2 Colles' fractures. A longer period of immobilization is inconvenient for the patient and unnecessary. Functional and anatomic results are equally good after 3 and after 5 weeks of immobilization.

▶ These authors contend that undisplaced Colles' fractures, and those with angulation but no comminution or shortening, can be successfully treated with only 3 weeks of immobilization. The final results show about 5 degrees of dorsal tilt on average, no shortening, and a 10% difference in strength (reported not to be statistically significant). Although these results appear to speak for themselves, I would like to see more functional data on these patients. Grip strength and motion are responsive measures of outcome after Colles' fracture, but may not be the most sensitive ones.[1] The end results may not be as similar as they seem. More to the point, despite these authors' contention that patients "did not seem to have more pain" after 3 weeks of immobilization than they did after 5 weeks, in my own practice I have found that many patients still have significant discomfort at 3 weeks. I believe that with undisplaced or minimally angulated, noncomminuted fractures, immobilization should continue until the fracture site is no longer tender.

P.C. Amadio, M.D.

Reference

1. Amadio PC, Silverstein MD, Ilstrup DM, et al: Outcome after Colles fracture: The relative responsiveness of three questionnaires and physical examination measures. *J Hand Surg [Am]* 21:781–787, 1996.

Corrective Osteotomies After Injuries of the Distal Radial Physis in Children
Hove LM, Engesæter LB (Haukeland Univ Hosp, Bergen, Norway)
J Hand Surg [Br] 22B:699–704, 1997
8–34

Background.—About 2% of all childhood fractures are physeal fractures of the distal radius. Growth disturbance is an uncommon complication but can cause reduced, painful wrist motion, loss of grip strength, and permanent disability. An experience with corrective osteotomy in 1 group of children is reported.

Methods and Findings.—Six children, aged 7–15 years, underwent corrective osteotomy of the distal forearm because of growth disturbance from posttraumatic closure of the distal radial physis. In 3 children, lengthening osteotomy of the radius was performed with grafts from the iliac crest. Osteotomies healed in a satisfactory position in all patients. Three had moderate malangulation of the radius and required ulnar shortening. The median postoperative palmar angulation of the distal radius was 4 degrees; the radial inclination, 22 degrees; and the ulnar variance, −2 mm. All children had complete pain relief after surgery. Total range of motion was 96% of the contralateral side.

Conclusions.—In children with growth disturbance from posttraumatic closure of the distal radial physis, some form of radial lengthening is recommended. The osteotomy must be wedged open to permit correction in 3 dimensions and realignment of both the distal radioulnar and radiocarpal joints. In young patients, intervention in childhood before the deformity becomes too severe is indicated.

▶ The title of this paper suggests that all 6 patients in this series developed distal radial deformities because of a posttraumatic growth disturbance, rather than by a malunion. Partial or complete premature physeal arrest is a relatively infrequent complication of distal radial physeal fractures. Less than 5% of such fractures go on to a premature physeal arrest. The potential for such a deformity to develop, however, mandates that such fractures be followed-up for a minimum of 6–12 months. In younger children (less than 13 years in girls and 14 in boys), my initial approach is to assess the size and extent of the premature physeal arrest and to excise it if possible. This is often preferable to repeated osteotomies. Distal radial osteotomies, as indicated in this paper, are reserved for patients with failed physeal bar excisions, successful excisions with residual deformity, or patients near skeletal maturity (girls more than 13, boys more than 14 years of age). In such circumstances, I agree with the treatment proposed by the authors. Epiphysiodesis of the ulna can be performed either through the same dorsal incision used for the radial osteotomy or through a small percutaneous incision over the dorsal ulnar physis. Like the authors, I find that distal radial osteotomies are preferable to techniques of external distraction lengthening.

W.J. Shaughnessy, M.D.

Long-term Results of Radioscapholunate Fusion Following Fractures of the Distal Radius
Nagy L, Büchler U (Univ of Bern, Switzerland)
J Hand Surg [Br] 22B:705–710, 1997   8–35

Introduction.—The role and indications for limited wrist arthrodesis are controversial and validation requires long-term studies that include late complications, document outcomes, and assess survivorship. A group of patients who had partial radioscapholunate wrist fusion were examined to determine the long-term results.

Methods.—There were 15 patients with radioscapholunate fusion for traumatic lesions of the radiocarpal junction who were studied for 8 years. Wrist fusion was performed on 5 patients because they had non-union or early progressive arthritis.

Results.—Eight of the 10 wrists with retained mobility continued to function satisfactorily. Pain was reported in 2 wrists for reasons other than secondary midcarpal arthritis. Patient satisfaction was comparable in the 2 groups, with the wrist score being better for wrists with residual motion. The number of preceding operations and the range of motion before partial fusion corresponded inversely with the survival of radioscapholunate partial wrist fusion. There was toleration of secondary midcarpal arthritis, if present, because it arose early. Technical mistakes and complications were strongly linked to failures.

Conclusion.—With functioning radioscapholunate fusion procedures, good results which proved durable over an 8-year period, were achieved in

7 of 15 patients. The currently unacceptable complication rates must be lowered drastically, however, before this procedure can be considered a reliable option. Patient selection and the techniques of fusion must also be improved upon. Better candidates for this procedure may be patients with fewer than 2 operations before radioscapholunate fusion, and patients with preoperative stiffness of the wrist. A better fixation device may address the high non-union rate.

▶ In the patient with a severe intra-articular fracture of the distal radius, who develops radiocarpal arthrosis and pain, radioscapholunate fusion may be a good alternative to total wrist fusion or wrist arthroplasty procedures. Büchler initially reported good results with this procedure, with a mean follow-up time of almost 2 years, in 1991. This article presents an 8-year follow-up study of these patients. Of 15 patients reviewed, 5 (33%) had undergone wrist fusion because of non-union or early arthrosis leading to pain. Of the 10 wrists not undergoing fusion, 8 were functioning well, with 2 out of 10 causing complaints of pain in the wrist. The authors discussed the significance of 4 non-unions secondary to radioscaphoid fusion not healing. These patients had associated painful instability in all instances. Salvage procedures were clinically unsuccessful.

Ultimately, good results were achieved in 7 out of the 15 cases at 8 years. These results were durable over this period in the face of heavy work. In this series, there was a very high complication rate, which the authors felt was secondary to technical problems.

E. Akelman, M.D.

The Different Types of Algodystrophy After Fracture of the Distal Radius: Predictive Criteria of Outcome After 1 Year
Laulan J, Bismuth J-P, Sicre G, et al (Centre Hospitalier Universitaire Trousseau, Tours, France)
J Hand Surg [Br] 22B:441–447, 1997   8–36

Introduction.—Algodystrophy (AD) is characterized by sensory, autonomic, and motor symptoms, and many authors consider the sympathetic nervous system to be involved in the induction and maintenance of the syndrome. The incidence of AD after fracture of the distal radius (FDR), although low (between 0.2% and 2.1%) in retrospective studies, has ranged from 25% to 37% in prospective clinical or radiographic studies performed at about 8 weeks. A prospective study was designed to identify early diagnostic and prognostic criteria for AD after FDR.

Methods.—During a 7-month period, all patients with FDR treated surgically were enrolled in the study. The 125 cases were evaluated using a clinical and radiographic score for AD at 1, 6, and 12 weeks. Twenty-two patients were lost to follow-up, leaving 103 FDRs for 1-year assessment. Parameters studied in clinical evaluation were diffuse spontaneous pain, abnormal pain elicited on examination, vasomotor and sudomotor

TABLE 3.—Performance of Clinical Scores in Predicting Active Algodystrophy With Sequelae at 1 Year

	Clinical scores > 7		
	1 week	6 weeks	12 weeks
Sensitivity	0.54	0.86	1
Specificity	0.81	0.93	0.94
PPV	0.30	0.75	0.74
NPV	0.92	0.96	1

Abbreviations: PPV, positive predictive value; NPV, negative predictive value.
(Courtesy of Laulan J, Bismuth J-P, Sicre G, et al: The different types of algodystrophy after fracture of the distal radius: Predictive criteria of outcome after 1 year. J Hand Surg [Br] 22B:441–447, 1997.)

dysfunction, trophic skin changes, and decreased range of motion of the finger joints. Radiographs were studied for generalized loss of density, patchy radiotranslucencies, subchondral radiotranslucencies, and loss of trabecular definition.

Results.—The patient group had a mean age of 54.8 years; 66% were women; 55% were retired or had sedentary occupations. Most FDRs were mixed fractures involving the metaphysis and epiphysis. Fractures were treated with K-wires in 55% of cases, external fixation in 33%, and osteosynthesis in 12%. Mobility at 1 year was rated as good in 39% of cases, moderate in 38%, and poor in 23%. Grip strengths for these rating categories were 64%, 23%, and 13%, respectively; radiographic results were 33%, 37%, and 30%, respectively. Four groups were distinguished at 1 year: definite AD with sequelae (active AD), definite AD without sequelae (transient AD), borderline AD, and absent AD. Patient satisfaction at 1 year was closely related to these categories. A clinical score greater than 7 at 6 weeks predicted 96% of active AD cases (Table 3). The presence of distal radioulnar joint pain was correlated with development of active AD, and active AD was more common in patients with a severe initial injury.

Conclusion.—The overall incidence of AD in these patients with FDRs was 26%; more than half of those affected (58%) had active AD with sequelae at 1 year. Treatment with calcitonin, started at 7.8 weeks, did not prevent sequelae.

▶ Although complex regional pain syndrome (CRPS) type 1—classic reflex sympathetic dystrophy or AD—remains a clinical diagnosis, specific pathophysiologic responses are demonstrable after distal radial fractures. The introduction of a semiquantitative scoring system for clinical and roentgenographic findings is a useful concept that would be strengthened by a patient-reported quality-of-life instrument.[1] The high incidence of CRPS in this series and the reports of Bickerstaff and Kanis[2] are of concern and a higher incidence than comparable published series regarding patients treated in the United States. When managing fractures of the distal radius, a high incidence of suspicion for CRPS is desirable, and early intervention in the presence of a dystrophic response or early CRPS is indicated. Either acute or delayed compression neuropathy of the median nerve and/or irritation of the superficial radial nerve may exacerbate or produce dystrophic symptoms or serve as a nociceptive focus using CRPS.

L.A. Koman, M.D.

References

1. Levine DW, Simmons BP, Koris MJ et al: A self-administered questionnaire for the assessment of severity of symptoms and functional status in carpal tunnel syndrome. *J Bone Joint Surg Am* 75A:1585–1592, 1993.
2. Bickerstaff DR, Kanis J: The natural history of post-traumatic algodystrophy. *J Bone Joint Surg Br* 73B(suppl II): 167, 1991.

Physiotherapy: An Overestimated Factor in After-Treatment of Fractures in the Distal Radius?
Oskarsson GV, Hjall A, Aaser P (Rikshopitalet, Oslo, Norway)
Arch Orthop Trauma Surg 116:373–375, 1997   8–37

Background.—After the standard 4–6 weeks of immobilization in a cast for Colles' fracture, systematic training is necessary for the patient to regain adequate wrist function. The benefit of supervised training compared with self-training is unclear. A few recent studies on this issue have reached inconsistent conclusions. The intention of this study was to emphasize the good functional outcome that can be achieved by self-training guided by careful instructions given by the surgeon, not to discredit the work done by physiotherapists.

Methods.—The effects of supervised training and self-training were compared in 110 patients treated for Colles' fracture. The mean patient age was 58 years. Supervised training by physiotherapists and self-training began 4–6 weeks after cast removal. Evaluations were performed at 10 and 35 weeks. The nondominant arm was estimated to be 15% weaker than the dominant arm.

Results.—The patients' self-assessed pain scores at 10 weeks were 6.0 for those who had supervised training and 4.6 for those who were self-trained. Of patients who had supervised training, 93% reported that the training was effective. No functional advantages were seen in patients who had supervised training, compared with self-trained patients.

Discussion.—Self-training guided by careful instructions by the surgeon can be as effective as training supervised by a physiotherapist for achieving good functional outcome after Colles' fracture. After typical distal radius fracture, only patients with severe stiffness and patients who cannot or will not undertake a self-training program should be referred for physiotherapy.

▶ A good point from this study is its suggestion that self-training can be as effective as physiotherapy in appropriate patients. Patients with severe stiffness and those who cannot perform a self-training program should be referred to a physiotherapist. Clinical judgement comes first.

P.B.J. Wu, M.D., M.P.H.

SUGGESTED READING

Nakamura R, Horii E, Imaeda T, et al: Ulnar styloid malunion with dislocation of the distal radioulnar joint. *J Hand Surg [Br]* 23B:173–175. 1998.
▶ The authors believe that a palmarly displaced and malunited ulnar styloid fracture might maintain the distal radioulnar joint dorsally displaced, with consequently restricted forearm rotation. Corrective osteotomy is helpful and perhaps necessary in such cases to allow reduction of the distal radioulnar joint. Ulnar shortening may be necessary as well, since relocation of the dorsally displaced ulnar may lead to ulnar impaction syndrome if the radius has shortened as a consequence of fracture.

V.R. Hentz, M.D.

Oskarsson GV, Aaser P, Hjall A: Do we underestimate the predictive value of the ulnar styloid affection in Colles fractures? *Arch Orthop Trauma Surg* 116:341–344, 1997.
▶ The importance of the ulnar styloid in distal radius fractures is often considered, yet the styloid itself is rarely treated. This study suggests the intuitively obvious, that the presence of an ulnar styloid fracture indicated a more severe injury to the carpus and soft tissues, and thus adversely affects outcome. The limitations of the study are many: (1) the use of a heterogenous group of "Colles' fractures" age 25–75 years, (2) the use of an arbitrary collection of radiographic variables, and (3) the comparison with classification systems, such as the Frykman and Older systems, that are useful for literature references but poor predictors of success. They are on the right track, however, and long-term prospective studies comparing similar types of fractures may provide further information.

A.L. Ladd, M.D.

Distal Radioulnar Joint

Triangular Fibrocartilage Complex Lesion in Distal Forearm Fractures of Children: Arthrographic Study [French]
De Gauzy JS, Kany J, Razafimbahoaka F, et al (CHU Purpan, Toulouse, France)
La Main 3:9–16, 1998   8–38

Introduction.—Distal forearm fractures are frequent in children. Arthrographic studies in adults with such fractures have revealed that they are frequently associated with triangular fibrocartilage complex (TFCC) tears. The goal of this study is to explore whether TFCC tears also occur in children with distal forearm fractures.

Material.—A prospective study was carried out from 1992 to 1994 in all children with displaced forearm fractures requiring reduction under general anesthesia. None had previous history of trauma to the same forearm.

Method.—Before reduction of the fracture, an arthrography of the radiocarpal joint was performed with an injection of 1–2 mm of contrast fluid under an image intensifier. Frontal and lateral views of the wrist were carried out immediately after the injection.

Results.—Ninety children, aged 4–15 years (mean, 10 years 2 months) were studied. There were 66 males and 24 females. Arthrographies showed a leakage of the contrast fluid to the distal radioulnar joint in 16 cases (18%). The tear was located centrally on the TFCC in 12 and on its ulnar border in 4. There was no significant correlation between the type of fracture and the presence of a tear, except in the 2 Galeazzi's fractures of the series, both had a tear. No specific treatment was adopted for the TFCC tears. Fourteen children underwent reduction and cast immobilisation, and 2 had an internal fixation because of an unstable reduction. Nine of these children were reviewed after 6 months. Eight had a normal wrist, and one had a palpable click during prosupination related to a non-union of the ulnar styloïd. A control MRI was performed in 4 children, with a normal aspect of the TFCC in 2, a heterogenous aspect of the tear site in one, and persistance of a tear in one.

Discussion.—TFCC lesions after a displaced distal forearm fracture seem to be as frequent in children as they are in adults. No study was performed in undisplaced fractures; therefore, the global incidence of those tears in distal forearm fractures remains unknown. These lesions were asymptomatic at 6 months and awareness of their existence has not modified the authors' choice of treatment.

▶ There does not seem to be any previous study of these TFCC tears in children and this work is very useful in this matter.

The first question which arises is that of the possible existence of congenital tears of the TFCC. The many works of Mikic,[1-5] including 38 fetal dissections, have failed to reveal any case of congenital perforations, but two reports by Weigl[6] and more recently by Tan[7] conclude to their existence. In Tan's study all congenital perforations (27/120 wrists) were located at the junction of the radial and middle third of the TFCC. It is noteworthy that of the 16 tears reported by the authors, 12 were located centrally.

The second question deals with the mechanism of these tears. This question is difficult to understand because tears have been found in all types of displaced distal forearm fractures, whether isolated radius or combined radius and ulna, with no significant correlation and regardless of the site of the fracture (metaphyseal, physeal or styloid). Their presence in Galeazzi's fractures (2 cases) and in isolated radial fractures (4/14) may seem logical, but they are more difficult to understand in distal fractures (7/48) or epiphyseal separation (1/3) of both bones, or any combination of fracture of one bone and epiphyseal separation of the other.

C. LeClercq, M.D.

References

1. Mikic Z, Sad N: Arthography of the wrist joint: An experimental study. *J Bone Joint Surg Am* 66:371–378, 1984.
2. Mikic Z: Age changes in the triangular fibrocartilage of the wrist joint. *J Anat* 126:367–384, 1978.
3. Mikic Z: Detailed anatomy of the articular disc of the distal radio ulnar joint. *Clin Orthop* 245:123–132, 1989.
4. Mikic Z, Somer L, Somer T: Histologic structure of the articular disk of the human distal radioulnar joint. *Clin Orthop* 275:29–36, 1992.
5. Mikic Z: The blood supply of the human distal radio ulnar joint and the microvasculature of its articular disk. *Clin Orthop* 275:19–28, 1992.
6. Weigl K, Spira E: The triangular fibrocartilage of the wrist joint. *Reconstr Surg Traumatol* 11:139–153, 1969.
7. Tan ABH, Tan SK, Yung SW, et al: Congenital perforations of the triangular fibrocartilage of the wrist. *J Hand Surg [Br]* 20:342–345, 1995.

The Utility of High-Resolution Magnetic Resonance Imaging in the Evaluation of the Triangular Fibrocartilage Complex of the Wrist
Potter HG, Asnis-Ernberg L, Weiland AJ, et al (Hosp for Special Surgery, New York)
J Bone Joint Surg Am 79-A:1675–1684, 1997   8–39

Introduction.—Tears of the triangular fibrocartilage complex of the wrist may not be readily apparent on physical examination because many other lesions may produce pain on the ulnar side. Arthrograms of the wrist have been used to detect these tears, but their ability to localize the tear and provide information about adjacent soft-tissue structures may be limited. The value of high-resolution MRI in the detection and localization of tears of the triangular fibrocartilage complex was prospectively studied.

Methods.—Seventy-seven patients, all with pain, ligamentous instability, and/or occult ganglia, were evaluated from January 1993 to April 1996. The MRI studies used a dedicated surface coil and 3-dimensional gradient-recalled techniques. Images were assessed for radial or ulnar avulsion, central defects, degenerative intrasubstance changes, joint fluids, and complex tears of the triangular fibrocartilage complex. If images revealed uniformly low signal intensity at both the radial and ulnar attachment, an articular disk was considered to be normal (Fig 1). Findings of MRI were compared with those of arthroscopy.

Results.—Fifty-nine of 77 patients appeared to have a tear of the triangular fibrocartilage complex at MRI; 57 cases were confirmed at arthroscopy. Fourteen of 21 partial tears identified at MRI were confirmed on arthroscopic examination. Twenty-nine tears were ulnar, 8 were radial (Fig 5), 9 were central, and 11 were complex. When arthroscopy was used as the standard, MRI had a sensitivity of 100%, a specificity of 90%, and an accuracy of 97% for detecting a tear of the triangular fibrocartilage complex of the wrist. In 53 of 57 tears, MRI provided accurate localization; sensitivity was 100%, specificity 75%, and accuracy 92%.

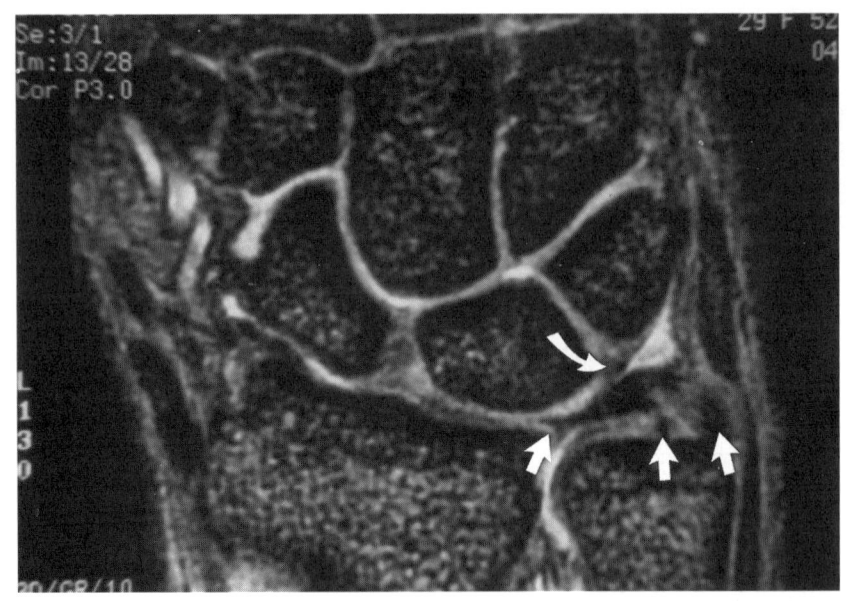

FIGURE 1.—Coronal gradient-echo image of a 31-year-old woman who had an occult ganglion of the wrist and no history of trauma. The image, made through the middle portion of the articular disk, demonstrates intact radial and ulnar attachments (*straight arrows*) and an intact lunotriquetral ligament (*curved arrow*). The triangular fibrocartilage complex was found to be intact on arthroscopic examination. (Courtesy of Potter HG, Asnis-Ernberg L, Weiland AJ, et al: The utility of high-resolution magnetic resonance imaging in the evaluation of the triangular fibrocartilage complex of the wrist. *J Bone Joint Surg Am* 79-A:1675–1684, 1997.)

Discussion.—Subtle morphologic changes in the triangular fibrocartilage complex can be detected if proper MRI technique is used. All images obtained in these patients used a 1.5-tesla superconducting magnet and either a 5-inch curved receive-only surface coil or quadrature design phased-array wrist coil. The coronal volumetric acquisition was centered over the proximal aspect of the lunate, and the slice thickness was 1 mm. No contrast medium was used.

▶ With MRI optimized for the wrist, including use of a 1.5 tesla MR machine, a specific surface coil for wrist imaging, a small field of view of 8 cm, and sections as thin as 1 mm with a 3-dimensional gradient echo sequence without interslice gap, excellent detection rates of triangular fibrocartilage complex tears can be achieved. As shown in this study, sensitivity was 100%, specificity was 90%, and accuracy was 97% for detection of 57 triangular fibrocartilage complex tears, confirmed by wrist arthroscopy.

G. Bergman, M.D.

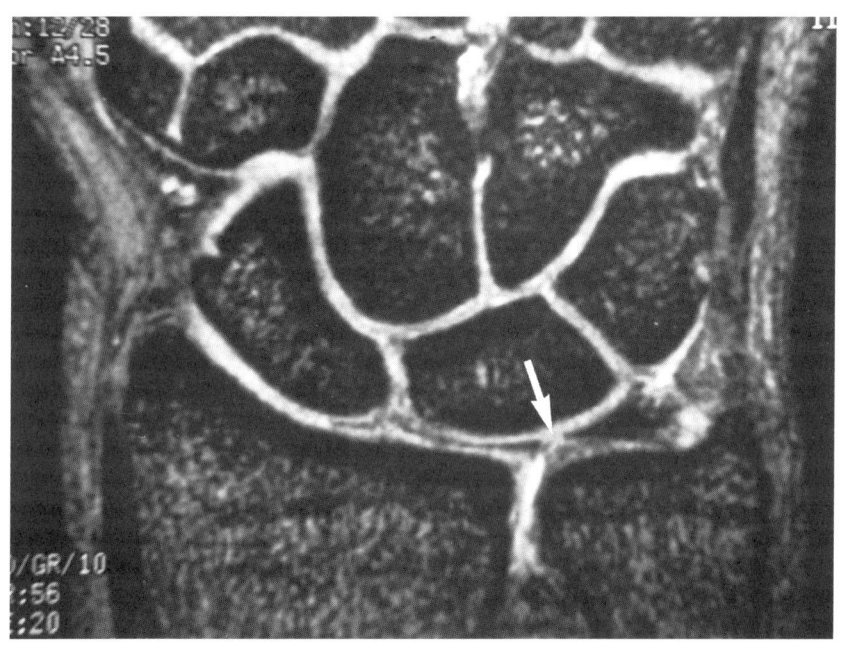

FIGURE 5.—Coronal gradient-echo image of a 46-year-old man who had had a previous twisting injury, demonstrating a radial detachment of the articular disk (*arrow*). The detachment was confirmed at the time of arthroscopy. (Courtesy of Potter HG, Asnis-Ernberg L, Weiland AJ, et al: The utility of high-resolution magnetic resonance imaging in the evaluation of the triangular fibrocartilage complex of the wrist. *J Bone Joint Surg Am* 79-A:1675–1684, 1997.)

The Interosseous Membrane and Its Influence on the Distal Radioulnar Joint: An Anatomical Investigation of the Distal Tract

Gabl M, Zimmermann R, Angermann P, et al (Univ Hosp, Innsbruck, Austria)
J Hand Surg [Br] 23B:179–182, 1998   8–40

Purpose.—Forearm rotation involves interaction of the radius, ulna, interosseous membrane, and proximal radioulnar joint with the distal radioulnar joint (DRUJ). Understanding of the causes of DRUJ instability requires analysis of all structures affecting this joint. An anatomic, histologic, and functional study of the interosseous membrane and its effects on the DRUJ is reported.

Methods and Findings.—Dissections and other studies were performed in 45 cadaver wrists. The distal tract of the interosseous membrane was found to extend from the radius proximally to the ulna distally. The distal tract's origin from the radius was 22 mm proximal to the distal dorsal corner of the sigmoid notch. At this site, central fibers were attached with fibrous cartilage, and superficial bundles were found mixed with periosteum. The tract was 8 mm in width, 31 mm in length, and 1 mm in thickness. The distal insertion was the capsule of the DRUJ, between the sheaths of the extensor digiti minimi and extensor carpi ulnaris tendons,

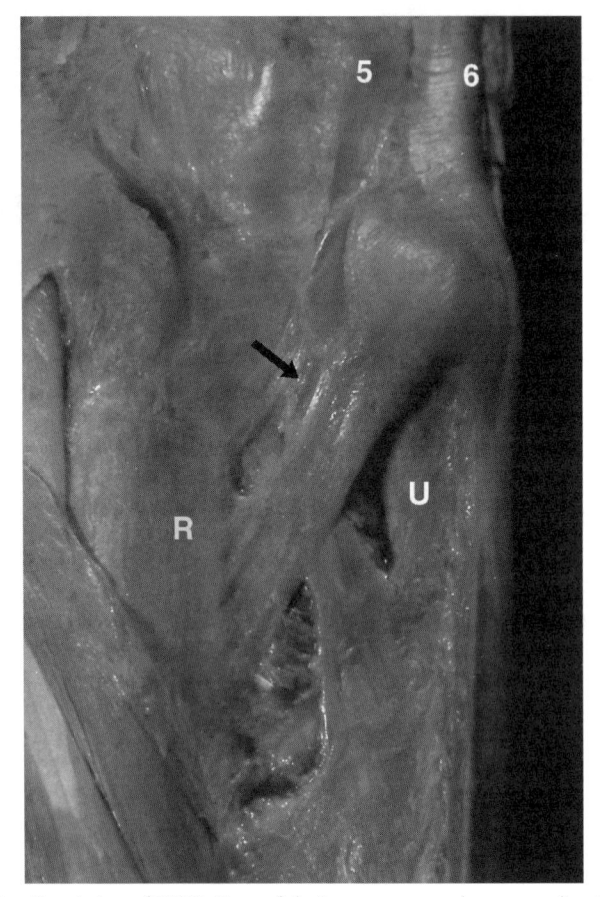

FIGURE 1.—Dorsal view of DRUJ: Tract of the interosseous membrane extending from the distal radius to the DRUJ (between ECU and EDM). A, the tract is taut in pronation. Distal tract of the interosseous membrane (*arrow*); 5 and 6, locations of EDM and ECU tendons. *Abbreviations: ECU*, extensor carpi ulnaris; *EDM*, extensor digiti minimi; *R*, radius; *U*, ulnar. (Courtesy of Gabl M, Zimmermann R, Angermann P, et al: The interosseous membrane and its influence on the distal radioulnar joint: An anatomical investigation of the distal tract. *J Hand Surg [Br]* 23B:179–182, 1998.)

with deep fibers inserting directly at the triangular fibrocartilage. Pronation made the tract taut, and supination made it loose (Fig 1, A). Functionally, the distal tract of the interosseous membrane strengthened the dorsal capsule of the DRUJ, protecting the ulnar head in a sling during pronation.

Conclusions.—The findings help to clarify how the interosseous membrane affects the DRUJ. The distal tract of the interosseous membrane inserts at the triangular fibrocartilage, thus serving as a major stabilizing unit. The distal tract also acts as an additional stabilizer of the DRUJ, supporting the ulnar head during pronation, when the DRUJ is not covered by the extensor digiti minimi and extensor carpi ulnaris.

▶ This is a very important article, which nicely demonstrates a consistently present band of fibers originating in the dorsal radial metaphysis, which appears to have a substantial reinforcing effect on the dorsal joint capsule of the distal radioulnar joint. It is interesting to note that, very often, a similar process can be observed on the volar aspect of the joint as well. Perhaps these fibers allow an imbrication of the dorsal radioulnar joint capsule to have some mechanical benefit in patients with dorsal subluxation of the ulna relative to the radius. The actual mechanical properties of this structure should be studied in detail, to further support the hypothesis of the authors.

R.A. Berger, M.D., Ph.D.

Chronic Palmar Distal Radio-Ulnar Dislocation: Treatment With Sauvé-Kapandji Technique [Spanish]
Olea AG, del Valle EB, Coscoyuela MT, et al (Grupo de Cirugía de la Mano de Madrid; Unidad de Cirugía de la Mano, Spain; Hosp Severo Ochoa, Leganés, Madrid; et al)
Rev Ortop Traum 41:344–349, 1997   8–41

Introduction.—Because few reports are available on the treatment of chronic palmar dislocations of the distal radioulnar joint, a procedure for managing such dislocations is discussed.

Methods.—Two men, aged 30 and 32 years, were diagnosed as having a palmar dislocation of the distal radioulnar joint 10 and 14 months after the injury. The lesion was missed at first because the patients showed more apparent lesions in the same extremity. The diagnosis was confirmed by a CAT scan. Both patients were treated by arthrodesis of the distal radioulnar joint and proximal ulnar pseudoarthrosis (Sauvé-Kapandji procedure).

Results.—The 2 patients were reviewed on an average of 3 years after the Sauvé-Kapandji procedure, and both recovered a painless full pronation and supination of the forearm.

Conclusion.—The Sauvé-Kapandji procedure can be an effective form of treatment for chronic palmar dislocations of the distal radioulnar joint.

▶ A palmar dislocation of the distal radioulnar joint is a rare injury, and diagnosis can be initially missed. However, it is unusual to have to treat a 12-month-old dislocation. A Sauvé-Kapandji procedure seems to be a reasonable treatment as there is definite distal radioulnar joint destruction after such a long delay of treatment. The main complication of an S-K procedure is the possibility of creating an unstable and painful proximal ulna stump. This can be avoided by an adequate surgical technique. It is very important not to disturb the static and dynamic structures that stabilize the ulna to the radius: pronator quadratus muscle (deep head), interosseous membrane, and FCU muscle insertions. The entrance of the screw should be placed anterior to the ECU (forearm in supination) to maintain the tendon dorsal to the pseudoarthrosis for added stabilization.

A. Lluch, M.D., Ph.D.

Suggested Reading

Lluch A, Garcia-Elias M: The Sauvé-Kapandji procedure: Technical considerations. *Orthop Surg Tech* 9:67–70, 1995.

The Role of Wrist Arthroscopy in the Management of Complex Triangular Fibrocartilage Tears: A Report on a Series of 124 Cases [French]
Fontes D (Clinique du Sport, Paris)
La Main 3:17–22, 1998
8–42

Objective.—The efficacy of arthroscopy in diagnosis and treatment of triangular fibrocartilage complex (TFCC) lesions is evaluated.

Method.—The experience of 1 arthroscopist between 1990 and 1996 was retrospectively reviewed. One hundred twenty four arthroscopies were directed to treatment of TFCC lesions. According to Palmer classification, 97 (78%) of these lesions were Class 1 (trauma) and 27 (22%) were Class 2 (degenerative).

In Class 1, mean patient age was 36.7 years. Class 1A lesions (central) represented 51.5% of cases; class 1B(ulnar avulsion), 17.5%; class 1C (distal avulsion), 5%; and class 1D (radial), 26%. Forty percent represented sport injuries, 28% were work injuries, and 32% were domestic accidents. Delay of treatment from onset was an average of 218 days. Ulnar variance was constantly positive in class 1A, 1B, and 1D and negative in class 1C. Class 1A was treated by central excision, 1B by styloid osteosynthesis or Poehling-Whipple direct suture, 1C by shaving, and 1D by either radial reinsertion (4 cases) or Whipple central excision (21 cases).

In Class 2, mean patient age was 53 years. The repartition was class 2A (6 cases), class 2C (3 cases), class 2D (14 cases) and class 2E (4 cases). Delay of treatment from onset was an average of 192 days. Mean positive variance was 1.5 mm. Treatment consisted of central débridement, shaving of synovial and chondral lesions plus a "wafer" procedure when protrusion of ulnar head demonstrated cartilage lesions.

Results.—According to Mayo Modified Wrist Score (100 points), good and excellent results were achieved in 84% of Class 1 and 63% of Class 2 cases.

Conclusion.—Ulnar shortening is only indicated in positive ulnar variance cases that are not responsive to primary endoscopic treatment. Arthroscopy is the best method for diagnosing and managing TFCC lesions.

▶ This article reviews a large series of arthroscopic treatment of TFCC lesions by 1 surgeon working in a sport clinic. If such treatment is of evident benefit in a population of sport-persons, one wonders if this experience could be transposed to the everyday larger group of patients on compensation who come in with the hand equivalent of "low-back pain".

G. Foucher, M.D.

Suggested Reading

Kapandji AI: Amélioration technique de l'opération Kapandji-Sauvé, dite "Technique III." *Ann Chir Main* 17:78–86, 1998.
▶ When A.I. Kapandji reports on a modification of M. Kapandji's (Sauvé-Kapandji procedure) one should pay attention. In this article, A. Kapandji describes his "Technique III." The principal differences relate to maintaining all possible connections between the proximal ulna and the extensor carpi ulnaris and its tendon sheath, removing cartilage from the radius and ulnar via a dorsal exposure, and a differently configured osteotomy. He reports on his initial 8 cases and believes they demonstrate better stability and faster recuperation.

V.R. Hentz, M.D.

9 Neuromuscular Disorders

An Implanted Upper-Extremity Neuroprosthesis: Follow-up of Five Patients

Kilgore KL, Peckham PH, Keith MW, et al (Case Western Reserve Univ, Cleveland, Ohio; Cleveland Veterans Affairs Med Ctr, Ohio; MetroHeatlh Med Ctr, Cleveland, Ohio)
J Bone Joint Surg Am 79-A:533–541, 1997 9–1

Objective.—Functional neuromuscular stimulation provides functional grasp patterns for tetraplegic patients. A report of the first 5 patients to receive the recently developed implantable systems with leads tunneled subcutaneously to the muscles was presented.

Methods.—The stimulator was implanted in 5 patients (2 women), aged 28–57 years, with spinal cord injuries below the fifth or sixth cervical nerve root (Fig 1). Additional surgeries included cross anastomoses of the extrinsic muscles to counter asynchronous motion of the fingers, tendon transfers, side-to-side tendon anastomoses, arthrodesis of the thumb joint, and rotational osteotomy of the radius. After implantation the patient was fitted with an above-the-elbow cast for 3 weeks for stabilization of electrodes. One to 2 months after surgery, a lateral and a palmar grasp pattern were programmed and tailored for each patient. Patterns were controlled by shoulder motion in 4 patients and wrist motion in 1. Each patient received 3 weeks of training and was then discharged to use the device at home. Patients were evaluated at 6 months and yearly thereafter. Grasp and pinch force were measured, and a 6-object grasp-release test was performed. The ability to perform activities of daily living was evaluated with and without the prosthesis. Frequency of patient use was monitored.

Results.—Patients were followed for an average of 4 years and 8 months. Patients had no active grasp before implantation or when the prosthesis was turned off. They were able to control the degree of grasp closure and grip strength and to use the prosthesis independently and regularly. Pinch strength ranged from 8 to 25 N. The patients had 22 operative procedures performed to facilitate use of the prosthesis.

Conclusion.—The implanted neuroprosthesis was safe and reliable and has been used for as long as 7 years.

FES System Components

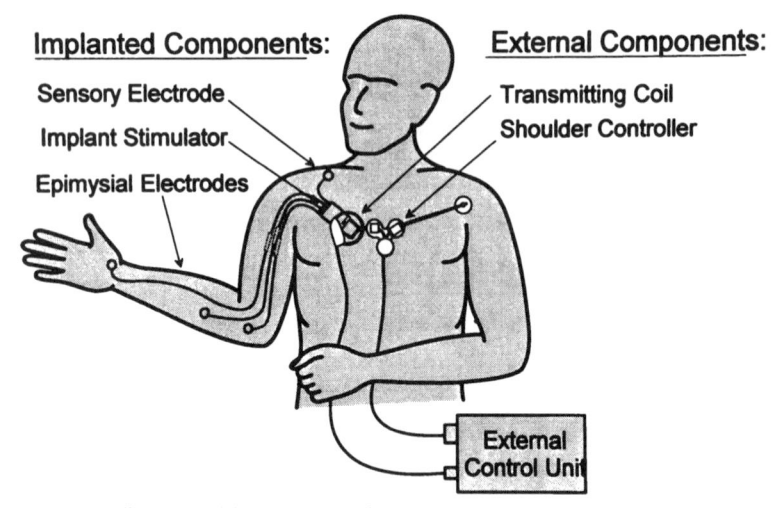

FIGURE 1.—Illustration of the components of the neuroprosthesis system. The implanted components include the stimulator, leads, connectors, and epimysial electrodes. The external components include the shoulder control unit, the transmitting coil, and the external control unit. The entire system is portable; the external control unit is usually placed in a bag on the back of the wheelchair. (Courtesy of Kilgore KL, Peckham PH, Keith MW, et al: An implanted upper-extremity neuroprosthesis: Follow-up of five patients. *J Bone Joint Surg Am* 79-A:533–541, 1997.)

▶ In July 1997, the United States Food and Drug Administration authorized release of this upper-extremity neuroprosthesis from its previous investigational-only status. As of the date of this review, about 60 patients have undergone implantation at sites around the world. The investigators in Cleveland have implanted the lion's share. In spite of the multicenter nature of the device, to date, only 2 patients have had to have all or several components of their systems explanted because of infection.

It has been exciting to see this technology evolve from a step-sister of functional neuromuscular stimulation for the lower extremity in the larger paraplegic population into a real product that has the potential for restoring useful hand function to a subset of our tetraplegic patients for whom, heretofore, we have had so little to offer. Every new technology evokes certain caveats from greying "experts." Mine is: Be extremely cautious if this procedure is your very first upper-extremity operation on a tetraplegic patient. How ironic that functional neuromuscular stimulation for the lower limb still languishes in the laboratory.

V.R. Hentz, M.D.

Ulnar Nerve Fascicle Transfer Onto the Biceps Muscle Nerve in C5-C6 or C5-C6-C7 Avulsion of the Brachial Plexus, Based on a Series of 18 Cases [French]

Loy S, Bhatia A, Asfazadourian H, et al (Hôpital Bichat, Paris; A-17 Mantri AC I, Pune, India)
Ann Chir Main 16:275–284, 1997   9–2

Objective.—Patients presenting an avulsion of C5-C6 and C5-C6-C7 plexus brachial roots are typically managed by neurotization or tendon transfer. A new technique for neurotization is discussed.

Method.—A new technique of neurotization was used that consists of sacrificing 2 fascicles of the ulnar nerve at the proximal arm level and suturing them directly to the motor branch of the biceps muscle. Among 18 patients, 8 (44%) were C5-C6, and 10 (56%) were C5-C6-C7 avulsions. The patients were aged from 17 to 41 years (mean age, 25 years), and the delay between injury and operation ranged from 4 months to 6 years (mean delay, 17 months). Seventeen patients were reviewed at follow-up times ranging from 6 to 56 months (mean time, 27.5 months.)

Results.—There were 3 patients where no muscle contraction was obtained. Ten patients reached a grade 3 or 4 biceps function and 4 patients achieved a grade 2 (according to the British Medical Council Research). In 7 (87.5%) of the 8 C5-C6 patients, recovery of elbow flexion was sufficient (1 requiring an additional Steindler transfer). In 4 (44.4%) of the 9 C5-C6-C7 patients, recovery of elbow flexion was sufficient but 4 (44.4%) needed additional Steindler transfer. No patient (except 1 lost early after operation) had any sensory or motor functional deficit in the ulnar nerve territory. At follow-up, the 2-point discrimination test was 3 to 5 mm in 3 patients. In 12 patients tested, the Semmes Weinstein monofilament test ranged between 1.65 and 3.61 grams.

Conclusion.—Ulnar nerve fascicle neurotization of the biceps motor branch is advisable early in C5-C6 avulsion. Elbow flexion predictably recovered against gravity in less than 6 months.

▶ This is a new and intriguing alternative treatment for the challenging issues of C5-C6 plexus avulsion. It could be interesting to compare, in an animal model, this method, which sacrifices some fascicles of an intact nerve, with the technique presented orally by Ulrich Mennen consisting of simply opening a perineurium window and performing an end-to-side anastomosis. Anyone care to try it?

G. Foucher, M.D.

▶ In 1994, Oberlin et al. introduced this technique in a preliminary report of 4 patients.[1] His series has now grown to 18, and other surgeons around the world have adopted this technique. This is a really wonderful addition to the surgical armamentarium. I now prefer it to intercostal or medial pectoral nerve transfer and have had very rewarding results (though in many fewer patients than Oberlin et al. report). It is technically much less difficult than the other described procedures. The speed of reinnervation exceeds all others. I have seen no lasting dysfunction in the donor ulnar nerve. It is absolutely necessary to have available a micro-sized nerve stimulator and a controller that allows very small current or duration signals in order to properly assess the ulnar nerve components. The disposable stimulators available in the United States are inadequate. Even at the lowest amplitude, the stimulator is too strong for the task.

V.R. Hentz, M.D.

Reference

1. Oberlin C, Beal D, Leechavengvonds S, et al: Nerve transfer to biceps muscle using a part of ulnar nerve for C5 C6 avulsion of the brachial plexus: Anatomical Study and report of 4 cases. *J Hand Surg [Am]* 19:232–237, 1994.

Significance of Elbow Extension in Reconstruction of Prehension With Reinnervated Free-Muscle Transfer Following Complete Brachial Plexus Avulsion
Doi K, Shigetomi M, Kaneko K, et al (Ogori Daiichi Gen Hosp, Japan)
Plast Reconstr Surg 100:364–372, 1997   9–3

Background.—Brachial plexus injuries are devastating injuries that are often seen in young, active individuals. Complex reconstruction using free-muscle transfer can provide strong, reliable motor recovery for finger function. The procedure involves 2 free-muscle transfers: first, transfer of the first free muscle neurotized by the spinal accessory nerve for elbow flexion and finger extension; and second, transfer of free muscle reinnervated by the fifth and sixth intercostal nerves for finger flexion and neurotization of the triceps brachii via its motor nerve by the third and fourth intercostal motor nerves to extend and stabilize the elbow. Suturing the sensory rami from the intercostal nerves to the median nerve restores hand sensibility.

Methods.—There were 31 patients with complete avulsion of the brachial plexus who had reconstruction of elbow extension by intercostal nerve transfer after reconstruction of prehension using a single or double free-muscle transfer. The mean patient age was 23 years.

Results.—Analysis of long-term results was completed in 24 patients. On serial electromyographic examination, reinnervation of the triceps muscle was showm to take longer than reinnervation of the transferred muscle. The ultimate strength of the triceps muscle was weak. No patient attained M5 grade, 2 attained M4 grade, 4 attained M3 grade, 8 attained M2 grade, 5 attained M1 grade, and 5 patients attained M0 grade. In spite of this weak recovery, 14 patients had useful functional recovery of the triceps muscle, with stabilization of the elbow joint against the transferred muscle acting as a simultaneous elbow flexor and wrist or finger extensor.

Discussion.—Elbow stability must be obtained to achieve voluntary finger function after free-muscle transfer. If the triceps muscle does not recover after intercostal nerve neurotization, transfer of the reinnervated infraspinatus to the triceps muscle may be performed to stabilize the elbow.

▶ In the ambulatory patient, absence of elbow extension is a reconstructive goal of relatively low priority. The effects of gravity serve to extend the elbow sufficiently for most patients. Doi and co-authors make the case for reconstruction of active elbow extension in the patient with complete brachial plexus palsy. They have extended to the brachial plexus patient what surgeons interested in improving upper extremity function in the tetraplegic patient have learned. That is, it is not necessary to reconstruct strong elbow extension. What is necessary is to reconstitute the stabilizing effect of the triceps muscle so that more distal transfers will function better.

In the case of the patient with complete brachial plexus palsy secondary to multiple avulsions, a muscle used to provide elbow flexion—if attached to a muscle distal to the elbow—can assist in regaining that function provided that the flexor effect of the transfer at the elbow can be checkreined. For example, a transfer for elbow flexion can be attached into the tendon of a wrist extensor. The transfer will flex the elbow preferentially unless the elbow extensor can be simultaneously activated. In this case, the power of the transfer will be directed toward the more distal function, e.g., wrist extension, which might, itself, activate a tenodesis-type finger flexor.

V.R. Hentz, M.D.

Anatomical Factors Predisposing to Focal Dystonia in the Musician's Hand: Principles, Theoretical Examples, Clinical Significance
Leijnse JNAL (Erasmus Univ, Rotterdam, The Netherlands)
J Biomech 30:659–669, 1997
9–4

Objective.—Repetitive use injuries in musicians are associated with hand difficulties, particularly when constraints on movement occur. Stretching of intertendinous connections, movement in the slack region of the connections, coactivation, and compensatory movements can increase muscle load. Model results from kinematic studies of finger movements with connected tendons and the model studies of the kinematics and the motor forces and stresses of the finger with lumbrical were discussed in terms of the analysis and treatment of focal dystonia complaints.

Methods.—Static forces in coupled fingers and relationship between motor forces and loads were analyzed using mathematical representations of anatomically interconnected muscles, end tendon forces, and external loads, coactivation motor forces and constants, or passive connection stiffness constants in an appropriately dimensioned coactivation matrix (Fig 1). Agonists and antagonists of a motor M can be expressed as a function of independent motor forces. Physiologic muscle load can be quantified by summing the muscle stress over the physiologic cross-sec-

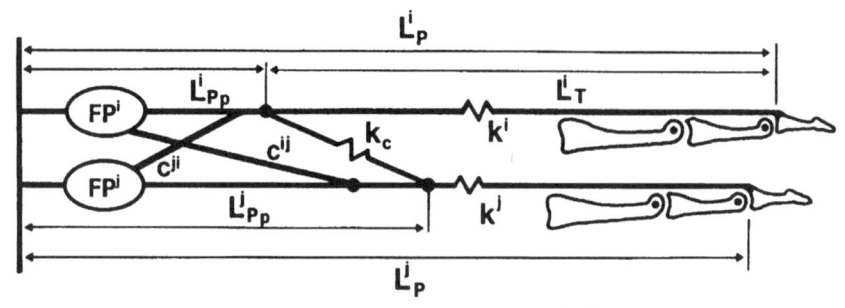

FIGURE 1.—Model of interconnected motors. *Abbreviations:* c^{ji}, c^{ij}: coactivations; k_c: stiffness of connection. (Reprinted from Leijnse JNAL: Anatomical factors predisposing to focal dystonia in the musician's hand: Principals, theoretical examples, clinical significance. *J Biomech* 30:659–669. Copyright 1997, with kind permission from Elsevier Science Ltd, The Boulevard, Langford Lane, Kidlington OX5 16B UK.)

tional area. Physiologic muscle load multiplied by the contraction speed of the entire fiber length yields the power per muscle volume.

Results.—Anatomical interconnections or constraints can increase the load on certain muscles and lead to focal dystonia. In the case of stretched connections, the extensor, lumbrical, and interossei are most strained. Certain unstretched connections can strain the interossei, resulting in compensatory movements that increase muscle load on larger body segments that become the main power source. Clinical applications included relief of flexion cramping; eliminating a sufficient number of constraints to allow less stressful movements by redesigning instruments, changing hand positions, and clearing intertendinous connections; treatment of focal dystonia by using less stretched connections; surgical removal of the connections; and correcting posture problems.

Conclusions.—Biomechanical and surgical solutions to focal dystonia, arising from results of a mathematical model measuring forces of anatomical interconnections, were presented.

▶ The functional consequences of tendinous interconnections among the fingers are thoroughly explored in this article. The robust theoretical analysis of the anatomy of the hand allows a clear illustration of the mechanical function of these interconnections. The way in which the author extrapolates these interpretations to clinical dystonia serves as an elegant tutorial on the mechanical interpretation of anatomical systems. This article should be read by all hand surgeons wishing to gain insight into the mechanical function of the complex tendinous system of the fingers.

F.J. Valero-Cuevas, Ph.D.

Piper's Palsy: A Focal Dystonia
Lederman RJ (Cleveland Clinic Found, Ohio)
Med Probl Perform Art 13:14–18, 1998

Introduction.—Focal dystonia is a rare but disabling disorder of instrumental musicians. This syndrome is described in 4 bagpipers.

Bagpipe Features.—The bagpipe melody is supplied through a single pipe with holes stopped by the right index through little fingers and the left index, middle, and ring fingers and thumb during playing. The left hand position is usually one of dorsiflexion at the wrist, flexion at the metacarpophalangeal joints, and extension at the interphalangeal joints. This creates considerable tension in the lumbricals and finger flexors. Stresses on the left hand are further potentiated by the fact that the left arm is draped over and supports the bag and weight of the instrument. Rapid finger movements are required, especially of the middle and ring fingers, for the embellishments that create special sounds of the bagpipes.

Patients.—Age range of 1 female and 3 male patients was 31–64 years; age at onset of dystonia was 27–49 years. All bagpipers had been playing from 13 to 45 years at onset of dystonia. The dystonic manifestations were similar for all 4 pipers and involved at least the left middle finger. The predominant dystonic manifestation was involuntary flexion in 3 patients. Onset was insidious and progressed over a 1- to 2-year period for 3 patients and a 3- to 5-year span for the fourth patient. Ability to perform was severely compromised in all patients. Treatment focus was on medication and measures (wrist splints and surgery) to alleviate presumed nerve entrapment. The most frequently used medications were nonsteroidal antiinflammatory drugs and muscle relaxants. Two of 3 patients treated with trihexyphenidyl had a modest response. One patient was able to play up to 8 hours when using trihexyphenidyl and 2 finger splints for the right hand, which he fashioned himself. Treatment with a series of botulinum toxin injections was partially helpful for 2 years in the female patient. She reduced her playing and no longer competes. One patient abandoned playing, and the remaining patient plays up to 1 hour daily and uses trihexyphenidyl before playing.

Conclusion.—Treatment of focal dystonia in bagpipers is suboptimal. Until better techniques are determined, the use of medication, botulinum toxin injections, mechanical aids, and technical retraining will have to suffice.

▶ This article may seem a bit esoteric to be included in the YEAR BOOK. After all, how many bagpipe players is one likely to see in a lifetime of practice? However, this illustrates one point quite well: Focal dystonia occurs in individuals who perform unusual movements with the hand in an excessively repetitive manner. Here are four patients with little in common other than that they play the bagpipes regularly. Yet they all developed a fairly rare movement disorder with almost identical characteristics. Dr. Lederman's review of focal dystonia nicely summarizes the current knowledge on the subject and is worth reading for this alone.

K.A. Bengtson, M.D.

Surgery of the Spastic Hand in Cerebral Palsy
Dahlin LB, Komoto-Tufvesson Y, Sälgeback S (Malmö Univ, Sweden)
J Hand Surg [Br] 23B:334–339, 1998   9–6

Objective.—About one third of children with hemiplegic cerebral palsy have spastic hemiplegia. These patients have not only a characteristic pattern of upper-extremity deformity, but also sensory impairments that adversely affect the results of reconstructive surgery. The surgical results appear to be closely related to the preoperative stereognosis, i.e., the ability to describe and recognize objects without seeing them. The results of reconstructive upper-extremity surgery in patients with spastic hemiplegic cerebral palsy are reported.

Methods.—The experience included 36 patients with cerebral palsy of the spastic hemiplegic type who underwent upper-extremity reconstructive surgery. The reconstruction was usually done in 2 stages, with a number of different operative procedures. The arm was kept in a cast for 6 weeks, followed by comprehensive occupational therapy. Follow-up evaluations, including assessment of stereognosis, were performed at 6 and 18 months postoperatively.

Results.—Gripping and grasping abilities were significantly improved at follow-up. Wrist supination and range of motion also improved in most patients, and the thumb-in-palm deformity was corrected or markedly improved. Stereognosis improved to a striking degree. The reconstruction met the patient's expectations in most cases.

Conclusions.—For patients with spastic hemiplegic cerebral palsy, upper-extremity reconstruction provides good results. Hand function is significantly improved for most patients. The improvement in stereognosis is unexpectedly high, perhaps as a result of functional cerebral reorganization induced by modified afferent inflow.

▶ This interesting article describing a study of older patients suggests that stereognosis may be improved by judicious surgery that positions the hand for prehension in certain cases of cerebral palsy. The keys to success in this type of surgery remain not only meticulous technique but also judicious case selection and the establishment of realistic expectations in the patient and the patient's parents. Some clinicians have used the help of psychologists in patient assessment and preparation; that, too, may be a reasonable adjunctive measure.

P.C. Amadio, M.D.

Rotator Cuff Repairs in Individuals With Paraplegia
Goldstein B, Young J, Escobedo EM (DVA Puget Sound Health Care System, Seattle; Univ of Washington, Seattle)
Am J Phys Med 76:316–322, 1997

Objective.—Shoulder pain and dysfunction can result in significant morbidity for patients with paraplegia as a result of spinal cord injury (SCI). Although treatment and outcomes of shoulder problems have been reported in individuals with SCI, no controlled studies have compared nonsurgical and surgical treatments of rotator cuff tears. The outcome of decompressive shoulder surgeries for rotator cuff repairs in patients with SCI were examined retrospectively.

Methods.—A computer search identified 5 male patients, aged 46 to 72, with SCI who had undergone rotator cuff repair since 1987.

Results.—All patients had shoulder pain, and 2 patients had received >3 steroid injections. Four patients (5 shoulders) had large tears and atrophy. One patient had a 2-cm tear of the supraspinatus tendon. The first 4 patients received 6 weeks of rehabilitation, and the last patient had 12 weeks of rehabilitation. The first 4 patients with large tears failed to have improved shoulder function. Three had a decreased range of motion, 1 had decreased pain, and 2 could no longer reach overhead. The fifth patient had improved strength and range of motion, and decreased pain after surgery.

Conclusion.—In this small series, SCI patients with atrophy, humeral head displacement, or large tears of the rotator cuff had poorer outcomes than those with smaller tears. Additional study of conservative treatment for these patients is needed.

▶ This study provides real experience to support the anecdotal notion that wheelchair patients do poorly after rotator cuff repair. Five of six shoulders by retrospective review did poorly, all of which had large tears or dysfunctional cuffs. A comment based on our own population at the Palo Alto VA Spinal Cord Unit: most symptomatic shoulders, including those with documented tears, improve with a well concerted rehabilitation program. Of those patients with continued pain after three months of therapy, few cuff tears found by magnetic resonance imaging are considered repairable, since a paraplegic typically has longstanding pathology with a large to massive tear. When a potential surgical candidate is chosen, even fewer patients are willing or able to comply with a very strict postoperative protocol. This prohibits active transfers and the use of a manual wheelchair for 10 to 12 weeks when we feel the cuff is capable of withstanding the abnormal forces seen with non-ambulators. This regimen is increasingly more difficult to carry out as managed care afflicts the VA health care system. Arthroscopic decompressions have proven very useful in these patients, with fewer constraints on compliance and regimen.

A.L. Ladd, M.D.

10 Arthritis

Proximal Interphalangeal Joint Denervation [French]
Foucher G, Long Pretz P (SOS Main, Strasbourg)
La Main 3:55–60, 1998   10–1

Objective.—Bouchard proximal interphalangeal (PIP) degenerative arthritis most frequently runs a benign course. A few patients with this condition, however, have intractable pain resistant to conservative treatment although keeping a functional range of motion.

Method.—According to the anatomical work of Schultz (1984), all the PIP innervation emanates from branches of the 2 palmar collateral nerves, at the proximal phalanx level. A resection of these palmar branches was performed through a modified Bruner approach, under metacarpal nerve block and on an outpatient basis. No postoperative immobilization was necessary. Twenty-six patients (mean age, 67 years) were operated on 34 joints. Two groups of patients were isolated according to follow-up protocol. Group 1 was composed of 11 patients (12 joints) reviewed after a mean follow-up of 6.5 years. Group 2 was composed of 15 patients (22 joints) reviewed after a mean follow-up of 26 months.

Results.—There was no postoperative complication except transitory distal paresthesia in a third of the patients. Pain improvement was assessed on the Visual Analogic Scale. Three joints were not improved and 2 indicated a recurrence. In the remaining 29 joints, mean improvement was 88%. Only 1 joint in group 1 lost 20% of its mobility at long-term follow-up.

Discussion.—In nodal Bouchard arthrosis with relevant pain and the preservation of more than 60 degrees of arc of motion, prosthesis implant is not a good solution to alleviate pain, as it usually results in a limited range of motion.

Conclusion.—PIP denervation in selected cases is a simple, safe, cheap operation, resulting in a mean pain improvement of 88% in 85% of operated joints.

▶ Guy Foucher is not a new-comer in the field of joint denervation; he described a refined technique of total wrist denervation in 1992.[1] Here he and his coworker utilize the work performed by Schultz et al. in 1984, who showed that innervation of the PIP joint was through a single articular branch, raising from the collateral nerve at mid-phalangeal level and entering the joint proximally together with the articular artery.[2] The authors state that at surgery they have severed all branches arising from the collateral nerve, from the web space to the PIP joint, except for the dorsal branch, because they found it difficult to decide which one was the articular branch. They fail to state whether the arterial articular branch was also severed. This is a theoretical problem for the joint blood supply. The authors do not comment on this, but only on radiographs performed on 9 operated joints. There was no mention of bone or joint necrosis.

The existence of two follow-up groups owes to the fact that after a successful outcome in the initial 10 patients (11 joints) there was a complete failure in the 11th patient. The authors abandoned the technique until they reviewed that patient at a later date and found out that pain relief had occurred after 3 months. A subsequent comprehensive review of all patients showed that pain relief was immediate in only 45% and occurred after 3 months in 55%. Finally, the authors state that, as expected, this operation did not have any beneficial effect on the degenerative process itself with radiological progression in 4 out of the 9 cases with available X-rays, and progression of a pre-existing clinodactyly in one out of 14.

Because of the favorable results of the procedure in 85% of patients, we feel it is useful in those cases with irretrievable pain and a good range of motion where the only other options were either abstention or a major procedure such as arthroplasty or arthrodesis with a significant reduction in the functional range of motion.

C. LeClercq, M.D.

References

1. Foucher G, Da Silva JB: Denervation of the wrist [French]. *Ann Chir Main Memb Super* 11:292–295, 1992.
2. Schultz RJ, Krishnamurthy, S, Johnston AD: A gross anatomic and histologic study of the innervation of the proximal interphalangeal joint. *J Hand Surg [Am]* 9:669–674, 1984.

▶ I have never tried PIP joint denervation, but on the basis of this article, I think I would be willing to give it a go the next time I have a patient with painful PIP arthritis with good range of motion.

P.C. Amadio, M.D.

Arthroscopic Evaluation and Treatment of Thumb Carpometacarpal Joints
Culp RW, Osterman AL (Philadelphia Hand Ctr, King of Prussia, Pa)
Atlas Hand Clin 2:23–28, 1997   10–2

Objective.—The anatomy of the carpometacarpal (CMC) joint as well as indications for and technical aspects of its evaluation were described.

Anatomy.—The thumb CMC joint is a 2-saddle joint with saddles perpendicular to each other. The joint is stabilized by 2 ligaments of which the palmar oblique is the more important. The first extensor compartment runs across the joint, the radial artery traverses the dorsal capsule, and the superficial branches of the radial nerve are located in subcutaneous tissue.

Indications.—Arthroscopic evaluation is indicated when conservative management fails or when loose bodies, acute fractures, osteoarthritis, or posttraumatic arthritic conditions are diagnosed.

> *Surgical Technique.*—With the arm at 90 degrees and the thumb in a traction tower with 5 pounds of traction applied, the joint is distended with saline and 2 portals are created. The joint is entered with a blunt obturator and cannula while the joint is continuously irrigated with saline via a small pump. The joint is investigated, the anterior oblique ligament is identified, any loose bodies are removed, arthritic changes are debrided and/or drilled, and a thumb spica splint is applied.

Discussion.—Arthroscopic evaluation is less invasive; it can detect cartilage damage and loose bodies before they appear on radiographs, resulting in less postoperative pain and stiffness.

Conclusion.—Arthroscopy is a useful tool for evaluating and treating the CMC joint of the thumb.

▶ This article provides a highly illustrated and succinct description of arthroscopy of the thumb CMC joint. Although the technique is still in its infancy and the procedures that can best be done by this technique are still to be worked out, the authors give the reader a clear idea of what to do and how to do it.

L.B. Lane, M.D.

Portals for Arthroscopy of the Trapeziometacarpal Joint
Gonzalez MH, Kemmler J, Weinzweig N, et al (Univ of Illinois at Chicago)
J Hand Surg [Br] 22B:574–575, 1997
10–3

Objective.—The locations and positions of subcutaneous structures of the trapeziometacarpal (TM) joint have not been studied. Cadaver hands were dissected to study the relationships of the tendons, nerves, and arteries around the TM joint.

Methods.—The extensor pollicis longus (EPL), extensor pollicis brevis (EPB), and abductor pollicis longus (APL) tendons were identified, the radial nerve was followed to the joint line, and the distances of the radial nerve to the EPL, EPB, and APL tendons were measured in 11 cadaver hands. Distances of the radial artery from the radial edge of the EPB tendon and the ulnar edge of the EPL tendon were recorded.

Results.—Specimen radial nerves had 2–5 branches. Seven hands had 1 or 2 branches of the radial nerve lying dorsal or dorsal and radial to the EPL tendon. Five hands had 1 or 2 branches dorsal to the EPB tendon or a branch radial to the tendon. Four specimens had 1 or 2 branches dorsal to the APL tendon. Whereas the radial artery crossed deep to the EPL and the EPB tendons in all hands, at the level of the joint line it was within 1 mm of the EPL in 7 specimens and within 2–8 mm radial to the radial edge of the tendon in 4 specimens. At the level of the joint line, the artery was ulnar to the EPB tendon at a distance ranging from 4 to 17 mm. At joint level, no neurovascular structures were found 0–6 mm radial to the radial edge of the APL tendon and 0–4 mm ulnar to the EPB tendon.

Conclusion.—There are a large number of anatomical variations in structures around the TM joint.

▶ This is an anatomical study with clinical application. The authors try to clarify the "safe entry points" for arthroscopy of the TM joint. With 11 fresh frozen cadaver hands, the authors have a limited sample size. Even so, they found a large number of anatomical variations in these few hands. Other anatomical studies evaluating the radial nerve and artery also found considerable anatomical variation in this area. Although the authors conclude that the safe areas are just palmarradial to the APL tendon and just ulnar to the EPB tendon, they also recommend blunt dissection to expose the capsule because of the "close proximity of the neurovascular structures." The authors have confirmed what other writers have also described: a great number of important structures coursing through this area.

The surgeon who proposes to perform arthroscopy of the TM joint should proceed with caution, as there is *no* truly "safe" entry point, only those made safe by careful dissection and delicate surgical technique. Readers who are interested in arthroscopy of the TM joint are urged to read the article written by Culp and Osterman, (Abstract 10–2) which provides a good description of the surgical technique.

L.B. Lane, M.D.

De la Caffinière Thumb Carpometacarpal Replacements: 93 Cases at 6 to 16 Years Follow-up
Chakrabarti AJ, Robinson AHN, Gallagher P (Norfolk and Norwich Hosp, Norwich, England)
J Hand Surg [Br] 22B:695–698, 1997   10–4

Objective.—The de la Caffinière prosthesis allows the establishment of a stable, pain-free, mobile joint and normal thumb length. Results of 93 sequential implants with an average follow-up of 11 years were reviewed.

Methods.—Between 1980 and 1989, 71 patients (9 men), aged 39–80 years, were implanted by 1 investigator with 93 de la Caffinière prostheses, 87 for osteoarthritis, 3 for rheumatoid arthritis, and 3 for posttraumatic arthritis. Patients were assessed by another investigator and followed radiologically to identify any loosening.

> *Technique.*—The trapeziometacarpal joint was exposed, avoiding the superficial radial nerve. About 5 mm of bone was resected and the shaft prepared with a rasp. The components were cemented into the cortical shell separately. In 21 joints, the trapezial component was cemented with the cup flange flush with the surface of the trapezium. Later, the cup was recessed and covered within the trapezium. In all joints, the cup was cemented in 50 degrees of abduction and 30 degrees of extension.

Results.—One patient was lost to follow-up. There were 55 living patients with 73 joint replacements available for review. There were 11 failures (12%) requiring revision, 9 as a result of aseptic loosening and 2 because of cup breakage. Survival at 16 years was 89%. Men under age 65 had the highest failure rate. There were 12 perioperative complications, including 3 superficial wound infections, 6 hypersensitive scars, 1 dislocation, and 2 cases of cup breakage. The mean time to failure was 3 years. Only 2 patients were dissatisfied.
Conclusion.—The de la Caffinière prosthesis provides a satisfactory treatment and good pain relief for carpometacarpal arthritis. Because working-age men have the highest failure rate, the prosthesis should be used with caution in this subgroup.

▶ This is the first long-term report of a large series of cemented carpometacarpal prostheses. Interestingly, implant survival is about that of total hip arthroplasty, deemed by nearly all as a very successful procedure. In this series, failures, if they occurred, came early, with loosening of the carpal component. Men under 65 years of age and, presumably, working, experienced a relatively high failure rate. After the authors had made some modifications, such as fully recessing the trapezial component within the bone, the frequency of failure diminished.

If the incidence of published reports is any indication, this has not been a popular substutute for either fusion or interposition arthroplasty for hand surgeons in the United States. There are probably many reasons for this, including influential publications and other biases. For example, hand surgeons seem to resist the willful exposure to the pungent odor of polymethylmethacralate.

Cement seems to be a separating point between the "big-bone boys" and the "little-bone boys," at least in my hospital. Probably, the most logical reason is that essentially all these procedures please the patient by relieving the pain. (See Abstract 10–5.) A few percentage points of difference in pinch strength or mobility are unlikely to prompt a surgeon to alter a technique with which that surgeon is already comfortable.

V.R. Hentz, M.D.

Trapeziectomy Alone, With Tendon Interposition or With Ligament Reconstruction? A Randomized Prospective Study
Davis TRC, Brady O, Barton NJ, et al (Nottingham and Derbyshire Royal Infirmary, Derby, England)
J Hand Surg [Br] 22B:689–694, 1997

Objective.—The results of trapeziectomy alone (T), trapeziectomy with soft tissue procedures (T + STI), and trapeziectomy with ligament reconstruction (T + LRTI) were compared in a randomized, prospective study.
Methods.—Between 1992 and 1994, 76 women were randomly allocated to T (30 patients), T + STI (23 patients), or T + LRTI (23 patients).

Technique.—The trapezium and carpometacarpal joint were exposed through a triradiate dorsoradial incision while protecting the superficial branches of the radial nerve. The palmaris longus tendon was rolled into a ball and sutured to the palmar capsule for the T + STI procedure. For the T + LRTI procedure, the metacarpal at the base of the thumb was resected, and a canal was made through the radial cortex. The ulnar half of the flexor carpi radialis tendon was freed, while preserving its insertion on to the base of the second metacarpal, and inserted through the thumb metacarpal base. The rest of the tendon was rolled into a ball and sutured to the palmar capsule. The thumbs were stabilized in 30-degree palmar abduction for 4 weeks using a Kirschner wire and for 6 weeks with a splint. Patients were reviewed at 3 and 12 months.

Results.—Pain levels, functional disability, range of movement, hand grip, thumb stiffness and weakness, and thumb pinch strength were similar in all groups at baseline and at 12 months. Complications in the T group included 1 wound infection, 1 pin track infection, 5 cases of radio neuritis, and 1 case of palmar neuritis. In the T + STI group, there was 1 pin track infection, 1 case of radial neuritis, 2 cases of palmar median neuritis, 5 cases of flexor carpi radialis/palmaris longus pulling, 1 case of scar tenderness, and 2 cases of reflex sympathetic dystrophy. In the T + LRTI group, there was 1 pin track infection, 1 case of radial neuritis, 2 cases of palmar median neuritis, 5 cases of flexor carpi radialis/palmaris longus pulling, 1 case of scar tenderness, and 2 cases of reflex sympathetic dystrophy.
Conclusion.—Trapeziectomy, whether alone or with tendon interposition or ligament reconstruction, yields similar functional, pain, range of movement, and strength results at 1 year.

▶ The abstract speaks for itself. The follow-up is short term (maximum, 1 year) and the numbers in each group are small. Small and perhaps statistically significant differences might be masked. Are these likely to be clinically significant differences? Probably not. It is unusual to see such patients after more than 1 year, unless the surgeon is particular interested in an outcome or the patient returns for treatment of the other hand. I see very few patients who come to me asking for revision of basal joint arthroplasty performed by another surgeon, compared with other clinical problems.

This is another example of the old surgical adage that if a number of procedures are promoted for the same problem, 1 of 2 circumstances exist. Either they all work well or none of them work well.

V.R. Hentz, M.D.

Cemented and Non-Cemented Replacements of the Trapeziometacarpal Joint
Wachtl SW, Guggenheim PR, Sennwald GR (Chirurgie St Leonhard, St Gallen, Switzerland)
J Bone Joint Surg Br 80-B:121–125, 1998 10–6

Background.—Movement of the thumb places considerable forces upon the trapeziometacarpal joint. Thus, prostheses for this joint must be strong enough to withstand these forces (up to 200 kg of applied force during pinch) without migration. Ball-and-socket prostheses have been used in other areas of the body and provide mobility, stability, and strength. These authors evaluated 2 ball-and-socket prostheses for their utility in replacement of the trapeziometacarpal joint.

Methods.—During 7 years, 88 trapeziometacarpal arthroplasties were performed in 84 patients (69 women and 15 men; mean age 61 years) with primary osteoarthritis, rheumatoid arthritis, or posttraumatic arthritis. In the first 4 years of the study, 43 joints were replaced with the de la Caffinière implant in which the prosthesis was cemented. In the last 3 years, 45 joints were replaced with the cementless Ledoux implant. Pain was graded on a 4-point scale, and wrist strength was measured by a dynamometer and compared with that on the contralateral wrist. Radiographs were used to assess cup migration, stem loosening, and osteolysis.

Findings.—Overall, 28 prostheses dislocated or became loose (18 Ledoux, 10 de la Caffinière) and required reoperation (mean of 8.9 months later for Ledoux, mean of 39.2 months later for de la Caffinière). Sixty-one prostheses survived in situ; 26 of the 28 surviving Ledoux implants were examined at a mean follow-up of 25.3 months, and 25 of the 33 surviving de la Caffinière implants were examined at a mean follow–up of 63.5 months. Pain scores with the Ledoux implant were: no pain, 23%; pain during loading, 50%; pain during movement, 19%; and pain at rest, 8%. Corresponding scores for the de la Caffinière implant were 44%, 48%, 4%, and 4%. Cup migration was substantial in both groups (46% of the Ledoux implants and 28% of the de la Caffinière cups), as was stem migration (15% of Ledoux stems and 24% of the de la Caffinière stems). Osteolysis in zones 1, 2, 3, 4, and 5 occurred in 85%, 42%, 15%, 69%, and 62% of the Ledoux implants and in 56%, 40%, 24%, 88%, and 28% of the de la Caffinière implants, respectively. The survival rate for the

Ledoux implant was 58.9% at 16 months and for the de la Caffinière implant survival was 66.4% at 68 months.

Conclusions.—Both ball-and-socket prostheses gave disappointing results when used for trapeziometacarpal joint replacement. Factors that argue against their use in this situation include that such implants do not mimic the anatomy of the trapeziometacarpal joint, because the first metacarpal is lateral to the trapezium. Also, their spherical design does not allow normal translation of shear forces. Furthermore, the stress induced by the implants can overwhelm the stress tolerance of cancellous bone, causing loosening and failure. Thus, ball-and-socket joints are not suitable for use in trapeziometacarpal joint replacement.

▶ It seems clear that constrained ball-and-socket replacements are not adequate substitutes for the saddle articulation of the thumb carpometacarpal joint. At Mayo, we are experimenting with an unconstrained design that mimics the normal saddle articulation. Such an implant clearly performs better in cadaver simulations; whether it will do so in vivo remains to be proven. In the meantime, the old standby trapezium excision, with interposition and ligament reconstruction by one's method of choice, remains the benchmark, as it has, remarkably, for nearly 50 years.

P.C. Amadio, M.D.

Radiological Course of Cemented and Uncemented Trapeziometacarpal Prostheses [French]
Wachtl SW, Guggenheim PR, Sennwald GR (Spital Altstätten, France; Chirurgie St Leonhard, Gallen, France; Berit Paracelsus Klinik, Niederteufen, France)
Ann Chir Main 16:222–228, 1997   10–7

Objective.—Some authors rely on prostheses to solve the problem of first carpometacarpal joint (CMCJ) arthritis. The authors compare the radiological evolution of 2 types of devices, 1 cemented (De la Caffinière) and 1 non-cemented (Ledoux).

Method.—Eighty-eight prostheses were implanted in 84 patients between 1988 and 1994. Of 45 non-cemented prostheses (group 1) there were 4 luxations and 14 loosenings, leading to 17 reoperations after a mean interval of 9 months. Of 43 cemented prostheses (group 2), 1 luxation and 9 loosenings led to 10 reoperations after a mean interval of 39 months. Of the 61 nonrevised implants, 51 were reviewed, 26 in group 1 (mean follow-up, 25 months) and 25 in group 2 (mean follow-up, 63.5 months).

Results.—The "survival rate" of the prosthesis was significantly different in the 2 groups (59% at 16 months in group 1 vs. 66% at 68 months in group 2). There was no statistical difference for pain (absent in 23% of group 1 vs. 44% in group 2), mobility or strength. Radiologic loosening was defined by osteolysis around the stem and metacarpal migration greater than 1% and for the cup by a 5-degree change of the angle between the axis of the cup and the second metacarpal. Loosening was observed in 15% of stems and 46% of cups in group 1 vs. 24% of stems and 28% of cups in group 2.

Conclusion.—A spherical prosthesis fixed in the trapezium is inadequate for first CMCJ arthroplasty.

▶ Many different devices have been proposed for first CMCJ arthropasty. This article focuses on the huge rate of loosening in both cemented and noncemented prosthesis with a revision rate of 23% and 38%, respectively. A major issue that is not even alluded to, is the technical difficulty of such revisions, mainly after cemented implants. When these figures are compared to the low rate of complication of trapezectomy with or without ligamentoplasty and soft tissue interposition (anchovy procedure), one could propose, at least, to reduce the place for such expansive and sophisticated implants.

G. Foucher, M.D.

▶ This article demonstrated a high incidence of both metacarpal shaft and trapezial cup prosthetic loosening. Because the results of soft tissue arthroplasty or fusions are so good, I do not see a need for use of a prosthesis for the CMCJ.

J.M. Failla, M.D.

First Metacarpal Osteotomy for Trapeziometacarpal Osteoarthritis
Hobby JL, Lyall HA, Meggitt BF (Addenbrooke's Hosp, Cambridge, England)
J Bone Joint Surg Br 80B:508–512, 1998
10–8

Introduction.—Trapeziometacarpal joint osteoarthritis is a painful condition that can cause adduction deformity of the thumb. Among the wide range of proposed operations, the simple technique of first metacarpal osteotomy has received little consideration. Long-term results of first metacarpal osteotomy in patients with trapeziometacarpal osteoarthritis are presented.

Methods.—The retrospective analysis included 41 thumbs of 33 patients with trapeziometacarpal osteoarthritis. There were 32 women and 9 men, average age 57. Mean follow-up was 7 years, with all patients evaluated by an independent surgeon. All patients underwent surgery because of pain that interfered with daily activities and that did not improve with conservative treatment. Abduction-extension osteotomy of the first metacarpal was performed using the technique of Wilson (Fig 1).

Results.—Fifty-one percent of thumbs were pain free, and 29% had discomfort only with heavy use. Ninety-three percent of patients reported improved hand function. Grip and pinch strength were normal in 82% of cases, including restoration of thumb abduction. The symptomatic results were equally good in patients with grade 2 and in patients with grade 3

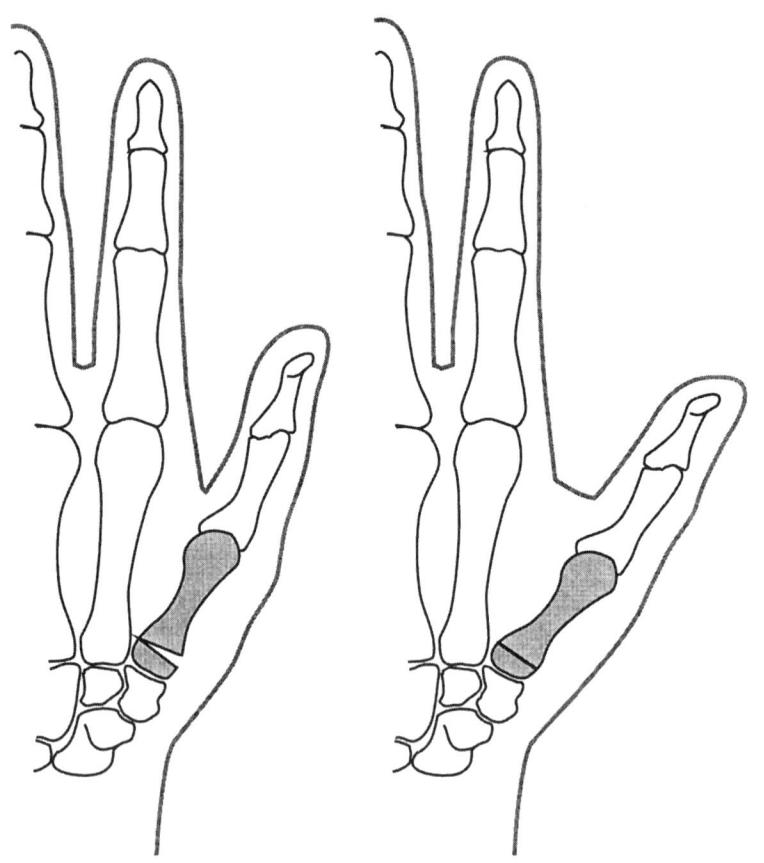

FIGURE 1.—Basal osteotomy corrects adduction contracture, restoring the first web space and reducing the tendency for the action of flexor and extensor pollicis longus to sublux the carpometacarpal joint. (Courtesy of Hobby JL, Lyall HA, Meggitt BF: First metacarpal osteotomy for trapeziometacarpal osteoarthritis. *J Bone Joint Surg Br* 80B:508–512, 1998.)

degenerative changes. The overall results were rated excellent in 18 hands, good in 12, and poor in 11.

Conclusions.—First metacarpal osteotomy is a simple procedure for pain relief in patients with trapeziometacarpal osteoarthritis. The technique provides correction of adduction contracture and restores grip strength and pinch strength, with few complications. Though useful in patients with early and moderate trapeziometacarpal osteoarthritis, this procedure is not indicated for those with severe disease or pantrapezial osteoarthritis.

▶ First metacarpal osteotomy has been largely underused, despite the excellent results demonstrated by the developer of the procedure, J.N. Wilson, in 1973. It has been my experience that the osteotomy is of limited benefit in relieving pain in pantrapezial degenerative disease, but that in lower grades of arthritis, where perhaps the degenerative disease is more focally localized, the technique has potential efficacy. It is unclear exactly why the osteotomy is beneficial in these patients, but the reason may be related to periarticular denervation as well as to realignment of the loads of the joint away from the degenerative foci. In cases of advanced or pantrapezial degenerative disease, the procedure still has a place, if the patients have an adduction contracture.

R.A. Berger, M.D., Ph.D.

Arthroscopic Synovectomy of the Rheumatoid Wrist: A 3.8 Year Follow-up
Adolfsson L, Frisén M (Univ Hosp, Linköping, Sweden)
J Hand Surg [Br] 22B:711-713, 1997   10-9

Objective.—Whether there is a long-term benefit of surgical synovectomy for joints affected by rheumatoid arthritis is controversial. Furthermore, there are no studies comparing arthroscopic synovectomy with open synovectomy. The long-term outcome after arthroscopic synovectomy was evaluated prospectively.

Methods.—The Whipple technique, including a traction device, a 2.4-mm-diameter arthroscopic, continuous irrigation, and a motorized shaver system, was performed on 24 wrists in 19 patients (3 men), whose average age was 46 years. Four dorsal and 1 radial portals were used to visualize the radiocarpal and midcarpal space, and another portal for the distal radioulnar joint was used in patients with intact triangular fibrocartilage. The average duration of surgery was 50 minutes. Range of motion was measured preoperatively and at an average of 3.8 years. Patients' subjective assessments of symptoms and function were obtained and compared with that of the normal wrist.

Results.—Seventeen patients improved. No long-term results of arthroscopic synovectomy have been published. Improvements in symptoms and function lasting an average of 3.8 years after arthroscopic synovectomy were documented. The minimally invasive procedure allows immediate mobilization, probably because the technique reduces postoperative pain. Because radiography shows an increased risk of further degeneration if significant arthritic damage is present at surgery, early synovectomy may decrease joint destruction. Other studies have found no link between early synovectomy and long-term radiographic appearance.

Conclusions.—That radiographic findings and clinical results were not correlated would suggest that wrist arthroscopic synovectomy should be performed on patients with Larson-Dahle-Eek radiologic index stage 0 to III arthritis. Arthroscopic synovectomy does not affect the long-term outcome of the rheumatoid wrist.

▶ These authors have done an excellent job in following up 24 wrists in 19 patients who initially were seen in 1993.[1] In their previously designed scoring system where 80 points is a maximum value for a normal wrist, patients showed an improved overall score from 43 to 55 at 3.8 years. Seventeen of the 24 wrists had improved, 5 were unchanged, and 2 were worse, according to the score. Arthroscopic synovectomy in the rheumatoid wrist reduces pain and improves wrist function in the majority of these patients. Of interest, radiographic progress of arthritic degeneration appeared to be less common in patients with no or very early changes of cartilage damage at the time of initial surgery. However, no correlation could be found between x-ray changes, range of motion, and subjective assessment of wrist function in their study.

E. Akelman, M.D.

Reference

1. Adolfsson L, Nylander G: Arthroscopic synovectomy of the rheumatoid wrist. *J Hand Surg [Br]* 18B:92–96, 1993.

Evolution of Surgical Indications in Treatment of Rheumatoid Arthritis of the Wrist: Experience Based on 603 Cases Operated From 1968–1994 [French]
Allieu Y (Hôpital Lapeyronie, Montpellier, France)
Ann Chir Main 16:179–197, 1997
10–10

Introduction.—The surgical experience of a single surgeon in a consecutive series of 603 patients with rheumatoid arthritis was described. The surgeon relates the evolution of his experience with the surgical treatment of wrists from 1968 to 1994.

Findings.—Therapeutic indications for surgery changed over time after a retrospective review of long-term results. A distinction was made between arthrodesis and arthroplasty of the wrist and conservative surgery, a combination of dorsal synovectomy and reaxation stabilization of the wrist. Five-year follow-up of conservative surgery showed that the disease progresses despite synovectomy. Reaxation stabilization using soft tissue (extensor retinaculum and tendon transfer) was not adequate to stabilize the wrist. Partial radiocarpal arthrodesis was needed most of the time (when the carpus demonstrated a medial translation or was performed early in potentially progressive forms) to stabilize the wrist. The Swanson implant was used to perform 70 arthroplasties from 1973 to 1988. Long-term follow-up revealed several complications that progressed over time. The Swanson implant was dropped in 1988. Twelve patients underwent wrist arthroplasty from 1979 to 1984 using Jackson's technique, which consisted of resection-interposition of a silastic sheath. This approach was abandoned in 1984 because of variable and unpredictable outcomes. Arthroplasties are no longer performed. Total wrist arthrodesis are performed with increasing frequency.

Conclusions.—Long-term follow-up of wrist surgeries is important in patients with rheumatoid arthritis.

▶ This article is valuable because the large number of patients confirms that wrist synovectomy and soft tissue realignment eventually fail with time because soft tissue repairs attenuate and wrist degeneration progresses. The author's conclusion is that radiolunate fusion will hold up better. This procedure will also correct ulnar translation and radial deviation deformities of the carpus; however, with time the midcarpal joint will eventually degenerate as well. The author does not address the incidence of midcarpal or radioscaphoid progressive degeneration with time. The value of this procedure may be to buy time, conserve some wrist motion, and to realign the carpus, before metacarpophalangeal MP joint arthroplasty. Whether total wrist fusion is better could be checked in an outcome study.

Regarding arthroplasty, the author also confirms the high incidence of complications with the Swanson silicone wrist and the lack of indications for this type of reconstruction. There is no mention of other total joint arthroplasty technique which may be indicated in some cases.

J.M. Failla, M.D.

Total Wrist Arthroplasty: A Quantitative Review of the Last 30 Years
Costi J, Krishnan J, Pearcy M (Repatriation Gen Hosp, Adelaide, Australia)
J Rheumatol 25:451–458, 1998   10–11

Introduction.—The original Swanson wrist prosthesis was a simple one-piece flexible silicone hinge. It gave way to implants consisting of radial and metacarpal stems with an articulating bearing surface, i.e., the Volz and Meuli prostheses. Current "third-generation" wrist prostheses use offset articulating surfaces to approximate the instant center of the wrist joint in the anteroposterior and lateral planes of motion. These include the Trispherical, Biaxial, and MWPIII total wrist arthroplasty prostheses (Figs 4, 5, and 6). Thirty years of published experience with various types of total wrist arthroplasties were reviewed.

Findings.—Experience with the original Swanson prosthesis showed high rates of fracture and surgical revision after 55 months' follow-up, with most fractures occurring at the junction of the distal stem and barrel. Initial experience with the second-generation Volz prosthesis revealed problems with a postoperative resting stance of ulnar deviation. This resulted from radial shift of the axis of the prosthesis relative to that of the normal wrist. Ulnar deviation was eliminated by a design modification, but subsequent experience revealed problems with bone resorption under the collar of the radial component, along with metacarpal loosening. These complications were most likely to occur in patients with posttraumatic degenerative joint disease. Still, the Volz prosthesis provided better results than the Meuli prosthesis, which was associated with revision rates of greater than 30%.

At the time of this review, few studies of the third-generation prostheses had been published. There were no fractures with any of these prostheses. Reported revision rates in this limited experience were up to 6% with the

Trispherical

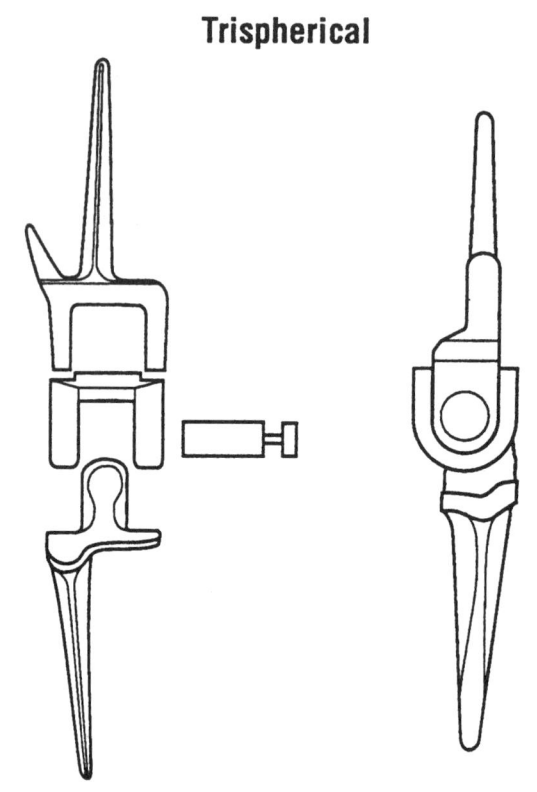

FIGURE 4.—Trispherical TWA prosthesis. (Courtesy of Costi J, Krishnan J, Pearcy M: Total wrist arthroplasty: A quantitative review of the last 30 years. *J Rheumatol* 25:451–458, 1998.)

Trispherical prosthesis, up to 17% with the Biaxial prosthesis, and 22% in 1 study of the MWPIII prosthesis.

Discussion.—Good clinical results have yet to be demonstrated with total wrist arthroplasty. Although few studies have been completed, the third-generation prostheses—with their closer approximation of the center of rotation of the wrist—have given promising initial results. One factor complicating comparison of the various prostheses has been the differing outcome measures used.

Biax

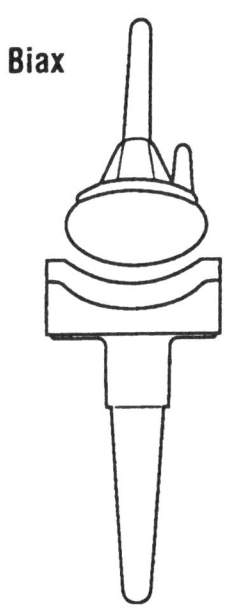

FIGURE 5.—BIAX TWA prosthesis. (Courtesy of Costi J, Krishnan J, Pearcy M: Total wrist arthroplasty: A quantitative review of the last 30 years. *J Rheumatol* 25:451–458, 1998.)

▶ The development of total wrist arthroplasty has been difficult. There is a strong need, and yet the perfect design has not been achieved. Outstanding results have been obtained in a small percentage of cases. Developers continue to seek a more perfect implant to satisfy the functional need for motion, particularly in patients with rheumatoid arthritis who have limited function in other upper extremity joints.

R.D. Beckenbaugh, M.D.

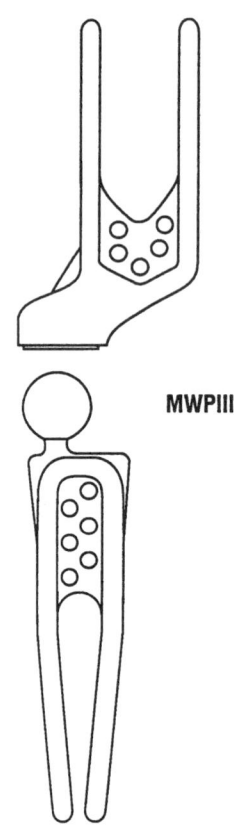

FIGURE 6.—MWPIII TWA prosthesis. (Courtesy of Costi J, Krishnan J, Pearcy M: Total wrist arthroplasty: A quantitative review of the last 30 years. *J Rheumatol* 25:451–458, 1998.)

Does Wrist Fusion Cause Destruction of the First Carpometacarpal Joint in Rheumatoid Arthritis? 18 Patients Followed for 2–6 Years

Belt EA, Kaarela K, Kautiainen HJ, et al (Rheumatism Found Hosp, Heinola, Finland; Tampere Univ, Finland)
Acta Orthop Scand 68:352–354, 1997   10–12

Objective.—Destruction of the wrist joint is common in patients with rheumatoid arthritis (RA). Concomitant erosions and destruction of the first carpometacarpal (CMC I) joint, which can cause thumb deformities, have not been fully described. After wrist fusion, stress on the thumb joint may be magnified. The destruction of the CMC I joint after total wrist fusion in patients with RA was assessed radiographically.

Methods.—Eighteen patients with RA (15 women), aged 34–65 years, having wrist fusion were followed for 2–6 years. Destruction of the CMC I joint was defined as grade 0 if bony outlines were intact and joint space was normal, grade 1 for erosion of less than 1 mm or joint space narrowing, grade 2 for 1 or more erosions of more than 1 mm, grade 3 for marked erosions, grade 4 for severe erosions, and grade 5 for destruction of bony outlines.

Results.—The average Larsen grade for CMC I joints was 0.9 before fusion and 2.5 at follow-up compared with 0.8 and 1.3, respectively, in control hands. At follow-up, control and fused hands were significantly different.

Conclusion.—Destruction of the CMC I joint was rapid and significant 2–6 years after fusion.

▶ This small study suggests that wrist fusion in patients with RA hastens *radiographic* destruction of the thumb CMC I joint. This is not surprising. We know that fusion of a joint places additional stress on the joints immediately proximal and distal to the fusion. That an underlying disease process is already affecting such joints speeds the process. The question that was not addressed by this study is the clinical effect of the radiographic changes. A large number of patients with radiographic changes of osteoarthritis of the thumb CMC I joint are not impaired functionally and are asymptomatic. What we, as surgeons, really want to know is whether the more rapid radiographic destruction of the thumb CMC I joint results in symptoms and functional impairment.

E.R. North, M.D.

Bone Scintigraphy of the Hands in Early Stage Lupus Erythematosus and Rheumatoid Arthritis
Van de Wiele C, Van den Bosch F, Mielants H, et al (Univ Hosp of Gent, Belgium)
J Rheumatol 24:1916–1921, 1997   10–13

Background.—The early joint symptoms of systemic lupus erythematosus (SLE), rheumatoid arthritis (RA), systemic sclerosis (SSc), and dermatomyositis-polymyositis (DM-PM) are often similar. Diagnosis of SSc and DM-PM is relatively easy because of the characteristic involvement of skin and muscles, but the differential diagnosis between SLE and RA in early-stage disease is difficult when clinical characteristics of SLE have not developed. A retrospective study evaluated the discriminatory value of bone scintigraphy in differentiating early stage SLE and RA.

Methods.—Between 1986 and 1994, 19 patients with early SLE and 20 with early RA were seen for symmetrical polyarticular complaints involving the hands and finger joints. Symptoms in both groups were of less than 3 months' duration. Nine patients with SLE had arthralgia in the absence of synovitis (group A) and 10 had clinical synovitis in the absence of arthralgia (group B). All 39 patients underwent a complete diagnostic investigation and were examined with standard whole-body bone scintigraphy and spot images of the hands. The bone scintigraphic studies were evaluated by 2 nuclear physicians blinded to clinical findings and other studies.

Results.—All 19 patients with SLE had normal radiographs of the hands. Bone scintigraphy showed diffuse, mildly increased juxta-articular tracer accumulation in 3 group A and 6 group B patients. Radiographs were also normal in patients with RA, but all 20 had foci of moderately to markedly increased subchondral tracer accumulation which corresponded with sites of clinical synovitis. All 19 patients with SLE were positive for antinuclear antibodies and 6 were anti-DNA negative. In the RA group, 7 of 20 patients were antinuclear antibodies positive and all 20 were anti-DNA negative.

Discussion.—Radiographs are often normal in both early-stage SLE and early-stage RA. Bone scintigraphy may be helpful in differentiating SLE from RA at this disease stage. Patients with SLE had either normal or diffuse mildly increased tracer accumulation, whereas those with RA had multifocal moderately to markedly increased tracer accumulation.

▶ Patients with early RA and essentially normal standard radiographs will have abnormal uptake on ^{99}Tc scintigraphy. Patients with early SLE will also have normal radiographs but will have scintigraphic results different from those of patients with RA. The patient with RA might benefit from proceeding directly to more potent medications, or perhaps to very early synovectomy.

V.R. Hentz, M.D.

Suggested Reading

Allieu Y: Development of surgical indications in the treatment of rheumatoid wrist: Report on experience based on 603 surgical cases, 1968–1994 [French]. *Ann Chir Main Memb Super* 16:179–197, 1997.
▶ This is a fascinating review of a single surgeon's extensive experience with the rheumatoid wrist—more than 600 cases—over a 30-year period. The lessons learned deserve repeating. Synovectomy is a temporizing procedure; recurrence of synovitis and disease progression are not likely despite early intervention. Soft-tissue realignments are unreliable. Arthroplasty has been gradually supplanted by radiolunate arthrodesis and total wrist arthrodesis due to the high rate of complications and failures. The simplicity of the message is a telling reminder of how far we still have to go in both our understanding and mastery of this frustrating and challenging disease.

P.C. Amadio, M.D.

Belt EA, Kaarela K, Lehto MUK: Destruction and reconstruction of hand joints in rheumatoid arthritis: A 20 year follow up study. *J Rheumatol* 25:459–461, 1998.
▶ This fascinating studied followed 83 patients for 20 years after their initial diagnosis with rheumatoid arthritis. Half ultimately had wrist fusions, a half dozen had metacarpophalangeal arthroplasties, and just 1 had thumb carpometacarpal surgery. A handful of finger joint fusions were done, and no proximal interphalangeal arthroplasties were performed. Hand function was not assessed, so we don't know whether the operated patients were better off or whether other, unoperated functional impairments existed. Nonetheless, this paper un-

derlines the fact that the main disability with rheumatoid arthritis in the hand is at the wrist level. Better solutions at this level, which could reduce the need for arthrodesis, would be welcome.

P.C. Amadio, M.D.

Gendi NST, Axon JMC, Carr AJ, et al: Synovectomy of the elbow and radial head excision in rheumatoid arthritis: Predictive factors and long-term outcome. *J Bone Joint Surg Br* 79B:918–923, 1997.
▶ A total of 171 patients with rheumatoid arthritis were followed for 5–25 years after elbow synovectomy and radial head excision. Although the short-term results were good, survivor analysis showed that eventually 80% of patients were candidates for further elbow surgery. Predictors of a better result from synovectomy and radial head excision were worse forearm rotation and better elbow flexion/extension, with a shorter duration of symptoms. Patients with a forearm rotation are less than 80 degrees and a flexion/extension arc over 60 degrees had just a 6% risk of failure in the long term.

P.C. Amadio, M.D.

Schneeberger AG, Adams R, Morrey BF: Semiconstrained total elbow replacement for the treatment of post-traumatic osteoarthrosis. *J Bone Joint Surg Am* 79-A:1211–1222, 1997.
▶ The May group report the 2- to 12-year follow-up of the Coonrad-Morrey semiconstrained elbow prosthesis in 41 nonrheumatoid elbows. As expected, the population is young and active. Also as expected, the complication rate is high: 27% reported as experiencing major complications, with 22% (of the series) requiring revision. The highest rate of failure was in patients with severe preoperative deformity. The authors stress the likelihood of failure in noncompliant patients—also an expected result. This includes, however, repetitively lifting 10 kg: an infant, for example. Experience with total hip replacements in young people indicates that most are "noncompliant" by traditional standards, and we should expect no different from young patients with posttraumatic arthritis of the elbow. This study permits us to add replacement to the rather few options available—all with high complication rates and varying success—as long as the patient understands and the surgeon anticipates the associated problems with elbow replacement in this population.

A.L. Ladd, M.D.

11 Tumors

Reconstruction of the Distal Aspect of the Radius With Use of an Osteoarticular Allograft After Excision of a Skeletal Tumor
Kocher MS, Gebhardt MC, Mankin HJ (Harvard Med School, Boston)
J Bone Joint Surg Am 80-A:407–419, 1998   11–1

Background.—Skeletal neoplasms often occur at the distal radius, and in some cases resection is indicated. Reconstruction of the wrist in such cases must consider the functional demands of the hand, the long-term results (because many patients are young), the limited surrounding soft

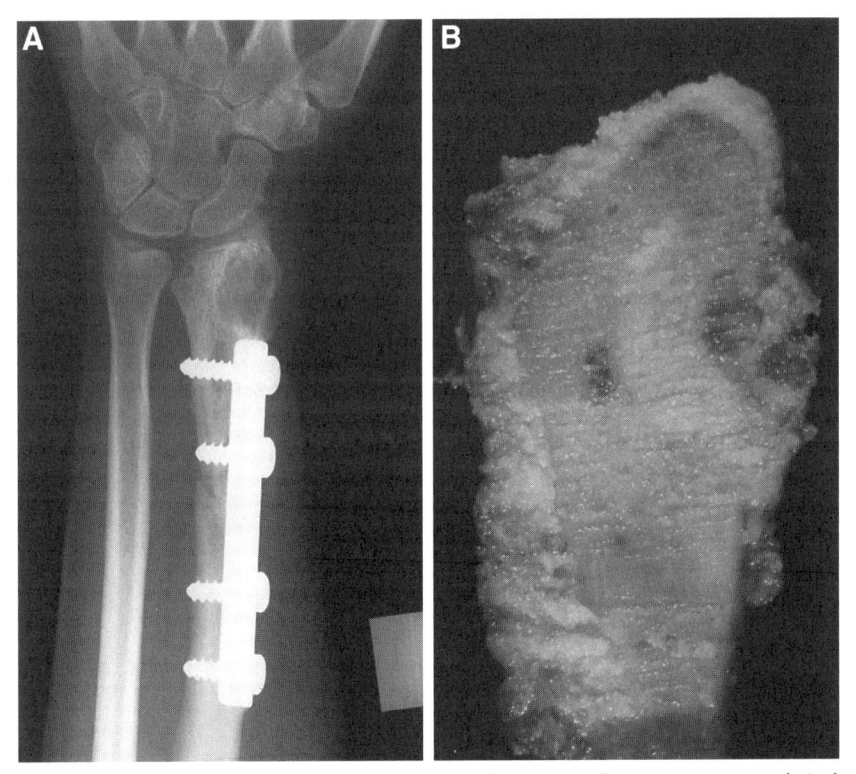

FIGURE 3.—**A**, radiograph showing a recurrent multifocal giant–cell tumor in a nonvascularized autogenous graft from the fibula. **B**, gross pathological specimen with the tumor. (Courtesy of Kocher MS, Gebhardt MC, Mankin HJ: Reconstruction of the distal aspect of the radius with use of an osteoarticular allograft after excision of a skeletal tumor. *J Bone Joint Surg Am* 80-A:407–419, 1998.)

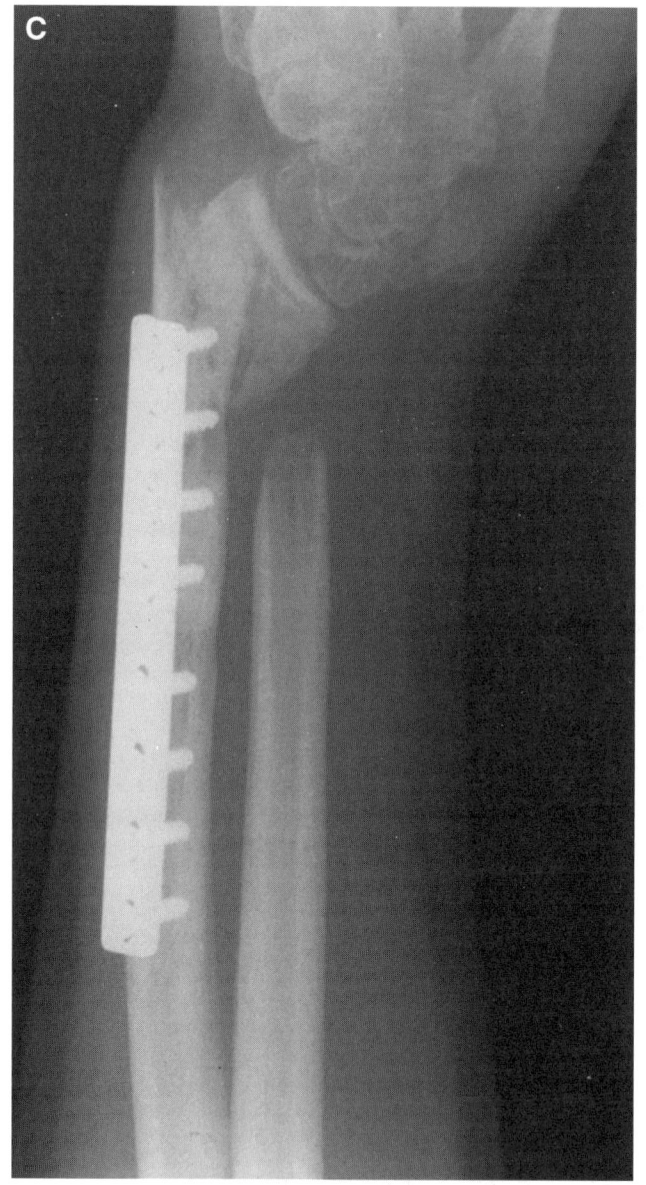

FIGURE 1, C.—Radiograph showing a fracture of the osteoarticular allograft 10 months after the reconstruction. (Courtesy of Kocher MS, Gebhardt MC, Mankin HJ: Reconstruction of the distal aspect of the radius with use of an osteoarticular allograft after excision of a skeletal tumor. *J Bone Joint Surg Am* 80-A:407–419, 1998.)

tissue, and the nerves and tendons in this area. These authors report their experience with the use of osteoarticular allografts to reconstruct the digital aspect of the radius after the excision of skeletal neoplasms.

Methods.—Over 19 years, 24 cadaveric osteoarticular allografts were implanted in 24 patients (13 women and 11 men; mean age, 31.5 years). Patients had undergone distal radius surgery for giant–cell tumor (n = 20; 9 recurrent lesions and 11 extracompartmental primary lesions with extension through the cortex or subchondral bone), desmoplastic fibroma (n = 2), chondrosarcoma (n = 1), or angiosarcoma (n = 1). The radiocarpal ligaments were also reconstructed and internal fixation was used. Average follow-up was 10.9 years (minimum of 2 years).

Findings.—In 2 patients the neoplasm recurred, 1 with a primary giant-cell tumor (Fig 3, A and B) and 1 with a desmoplastic fibroma (the latter patient had an above-the-elbow amputation). Eight patients required revision because of fracture (4 patients), wrist pain (2 patients), tumor recurrence (1 patient), or volar dislocation of the carpus (1 patient). Revisions were undertaken a mean of 8.1 years (range 0.8–17.8 years) after initial surgery and consisted of 7 arthrodeses and 1 amputation. In the 16 patients with a surviving allograft, pain occurred in association with moderate activities (4 cases) or severe (9 cases), and some patients had limitations in moderate activities (4 cases) or strenuous (9 cases). Range of motion averaged 36 degrees of dorsiflexion, 21 degrees of volar flexion, 16 degrees of radial deviation, 15 degrees of ulnar deviation, 58 degrees of supination, and 72 degrees of pronation. Although allografts survived in these 16 patients, they nonetheless had complications. In 4 patients, ulnocarpal impaction required excision of the distal ulna. In 4 patients, hardware had to be removed because of pain. Two patients experienced rupture of the extensor pollicis longus tendon, for which the extensor indicis proprius tendon was transferred. In 2 patients, the allograft fractured, requiring open reduction and internal fixation (Fig 1, C). One patient experienced volar dislocation of the carpus that required closed reduction. And 1 patient underwent excision of a ganglion of the dorsal aspect of the wrist.

Conclusions.—The rate of neoplasm recurrence after an osteoarticular allograft was low (2 of 24 patients, or 8%), particularly for giant–cell tumors (1 of 20 patients, or 5%). Function was restored in these wrists, with a moderate range of motion and relatively little pain while performing moderate activities. However, 8 of 24 allografts (33%) had to be revised. Nonetheless, osteoarticular allografts are a good solution for reconstruction of the distal aspect of the radius after skeletal tumor excision.

▶ This paper extends the series of distal radius allografts from the Massachusetts General Hospital (Smith et al). A total of 24 cases have been done, none since 1993, although the series eligibility date extended to 1996, according to the Methods section. Only 4 cases have been done this way since 1988. Although the authors express enthusiasm for this method of reconstruction, one must wonder whether there has been a change in their referral pattern, so they are seeing fewer eligible cases, or whether they now use other alternatives more often, such as curettage and methacrylate packing or fibular grafting. The results reported are somewhat worse than those that we have seen at Mayo Clinic with fibular grafting. We have not had any significant fibular donor site morbidity. Union can be speeded by vascularized fibula grafting with arthrodesis. Interestingly, although nonunion is clearly a problem with allografts, time to union is not discussed here. Prolonged immobilization while one waits for allograft union is also a factor of morbidity for the surgeon to consider. I would agree with these authors that allografting is an option for distal radius reconstruction, but, unless the patient refuses autograft, it would not be my first choice.

P.C. Amadio, M.D.

Vascularized Bone Grafts in the Treatment of Juxta-Articular Giant-Cell Tumors of the Bone
Kumta SM, Leung PC, Yip K, et al (Chinese Univ of Hong Kong)
J Reconstr Microsurg 14:185–190, 1998   11–2

Background.—One of the techniques used to treat giant-cell tumor of the bone is to resect the tumor *en bloc* while maintaining a thin shell of cartilage and subchondral bone. This defect must be replaced with tissue that will support the overlying cartilage and thus prevent its collapse. Vascularized bone grafts can be used for this purpose, and their use in patients with giant-cell tumor of the extremity was assessed.

Methods.—Thirty-four men and 4 women (mean age, 27 years) with giant-cell tumors of the distal radius (n = 18), proximal tibia (n = 8), proximal humerus (n = 8), proximal femur (n = 4), and calcaneus (n = 1) received vascular bone grafts to fill the postsurgical defect. In the case of giant-cell tumors of the distal radius, the tumor's position tends to disrupt the normal articulation. Thus in 3 of these 18 patients, the distal end of the radius was resected and replaced with a vascularized graft from the fibula. In the other 15 patients, a vascularized graft from the iliac crest was used (Fig 1). There is more cancellous bone in the iliac crest than in the fibula, and union seems to occur earlier with cancellous bone than with cortical bone. Furthermore, the vascularized iliac crest bone graft can also be used to reconstruct the radial side of the wrist joint (Fig 2, C). Follow-up ranged from 2 to 12 years for patients with giant-cell tumor of the distal radius.

Findings.—Of the 18 patients with distal radius involvement, all but 1 (94%) experienced union with the graft; this patient was reoperated and received a cancellous bone graft, after which union was achieved. Five patients (28%) had carpal subluxation, although the wrist was painless and there was functional range of movement. Two of these 5 patients (11% of total cases) showed degenerative changes, including 1 case of spontaneous radiocarpal fusion. Nonetheless, in all but 1 patient (94%) the wrist was pain-free and patients were satisfied with their range of motion. In 10 (56%) patients overall function was excellent and in 5

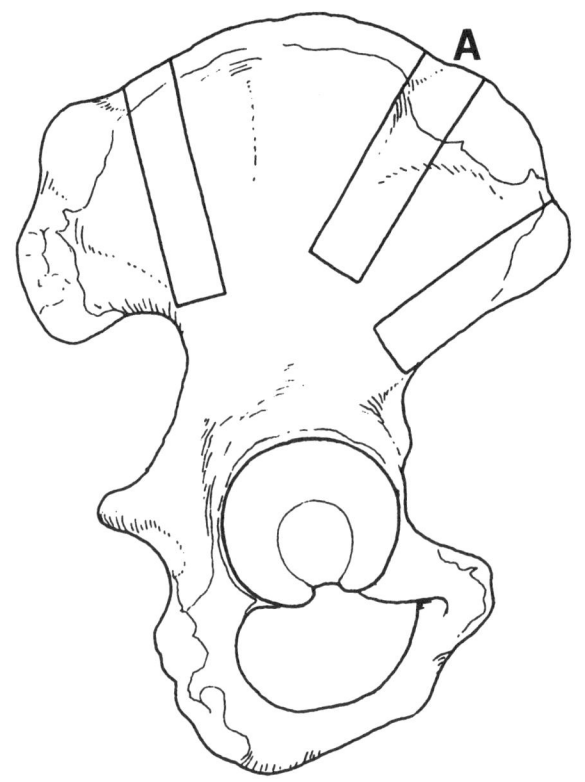

FIGURE 1.—Diagram of iliac crest, showing *A* as the most suitable area for harvesting a graft to replace the distal radius. (Reprinted with permission from *Journal of Reconstructive Microsurgery*, from Kumta SM, Leung PC, Yip K, et al: Vascularized bone grafts in the treatment of juxta-articular giant-cell tumors of the bone. *J Reconstr Microsurg* 14:185–190. Copyright 1998, Thieme Medical Publishers, Inc.)

(28%) it was good; the 3 (17%) patients with a fibular graft had fair scores. Overall, joint subluxation and degenerative changes were rated excellent or good in 11 (28%) of the patients, joint motion was rated excellent or good in 16 (41%) and joint stability was excellent or good in 12 (31%). Of the remaining 21 patients with juxta-articular grafts at other sites, 17 (81%) had excellent results and 3 (14%) had good results. Only 1 (5%) patient developed infection with complications and a subsequent poor result. Tumor recurred locally in 3 patients, twice in the proximal tibia at 16 and 23 months, and once in the proximal femur at 3 years.

Conclusions.—The subchondral bone and overlying articular cartilage were well supported by the vascularized bone grafts used. The tumor site was widely resected, yet joint function was not sacrificed, and many tumors did not recur. In particular, the vascularized iliac crest graft provided excellent or good results in reconstructions of the distal radius. One shortcoming of this method is that subluxation is likely because there is no

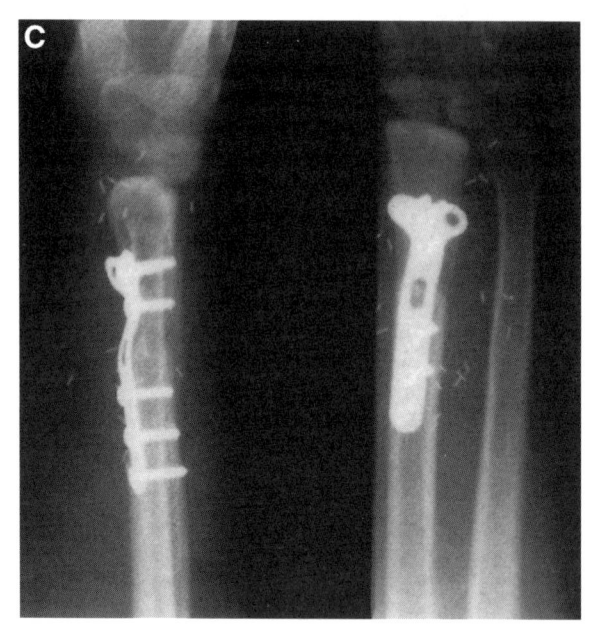

FIGURE 2, C.—Successful iliac graft replacement after surgery for a giant-cell tumor affecting the distal radius. (Reprinted with permission from *Journal of Reconstructive Microsurgery*, from Kumta SM, Leung PC, Yip K, et al: Vascularized bone grafts in the treatment of juxta-articular giant-cell tumors of the bone. *J Reconstr Microsurg* 14:185–190. Copyright 1998, Thieme Medical Publishers, Inc.)

articular surface for reconstructing the joint. However, none of the patients who had subluxation had unacceptable wrist motion.

▶ The use of vascularized iliac crest to replace the distal radius may be worth a longer look. The oncological results here are similar to those reported elsewhere: wide excision of giant cell tumor of bone results in low recurrence rates. Whether such an aggressive approach is necessary in all cases is another matter; the indications for wide excision and vascularized grafting vs. bone sparing options such as curettage and cementation were not discussed.

P.C. Amadio, M.D.

Treatment of Carpal and Digital Ganglions by Simple Aspiration, or Aspiration and Injection of Corticosteroid and/or Hyaluronidase
Seki JT, Bell MSG (Univ of Ottawa, Ont)
Can J Plast Surg 5:233–237, 1997   11–3

Background.—Conservative treatments advocated for carpal and digital ganglia include manual rupture, needle aspiration with or without injection of corticosteroids, and sclerosing agents. The success rates of these treatments vary, indicating that none is a definitive approach. The outcomes associated with simple aspiration and with aspiration and injection of corticosteroid or hyaluronidase were reported.

Methods and Findings.—The outcomes of 178 carpal and digital ganglion cysts in 174 patients, treated between 1987 and 1995, were analyzed retrospectively. The cumulative cure rates in 106 ganglia undergoing 1, 2, or 3 treatments with aspiration and triamcinolone acetonide injection were 45.3%, 52.2%, and 56.5%, respectively. Seventeen of 23 ganglia treated with combined triamcinolone acetonide and hyaluronidase recurred, yielding success rates of 17.4% and 26.1%, respectively, after 2 or 3 treatments. Simple aspiration performed in 26 ganglia (23 of which were volar digital ganglia) yielded success rates of 61.5% and 69.2% after 1 or 2 treatments, respectively. Overall, the success rate after a maximum of 3 treatments was 52.8%, regardless of treatment type and anatomic location of the ganglia.

Conclusions.—Given that the spontaneous regression rates of carpal and digital ganglia range from 38% to 58%, the outcomes of conservative treatment in this series are relatively poor. However, the current authors believe that surgery is too invasive for the treatment of these benign lesions and should never be advocated for a primary lesion. Further research on conservative treatments is planned.

▶ This is very helpful information, contradicting what many surgeons still say: "Let's just take it out, since injection won't cure it." Because of the proximity of the radial artery, and the high incidence of several small stalks from the radio-carpal joint that preclude elimination of the cyst by a single puncture, I do not aspirate palmar-radial wrist ganglia. The authors show a higher incidence of cure for digital ganglia than for wrist ganglia, and this is consistent with my experience. Simple aspiration with or without steroid yielded approximately 80% success, which is excellent and justifies injection as the first-line treatment. There is a smaller chance of cure (50%) for wrist ganglia. However, many of these patients are still happy, although the ganglion returns after injection, because it is smaller and less painful.

J.M. Failla, M.D.

The Use of Skeletal Traction in the Treatment of Severe Primary Dupuytren's Disease
Citron N, Messina JC (Nelson Hosp, London)
J Bone Joint Surg Br 80-B:126–129, 1998   11–4

Objective.—Various splinting and traction techniques have been attempted to correct problems caused by severe Dupuytren's disease of the hand. Early results of treatment by traction of patients with severe flexion deformities of the fingers as a result of Dupuytren's disease are described.

Methods.—Records of 13 consecutive male patients, aged 44–73, with Dupuytren's disease (Tubiana grades III and IV) of 18 fingers were reviewed retrospectively. Ten patients had a positive family history, a history

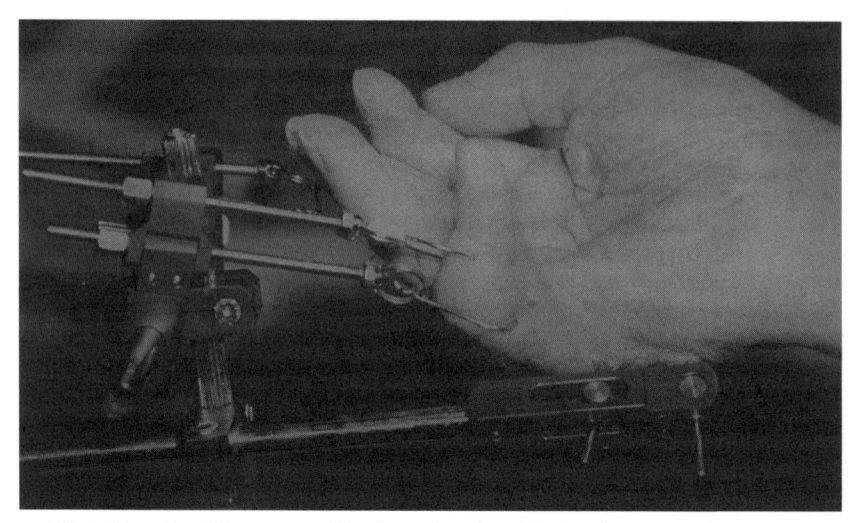

FIGURE 1.—The TEC apparatus. The device is anchored in the fifth metacarpal by two strong threaded pins. Traction is applied by turning the screws on the threaded rods attached to the skeletal traction rings. (Courtesy of Citron N, Messina JC: The use of skeletal traction in the treatment of severe primary Dupuytren's disease. *J Bone Joint Surg Br* 80-B:126–129, 1998).

of heavy alcohol use, or both. Twelve patients had skeletal distraction and fasciotomy. Two types of fixators were used to apply traction. The "Tecnica di Estensione Continua" (TEC) apparatus provides longitudinal traction to several fingers simultaneously and to various joints independently (Fig 1). The Verona fixator applies angular corrective force and distraction on 1 joint at a time. It was used on the PIP joint (Fig 2). The fixator was applied, and then the hand was rested for 2–3 days to allow pain and swelling to subside. Distraction was then maximally applied until correction or for 4 weeks. The fasciotomy was then performed.

Results.—Patients were observed for an average of 18 months. The average extension deficit improved to 39 degrees from 139 degrees, the PIP joint improved to 29 degrees from 80 degrees, and the mean total range of active movement increased to 202 degrees from 162 degrees for grade III and to 150 degrees from 96 degrees for grade IV deformities. Average range of movement increased to 175 degrees from 123 degrees. There were 2 recurrences. An extension contracture developed in 1 patient as a result of adhesions to the flexor tendon. This patient was treated with a 2-stage graft. Algodystrophy with joint stiffness, pain, and autonomic dysfunction appeared in 5 patients.

Conclusion.—Although there was a high incidence of complications in this group of patients with Dupuytren's disease, corrective external fixation may be appropriate for cooperative patients with severe disease. This treatment is, however, only one component of a carefully planned comprehensive treatment program.

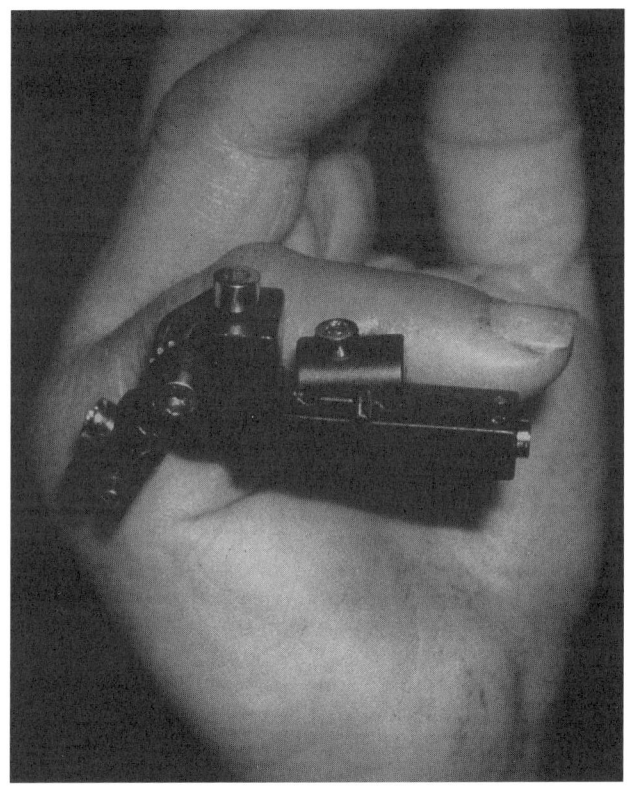

FIGURE 2.—The Verona apparatus. The device is anchored by two threaded pins in the bone on each side of the PIP joint. The patient uses a small Allen key to turn a worm gear and apply a corrective force. (Courtesy of Citron N, Messina JC: The use of skeletal traction in the treatment of severe primary Dupuytren's disease. *J Bone Joint Surg Br* 80-B:126–129, 1998).

▶ Progressive preoperative distraction is a useful adjunct to the management of severe contractures. Both of these techniques seem useful.

P.C. Amadio, M.D.

The Mechanical Properties of the Palmar Aponeurosis and Their Significance for the Pathogenesis of Dupuytren's Contracture
Millesi H, Reihsner R, Eberhard D, et al (Ludwig Boltzmann Inst for Experimental Plastic Surgery, Vienna)
J Hand Surg [Br] 22B:510–517, 1997   11–5

Objective.—The biomechanical properties of tendons and skin are well known. Whereas collagen fibers are wavy under low strain, this waviness is lost when the tissue is strained beyond 3%. The biomechanical behavior of tissues from different groups of patients with Dupuytren's contracture (DC) was investigated and compared with that of normal palmar aponeurosis (NPA) and normal tendons (NT) from patients without Dupuytren's disease.

Methods.—Normal tendons were excised from patients with carpal tunnel syndrome, as well as a segment of NPA. The total palmar aponeurosis was excised from patients with Dupuytren's disease, including a segment of normal palmar aponeurosis (ANPA), thickened fiber bundles (THFB), and cords or contracture bands (CB). Uniaxial biomechanical tensile testing performed included residual strain, hysteresis loop, recovery time between tests, load relaxation tests, inverse relation at strain levels before and after partial unloading, retardation, and inverse retardation.

Results.—The residual strain and relaxation and inverse relaxation values were lower for NT, but the hysteresis loop was larger, particularly at higher strain levels. In patients with DC, the value of biomechanical measures increased from ANPA to THFB to CB, even at lower strain levels. The recovery times of NT, NPA, ANPA, and THFB were significantly lower than for CB. Residual strain and the hysteresis loop were significantly increased in ANPA compared with NPA results.

Conclusions.—Biomechanical changes can be detected in ANPA even before the cellular proliferation leading to DC occurs. These changes appear to be related to structural changes in the elastin network that result in more viscoelastic behavior. The sudden increase in the mechanical recovery time in CB is characteristic of occurrence of contracture.

▶ The authors have performed an elegant biomechanical study on the properties of the NPA and their significance to Dupuytren's disease. Normal palmar fascia, NT, THFB, and Dupuytren's cords were studied by loading to strain levels of 2.5%, 5%, or 10% and then unloading. The authors have carefully investigated a variety of biomechanical parameters including the area between loading and unloading curves (hysteresis loop); recovery time, which tests the load strain if a specimen is loaded immediately after unloading; load relaxation; inverse relaxation; retardation, which applies constant strain levels as a function of time; and inverse retardation.

The authors conclude that biomechanical changes occur before cellular proliferation in Dupuytren's disease. However, the data are somewhat conflicting in that the apparently normal fascia in Dupuytren's disease in 11 samples (of 33) have residual elongation. Therefore, it is not entirely clear from this data that apparently normal palmar fascia from Dupuytren's disease shows biomechanical properties which are totally consistent with developing pathology. The authors explain this by suggesting a link in apparently normal fascia to structural changes in the elastin network.

The final conclusions of this paper are clearly supported by the data presented. Specifically, changes in biomechanical parameters in thickened fiber bundles and Dupuytren's cords are the result of a shift from elastic to viscoelastic properties, and a large increase in mechanical recovery time occurs in Dupuytren's cords and goes along with the occurrence of DC.

The authors should be complimented on a detailed, thorough work.

M.A. Badalamente, Ph.D.

Percutaneous Fasciotomy for Dupuytren's Contracture: A 10-Year Review
Duthie RA, Chesney RB (Aberdeen Royal Hosps NHS Trust, Scotland)
J Hand Surg [Br] 22B:521–522, 1997   11–6

Introduction.—Percutaneous fasciotomy has long been used in the treatment of Dupuytren's contracture, but indications for the procedure have become limited. A nonselected group of 160 patients who underwent percutaneous fasciotomy for Dupuytren's contracture were reviewed for 10-year outcome.

Patients and Methods.—The patients, 141 males and 19 females, had been treated in 1981 and 1982. Lack of operating time was the reason that a more radical procedure was not undertaken. All patients had outpatient surgery under local anesthetic median and ulnar nerve block. Case notes of the 73 male and 9 female patients who were still alive at follow-up were examined. Data recorded included recurrent contractures, time to further operation, and the degree of fixed flexion deformity. Overall fixed flexion contracture was taken as the sum of deformities at the metacarpophalangeal and proximal interphalangeal joints.

Results.—The 82 patients alive at 10-year review had percutaneous fasciotomy for fixed flexion contracture in 109 digits. A mean preoperative overall deformity of 71 degrees improved to 22 degrees immediately after percutaneous fasciotomy. Twenty-eight patients (34%) had no further surgical intervention; their overall fixed flexion deformity at 10 years was 57 degrees. The remaining 54 patients (66%) subsequently underwent local radical fasciectomy at a mean of 60.4 months after the initial procedure; their mean overall fixed deformity at that time was 85%. The 2 groups did not differ significantly in degree of preoperative or postoperative contracture.

Conclusion.—Percutaneous fasciotomy is a safe and simple procedure with a low rate of complications. It remains particularly useful in cases not suitable for local radical fasciotomy. Patients who later required local radical fasciectomies had more aggressive disease but did have improvement for a considerable period after percutaneous fasciotomy.

▶ This understated article is only 1½ pages long. The authors demonstrate that percutaneous fasciotomy, if performed relatively early (average composite extensor lag at the metacarpophalangeal joint plus the proximal interphalangeal joint of 71 degrees), can result in about one third of the patients either needing or desiring no further surgery during the next 10 years and is associated with essentially no complications. There remains an important role for this procedure, one that warrants closer inspection in this era of managed care.

V.R. Hentz, M.D.

Suggested Reading

Dalrymple NC, Hayes J, Bessinger VJ, et al: MRI of multiple glomus tumors of the finger. *Skeletal Radiol* 26:664–666, 1997.
▶ MRI may be the most helpful modality in the diagnosis of glomus tumors of the terminal phalanx.

V.R. Hentz, M.D.

Jacoulet P, Faure P: Treatment of enchondromas of the hand with bone substitute: Preliminary report of five cases. *J Hand Surg [Br]* 22B:476–478, 1997.
▶ Five patients with solitary enchondroma were treated with curettage and calcium phosphate bone graft substitute. The authors correctly point out that the morbidity for this procedure is less than that of the traditional autograft, even if it is taken from the distal radius. Bone graft substitutes, when used as a filler, are useful and reasonable so long as one keeps in mind that they do not provide much structural integrity. There is no long-term result reported. However, the short term is encouraging.

L.K. Ruby, M.D.

Salamon A: Occurrence of myofibroblasts in recurrent Dupuytren's disease. *J Hand Surg [Br]* 22B:518–520, 1997.
▶ These authors have performed an ultrastructural study on tissue from recurrent Dupuytren's disease from 10 male patients. Myofibroblasts were found in 8 of 10 samples in recurrent Dupuytren's nodules. The authors' findings are in agreement with prior, although scant, literature which indicates that the pathobiology of recurrent Dupuytren's disease is similar to that seen in the initial phases of the disease. However, this study lacks certain details about the sites of recurrence in the 10 patients studied. It is unclear whether the sites studied are at the original location of initial disease or represent an extension of the disease to adjacent fingers. In addition, the authors have made no comment on how the age of the patients, duration of Dupuytren's disease, nor the preoperative severity are correlated, if at all, to the density of myofibroblasts present in the nodules.

M.A. Badalamente, Ph.D.

Varley GW, Needoff M, Davis TR, et al: Conservative management of wrist ganglia: Aspiration versus steroid infiltration. *J Hand Surg [Br]* 22:636–637, 1997.
▶ Important in this randomized study is the fact that the addition of steroid injection following aspiration of a ganglion seems to have no benefit over aspiration alone. The added benefit of aspiration, beyond a 33% success rate, is patient reassurance that the lesion is benign. This often results in the patient's choice to have no further treatment if the ganglion reappears.

R.A. Chase, M.D.

12 Congenital Problems

Operative Correction of Radial Club Hand: A Long-term Follow-up of Centralization of the Hand on the Ulna
Lamb DW, Scott H, Lam WL, et al (Princess Margaret Rose Orthopaedic Hosp, Edinburgh, Scotland)
J Hand Surg [Br] 22B:533–536, 1997   12–1

Objective.—Whereas centralization is the standard technique for treating radial club hand, there is little information about the long-term outcome of this surgery. The clinical and functional results of 21 centralizations for radial club hand in 17 patients treated between 1962 and 1975 were reviewed.

Methods.—Corrective ulnar osteotomy, centralization of the hand on the ulna, and tendon transfer were performed on 43 patients, aged 2–13 years, with 79 radial absences. In 34 cases, the records were sufficient for analysis. Thirteen pollicizations were performed. Upper-limb function was assessed using the Moberg "pick up" test and the Jebsen test. Patients filled out a questionnaire about family life, education, employment, recreation, transport, and self-care activities.

Results.—The forearm was between 50% and 66% of normal length. All patients could complete the Moberg and Jebsen tests. Grip strength was significantly diminished in pollicized hands (5.5 kg) and in nonpollicized hands (4.5 kg). The pinch grip test could not be performed. Of the 17 patients who answered the questionnaire, 2 had attended special schools; 17 had been employed full-time but 5 were now considered disabled; 10 were married, 2 were divorced, and 5 were single; 16 were driving; all managed self-care activities; all had recreational activities; 8 had occasional pain; and 1 complained of surgical scars.

Conclusions.—Overall function of the hand improved after pollicization, but grip strength was still significantly diminished. A pollicized index finger improved the cosmetic look of the hand.

▶ This brief article includes very useful information about the long-term results of centralization. The authors thoroughly studied 17 patients with 21 centralizations at least 21 years (average, 27 years) after their operation. Dr. Lamb's results are especially impressive, considering the average age at centralization of 6.5 years. The findings of the functional assessments and questionnaire provide the hand surgeon with valuable facts to pass along to parents of infants and children with radius deficiency.

The authors note that the distal ulnar physis did not fuse prematurely. This does not tell us, however, whether centralization affected the growth of the ulna, because, at least in mice, radiographic lucency in the region of the physis does not necessarily indicate that the physis is functioning normally.[1] The authors also note the common occurrence of spontaneous ulnocarpal fusion; this is not necessarily a negative outcome, because older children with ulnocarpal fusion after centralization are less likely to show recurrence of radial angulation when they undergo forearm lengthening by distraction osteogenesis.

M.A. James, M.D.

Reference

1. Barr SJ, Zaleske DJ: Physeal reconstruction with blocks of cartilage of varying developmental time. *J Pediatr Orthop* 12:766, 1992.

Evaluation of Five Different Incisions for Correction of Radial Dysplasia
Pilz SM, Muradin MSM, van der Meulen JJNM, et al (AZR Dijkzigt, Rotterdam, The Netherlands)
J Hand Surg [Br] 23B:183–185, 1998
12–2

Introduction.—A short forearm deviating to the radial side is the typical clinical picture of radial dysplasia, and has been described as "a profoundly abnormal hand joined to a poor limb by a bad wrist." The first incision was developed in 1894, which involved resection of the lunate and capitate and fixation of the distal ulna in the newly formed notch. About a century later, an S-shaped incision was developed, which extended on the dorsum from the base of the index finger over the ulnar side of the wrist and across the flexor aspect of the forearm to its radial border. Since then, other types of incisions were also developed. A retrospective evaluation was conducted of the 5 different incisions used for centralization from 1970 to 1996 in patients with radial dysplasia.

Methods.—There were 57 patients with 91 radial club hands seen in a 26-year period, and they were classified according to Bayne's classification system: 29 patients had type I deformity, 11 had type II, 12 had type III, and 39 had type IV. For the 33 patients treated by centralization, 5 different incisional approaches were chosen: the S-shaped incision, S-shaped incision with a dorsal transposition flap, the radial Z-plasty with an excision of the skin on the ulnar side, Z-plasty in the opposite direction, and the "bilobed" flap.

Results.—There were 16 centralizations done with the radial Z-plasty in combination with an ulnar excision. Four patients had 2 opposite Z-plasties that preserved wrist mobility as much as possible. Seven patients had the bilobed flap used in 1995 and 1996. No complications occurred before 1995 with the primary procedures. Venous congestion was seen in all 7 patients where the bilobed flap was used. Superficial necrosis of parts of the flap occurred in 4 of 7 patients. After the standard 8 weeks of cast immobilization, wound healing occurred spontaneously by delayed primary healing in all patients.

Conclusion.—The bilobed flap is currently used as the approach for centralization at the age of 6 months. Six months later, pollicization and opponensplasty can be done if necessary. The bilobed flap can give good access to exposure of the wrist and allows redistribution of the skin without waste. These are advantages that overrule the significant higher incidence of early complications.

▶ These authors present a very large series of patients with radial club hand treated with 5 different incisions. The incisions were classified into 2 groups, the far early flap group and the bilobed flap group. There were no healing problems in the first group. Despite problems with early venous congestion, the authors preferred the bilobed flap because of good exposure and judicious use of skin in coverage. They did not appreciate a learning curve, and combining this flap with a fixator for distraction may minimize the early complications.

J.A. Katarincic, M.D.

A Comparison of Patients With Different Types of Syndactyly
Kramer RC, Hildreth DH, Brinker MR, et al (Shriners Hosp for Children, Houston)
J Pediatr Orthop 18:233–238, 1998   12–3

Introduction.—Occurring at a rate of 1 per 2,000 to 2,500 live births, congenital upper-extremity syndactyly is a common feature, with 50% of cases being bilateral. Incomplete separation of digital rays during the 6th to 8th week of gestational development is the cause of congenital syndactyly. It can be an isolated entity or a syndrome. The functional results after syndactyly release by using a patient's nonoperated-on contralateral hand as a control has never been conducted. The functional outcome after syndactyly release was studied in patients with syndactyly resulting from Poland's syndrome and in patients with idiopathic forms of syndactyly.

Methods.—The retrospective study included patients with 1 involved hand and the control was the contralateral hand. During a 10-year period, 27 patients with only 1 hand involved underwent syndactyly release. The evaluation included 13 patients who had a total of 30 syndactyly releases. A detailed physical examination was conducted on each patient who also participated in occupational therapy.

Results.—In the Poland's syndrome group, statistically significant differences in function between the operated-on and control hands were noted, whereas with the idiopathic forms of syndactyly, the operated-on hands did not demonstrate significantly different function compared with the contralateral controls. Using the Minnesota Rate of Manipulation

Test, an average of 7.1 minutes was required to complete the test with the operated-on hands in the Poland's syndrome group compared with 5.3 minutes to complete the test with the control hands.

Conclusion.—More than syndactyly alone may be responsible for the functional deficits in hands affected by Poland's syndrome. Little postoperative functional deficit is a likely possibility with hands affected by idiopathic forms of syndactyly. There was poor fine-motor and functional ability with the affected hand in the children with Poland's syndrome. A prospective study should be conducted to confirm our results.

▶ The authors should be commended for trying to evaluate the functional results of their syndactyly releases. More of this information is needed in the evaluation of the multiple procedures reported for all types of congenital anomalies. The children with idiopathic syndactyly showed no statistically significant functional deficits postoperatively whereas the children with Poland's syndrome did, particularly in fine motor activity. The poorer function in the Poland's children is attributed to more than the syndactyly alone. The authors comment that comparison of preoperative and postoperative function would be even more valuable, and I would encourage them to pursue this.

J.A. Katarincic, M.D.

Ilizarov Distraction-Lengthening in Congenital Anomalies of the Upper Limb

Hülsbergen-Krüger S, Preisser P, Partecke B-D (Berufsgenossenschaftliches Unfallkrankenhaus, Hamburg, Germany)
J Hand Surg [Br] 23B:192–195, 1998   12–4

Introduction.—There are many advantages to the Ilizarov distraction-lengthening method used for the hand, forearm, and foot, including a remarkable lengthening of bone, avoidance of donor site morbidity, and achievement of additional soft tissue length with correction of multiplanar deformities. A review of patients on whom this method was used was conducted.

Methods.—Ilizarov distraction-lengthening was performed on 9 patients who had congenital anomalies. All patients had other procedures and were late cases. There were 5 patients with radial club hands, 3 with symbrachydactyly and 1 with camptodactyly. An extremely short forearm was the indication for treatment of a radial club hand with differences in forearm length ranging from 8 to 17 cm.

Results.—In the radial club hand, the average amount of lengthening was 5.8 cm with an average fixation time of 184 days. During lengthening, 1 patient had paresthesia of the superficial radial nerve. Flexion contractures of the elbow, wrist, and finger joints were performed in all 5 patients with radial club hand. Two patients with symbrachydactyly of the cleft-hand type achieved a pinch grip between a radial and an ulnar digit by lengthening the short ray. One failure occurred in a patient with the monodactyly type where an attempt was made to lengthen 3 transplanted proximal toe phalanges. There was also a failure in a patient with camptodactyly who had a soft tissue distraction.

Conclusion.—Pin infection is avoided by increasing the stability of frame construction with additional rings and linkage-bars. Pins should be fitted close to the frame without tension. Education on fixator hygiene must be given to patients. When distraction speed is too fast or when the device has been removed too early, fracture or pseudarthrosis of the newly formed bone can occur. Weekly X-rays must be taken to determine the optimum speed. With forearm lengthening, flexion contractures of the wrist and finger joints can occur.

▶ The authors report on the results of distraction lengthening in 9 patients. As with most other authors, they report a significant number of complications and offer suggestions on how to minimize problems. Although they show these operations are technically possible, I challenge the authors to show an improvement in the children's function to justify these surgeries.

J.A. Katarincic, M.D.

The Role of Metacarpophalangeal Pattern (MCPP) Profile Analysis in the Treatment of Triphalangeal Thumbs: Description of a Method and a Case Report
Zguricas J, Dijkstra PF, Hovius SER (Erasmus Univ, Rotterdam, The Netherlands; Academic Med Centre, Rotterdam, The Netherlands)
J Hand Surg [Br] 22B:631–635, 1997   12–5

Objective.—The metacarpophalangeal pattern (MCPP) profile analysis is a method of measuring the length of each of the 19 tubular bones of the hand and comparing the results against a standard that can be plotted on an MCPP plot. The use of MCPP profile analysis in the treatment of congenital hand deformities—specifically in the triphalangeal thumb—was reported.

Methods.—The bones are measured radiographically. A Q-score analysis (Q plot)—where Q is the log to the base 10 of the quotient of the length of the hand bone from a patient and the reference length for that bone—is constructed (Fig 1, B).

> *Case Report.*—An MCPP analysis, performed before surgery, showed a first metacarpal that was 50% too long, the proximal phalanx of the thumb that was 30% too long, and the distal phalanx of the thumb that was 20% too short. At surgery, the thumb was lengthened by using the extra phalanx length provided by means of reduction osteotomy and distal interphalangeal joint (DIP) arthrodesis. The reduction was calculated from the Q plot and measured bone lengths. The first metacarpal was reduced in

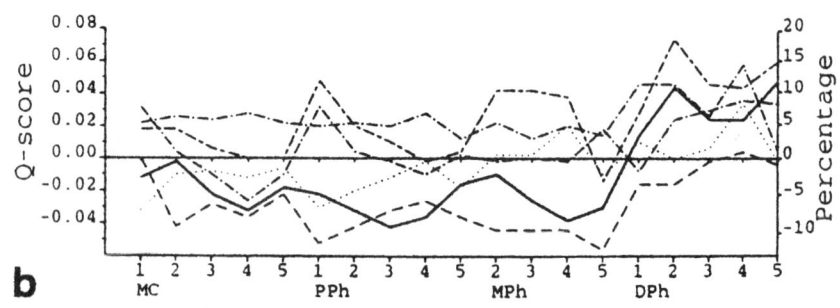

FIGURE 1, B.—Profiles of 6 different hands from 6 normal individuals; the *numbers* on the X axis represent the numbers of the hand bones; the *numbers* on the Y axis represent the percentage difference between the measured length of each individual bone from a patient and the reference length for that bone. The *zero line* represents the mean for the population. Note that there is no clear profile that can be distinguished and that all the measured values fluctuate within the normal range. (Courtesy of Zguricas J, Dijkstra PF, Hovius SER: The role of metacarpophalangeal pattern [MCPP] profile analysis in the treatment of triphalangeal thumbs: Description of a method and a case report. *J Hand Surg [Br]* 22B:631–635, 1997.)

length by 65%, making it 15% too short. The shortness compensated for the longer proximal phalanx, The new distal phalanx was 25% too long because of a slight malunion at the level of DIP arthrodesis.

Conclusion.—The MCPP profile analysis provides a simple, inexpensive method for calculating the correct architecture in a malformed hand. The Q plot takes 5 minutes per patient to generate. Additional studies should be conducted on larger numbers of patients to establish the utility of this method in patients with different hand malformations.

▶ MCPP profile analysis is the graphic representation of the relative lengths of the 19 different hand bones determined by radiographic and mathematical analysis of the hand. This article is the first on MCPP profile analysis to appear in the hand literature. The technique has the potential of being a significant contribution to reconstructive hand surgery.

Although MCPP profile analysis was first described in 1972 in *Radiology* and MCPP profile norms for the population were developed in 1991, it was not until very recently that the more general availability of personal computers and digitizers has enabled this method to be anything more than a research tool available only to a few surgeons. Although its use is still challenging for the average surgeon because of the mastery of technical details required, MCPP profile analysis can put into reproducible scientific terminology what gifted reconstructive hand surgeons like Littler and Buck-Gramko could create from their profound aesthetic understanding of the balance of the hand and the thumb.

If appropriately used, MCPP profile analysis can improve the ability of hand surgeons to plan preoperatively the reconstruction of triphalangeal thumbs and, potentially, other hand anomalies. It is recommended that the reader take note of this concept, as it may be of use.

L.B. Lane, M.D.

Suggested Reading

Anderson PJ, Hall CM, Smith PJ, et al: The hands in Pfeiffer syndrome. *J Hand Surg [Br]* 22B:537–540, 1997.

▶ The authors have collected 19 cases of this rare syndrome. Although the hand anomalies seen in these patients varied, hypoplasia or absence of the middle phalanx of the index or little finger was seen in the majority of patients. They propose that this finding is more useful in establishing the clinical diagnosis of this syndrome than the broad thumb originally described by Pfeiffer.

While this finding is interesting, it is likely to be incidental since, as the authors state, the definitive diagnosis of this syndrome is based on DNA analysis. Because only 3 of 19 patients had deformity sufficient to be referred to a hand surgeon, the information in this article is most likely to be useful to the geneticist.

M.A. James, M.D.

Cheng JCY, Wing-Man K, Shen WY, et al: A new look at the sequential development of elbow-ossification centers in children. *J Pediatr Orthop* 18:161–167, 1998.

▶ Most orthopedic surgeons grew up with the mnemonic *CRITOE* to remember the order of ossification of the bones at the elbow: Capitellum, Radial head, Internal (medial) epicondyle, Trochlea, Olecranon, and External (lateral) epicondyle. On average, these steps occur at ages 1, 5, 7, 9, 11, and 13 years, respectively. That data came from a U.S. study in the 1950s. This study of 1,500 Chinese children from Hong Kong suggests that the order and ages are not universally the same. The olecranon was found to ossify before the trochlea, and many of the ages were younger: 1, 5, 5, 9, 9, and 10 years for the capitellum, radius, medial epicondyle, olecranon, trochlea, and lateral epicondyle, respectively. It is possible that improved nutrition may have accelerated the ossification process over the years, or that ethnic variations exist.

P.C. Amadio, M.D.

Kamishima H, Minami A, Kato H, et al: Operative and histopathological study of the tendon sheath of the snapping digit in children. *J Jpn Soc Surg Hand* 987–990, 1998.

▶ This short article reports pathohistological difference between the tendon sheath of snapping digits in children and in adults. The authors concluded that the basic pathology of snapping digits in children is hyperplasia of the tendon sheath. Comparative histologic pictures of the tendon sheath in adults demonstrate degeneration. I just wonder if the degeneration of the tendon sheath could be a result of the previous injection of steroid, since inflammation is hardly observed there. At any rate, this pathohistological study distinctly differentiates the snapping digit of children from that of adults.

Y. Ueba, M.D., D.M.Sc.

13 Physical and Occupational Medicine

Cumulative Trauma Disorders in the Upper Extremities: Reliability of the Postural and Repetitive Risk-Factors Index
James CPA, Harburn KL, Kramer JF (Scarborough, Ont; Univ of Western Ont, London)
Arch Phys Med Rehabil 78:860–865, 1997   13–1

Purpose.—As the use of video display terminals (VDTs) has increased, so has the incidence of cumulative trauma disorders. Ergonomic improvements in the workplace are widely recommended as a means of preventing these disorders; however, it is not possible to draw any definitive conclusions regarding the contribution of ergonomic factors. There is currently no reliable, valid tool for assessing risky postures associated with VDT use. A measurement tool called the Postural and Repetitive Risk-Factors Index (PRRI) was tested for reliability.

Methods.—The PRRI involves techniques of video analysis of the postures and movements of the head, shoulder, and upper arm. It is based on the concept that movement behaviors are more important than workstation design. Video recordings were analyzed to identify those components of movement behavior thought to be risky, such as repetitiveness, awkward and static postures, and time spent therein. Two-hour videotaped assessments were performed on 2 separate days in 10 heavy users of VDTs in the banking industry. The PRRI criteria were used to assign a postural risk score to the subjects' movements. The test-retest reliability of the PRRI was calculated.

Results.—For any 1 session, the reliability coefficients for the PRRI scores met the minimum criteria for excellent reliability. Two-way analysis of variance also showed no significant difference between sessions. Analysis of the standard error of measurement suggested that a subject with a PRRI score of 25, when tested once on 1 day, would have to show a change of at least 8 points to confirm that a true change had occurred.

Conclusion.—This study demonstrates the reliability of the PRRI for evaluation of patients at risk of cumulative trauma disorders of the upper extremities. It appears to be a reliable measurement instrument that can be used at the job site to predict risk. Between-tester reliability remains to be established.

▶ This study shows that the PRRI proposed by the authors is reliable. It demonstrates that work site evaluations can be performed reliably with VCR cameras. Further study is needed to investigate the validity of this index for subjects with cumulative trauma disorders in the upper extremity.

P.B.J. Wu, M.D., M.P.H.

The Prevalence of Work-related Upper Limb Disorders in a Printing Factory
Trail IA (Wrightington Hosp NHS Trust, Wigan, England)
Occup Med 48:23–26, 1998   13-2

Introduction.—The relationship between problems of the upper limb and the workplace is complicated. The etiology, pathogenesis, and even existence of work-related upper limb disorders are controversial. Employees of a large printing company were evaluated to determine the value of a detailed medical and ergonomic assessment of the workplace in the prevention of work-related upper limb disorders.

Methods.—Workforce members completed a questionnaire regarding age, sex, occupation, length of employment, presence of upper limb problems, and workers' opinions as to how their upper limb problem started. All employees who reported upper limb problems were interviewed and underwent clinical examination. A thorough ergonomic evaluation of the workplace was undertaken, and recommendations were made regarding ergonomic changes. The three areas of concern were collating, knocking-up and jogging, and use of the guillotine. Recommendations included addition of upper limb evaluation to preplacement medical screening, education of employees, immediate medical assessment of any employees complaining of upper limb problems, and specific worksite modifications. Twelve months later all employees were given an identical questionnaire, and those who reported upper limb problems were examined.

Results.—Sixty-three of 179 employees completed the questionnaire. Of these, 44 underwent examination of the upper limbs. Of 38 employees involved in the knocking-up and jogging process, 15 had upper limb problems. Seven of 31 employees who worked on the guillotine and 3 of 5 operators who worked the Harris collator had upper limb problems. Twelve months after modifications were introduced, 61 of 170 employees returned questionnaires. Twenty-four employees working at the aforementioned problem work sites complained of upper limb problems.

Conclusion.—A reduction in the number of upper limb problems was realized at 12-month follow-up after recommended ergonomic changes were made in a printing factory. The prevalence of upper limb problems in the workplace can be controlled with appropriate ergonomic and medical input.

▶ The author states that this article is not intended to further clarify controversial issues regarding etiology, pathogenesis, or even the existence of work-related upper limb disorders. Thus, the reader should not interpret the findings as confirming work-related origins. Many of the upper extremity conditions and symptoms described in the article could have resulted from personal fitness issues, avocational activities, prior trauma, or metabolic conditions. Nevertheless, any program that succeeds in making the workplace more comfortable is to be applauded. Musculoskeletal complaints, regardless of origin, respond favorably to reduction in required level of physical demand, as demonstrated by the author. The observation that workplace modifications result in decreased reporting of symptoms does not confirm that such modifications are curative of specific, diagnosed conditions of the upper extremities, such as carpal tunnel syndrome.

P.A. Nathan, M.D.

Effects of Static Fingertip Loading on Carpal Tunnel Pressure
Rempel D, Keir PJ, Smutz WP, et al (Univ of California—San Francisco; NASA Ames Research Ctr, Moffet Field, Calif)
J Orthop Res 15:422–426, 1997

Background.—Although the pathophysiology of carpal tunnel syndrome has yet to be defined, it is suspected that increases in carpal tunnel pressure are involved. One of the ways to increase carpal tunnel pressure is to load the fingertips. This article assesses the effects of fingertip loading on changes in carpal tunnel pressure in normal subjects.

Methods.—A saline-filled catheter was inserted into the carpal tunnel of the nondominant hand in 15 healthy subjects (8 women and 7 men, 23 to 50 years old). The catheter was fitted to a pressure transducer that was kept level with the carpal tunnel by means of a jig for holding the arm and the transducer. Then, subjects used the tip of the index finger to press on a load cell with forces of 0, 6, 9, and 12 N. Ten different wrist positions were used: 15, 30, or 45 degrees of extension, the neutral position, 15, 30, or 45 degrees of flexion, 10 degrees of radial deviation, and 10 and 20 degrees of ulnar deviation.

Findings.—At all 10 wrist positions, fingertip loading significantly increased the carpal tunnel pressure over values with no loading. Even putting the wrist into the neutral position to start the study caused a mean increase in carpal tunnel pressure from 7.2 mm Hg before the study to 19.7, 44.6, 53.1, and 56.5 mm Hg with fingertip loads of 0, 6, 9, and 12, respectively (Fig 2). Both the fingertip force and the angle of the wrist had significant effects on carpal tunnel pressure. At all wrist positions, a

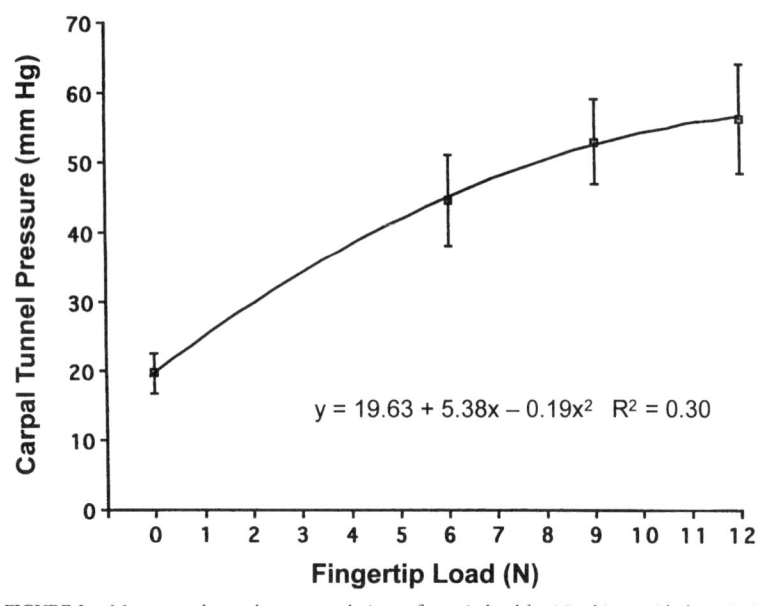

FIGURE 2.—Mean carpal tunnel pressure relative to fingertip load for 15 subjects with the wrist in the neutral position. *Error bars* represent standard error of the mean. The *line* represents a second-order polynomial fit of the data. (Courtesy of Rempel D, Keir PJ, Smutz WP, et al: Effects of static fingertip loading on carpal tunnel pressure. *J Orthop Res* 14:422–426, 1997.)

Equation shown in figure: $y = 19.63 + 5.38x - 0.19x^2$, $R^2 = 0.30$

fingertip force of 12N was associated with significantly greater carpal tunnel pressure than a force of 6N.

Conclusions.—Carpal tunnel pressure increased with any amount of fingertip loading and with any change of the wrist angle away from neutral. Effects of fingertip loading were stronger than those of wrist angle, indicating that fingertip loading forces (similar to those used in a pinch grip) are more important in determining pressures in the carpal tunnel.

▶ It is a quantum leap to establish a relationship between "sustained grip and pinch activities" and carpal tunnel syndrome from the authors' data on the relationship between fingertip loading and carpal tunnel pressures. The presented data suggest a methodology overly sensitive to slight fluctuations in carpal tunnel pressure. For instance, the mean baseline pressure in neutral before a subject assumes the "test posture" was 7.2 mm Hg which elevated to 19.7 mmHg when placed in the neutral test posture which was pronation. Earlier work presented by the authors showed higher pressures in the carpal tunnel in supination than in pronation. Many previous studies (referenced by the authors) in which carpal tunnel pressures were measured reported much lower carpal tunnel pressures when the forearm was supinated and the wrist was in neutral position. Therefore, the pressures in this study are all on the rather high side in comparison to what we are used to from the literature. In the study presented here, 10 degrees of radial deviation produced higher carpal tunnel pressures than *20* degrees of ulnar deviation with all fingertip loads applied producing an argument *against* all so-called ergonomically designed keyboards which avoid ulnar deviation. In fact, 10 degrees of ulnar deviation of the wrist produced *lower* carpal tunnel pressures than the neutral position with all forces applied to the fingertip. This experiment on 15 healthy subjects is interesting, but how it relates to any disease mechanism or aggravation is highly speculative.

R.M. Szabo, M.D., M.P.H.

Botulinum Toxin Does Not Reverse the Cortical Dysfunction Associated With Writer's Cramp: A PET Study
Ceballos-Baumann AO, Sheean G, Passingham RE, et al (Hammersmith Hosp, England; Inst of Neurology, London; Dept of Experimental Psychology, Oxford, England; et al)
Brain 120:571–582, 1997
13–4

Introduction.—Simple writer's cramp becomes a manifestation of focal arm dystonia if the involuntary muscle spasms also interfere with other actions. Activity in central motor pathways during writer's cramp can be studied noninvasively using $H_2^{15}O$-PET activation studies. Such studies on patients with idiopathic torsion dystonia previously demonstrated overactive striatum and frontal accessory areas and underactivity of the primary motor cortex and caudal supplementary motor area during volitional movement. To see if patients with writer's cramp showed a similar pattern, activation of the motor system was compared in healthy control subjects and patients with writer's cramp.

Methods.—The study included 2 men and 4 women with a mean age of 53 years, afflicted with writer's cramp. Five of the 6 were studied twice, before and after botulinum toxin. The 6 control subjects were 1 woman and 5 men, with a mean age of 47. All participants were right handed. Those with writer's cramp had no evidence of widespread dystonia. Both groups wrote a stereotyped word repetitively at a paced rate before and after treatment with botulinum toxin.

Results.—As in patients with idiopathic torsion dystonia, those with writer's cramp exhibited impaired activation of the contralateral primary motor cortex. Frontal association cortex, however, showed enhanced activation. Treatment with botulinum toxin improved writing and increased activation in parietal cortex and caudal supplementary motor area, but failed to improve the impaired activation of the primary motor cortex.

Discussion.—Impaired activation of primary motor cortex is involved in writer's cramp. Compared with normal control subjects, frontal association areas and parietal association areas in patients with writer's cramp showed greater activation.

Conclusion.—Treatment with botulinum toxin enhanced activation of parietal cortex and motor accessory areas, but the impaired activation of primary motor cortex was not normalized.

▶ The use of neuromuscular blockade with botulinum A toxin, 45% alcohol or phenol, has been documented in the management of posttraumatic spasticity. Currently, the use of botulinum A toxin is the primary modality for the management of dystonic posturing with pain, which includes writer's cramp. This study documents the efficacy of botulinum A toxin in writer's cramp, suggesting that alterations in movement strategy or cortical reorganization may be the mechanism involved. Our experience with botulinum A toxin in writer's cramp is mixed. All patients do not respond. However, in those patients who do respond, botulinum A toxin remains the treatment of choice for the management of dystonic writer's cramp.

L.A. Koman, M.D.

Instrument-specific Rates of Upper-Extremity Injuries in Music Students
Cayea D, Manchester RA (Univ of Rochester, NY)
Med Probl Perform Art 13:19–25, 1998   13–5

Introduction.—Musculoskeletal injuries of musicians have been reported with increasing frequency in the past decade. Most reports have described injury incidence rates for categories of musicians. Instrument-specific rates of upper-extremity problems caused by playing an instrument were assessed at a university-level music school in a longitudinal investigation of a single population.

Methods.—Data regarding all musculoskeletal problems of members of the prepaid student health plan were reviewed for academic years 1982–1983 through 1995–1996. Data were abstracted regarding upper-extremity musculoskeletal problems linked to playing of musical instruments. Instrument-specific rates (number of injuries per 100 performance major student years) were calculated.

Results.—During the 14-year observation period, students majoring in instrumental performance were seen for 513 performance-related injuries. The overall injury rate was 8.3. Instruments were categorized into low-, medium-, or high-rate tertiles based on their associated injury rates. Instruments in the low tertile (rate, 0–5.9) included all the brass instruments and the oboe and bassoon. Medium-injury-rate instruments (6.0–11.9) included all the bowed string instruments, the saxophone, clarinet, organ, flute, and percussion. The high-injury-rate instruments (12.0–18.0) included the piano, guitar, and harp. The overall injury rate was higher for female than for male musicians (8.9 vs. 5.9).

Conclusion.—Gender-specific data were not available for all 14 years; thus, sample size was small. This diminished the chance of finding smaller gender-specific differences. This is the first report of instrument-specific injury rates, so only broad comparisons can be made between these findings and results of trials assessing injury prevalence in groups of instruments. Musicians with the highest injury rates played string or keyboard instruments. The injury rate was significantly higher for female than for male musicians.

▶ This study improves on the previous epidemiologic studies of musicians' injuries. Cayea and Manchester follow a select group of musicians longitudinally over a 14-year period, relying on physician visit reports to establish diagnosis and frequency. Some previous studies have used patient self-report surveys to gather data on frequency and type of injury.[1,2] Others used the experience of a single physician.[3-5] This study uses medical records from visits to a student health service. Therefore, the data are not based on a layman's or patient's self-report or on the biases of a single clinician. The authors also report instrument-specific injury rates, which have not been studied before. Even though the literature on musicians' injuries has swelled over the last 15 years, the subject is still scantily studied, and well-performed studies such as this are highly welcomed.

K.A. Bengtson, M.D.

References

1. Fishbein M, Middlestadt SE, Ottati V, et al: Medical problems among ICSOM musicians: Overview of a national survey. *Med Probl Perform Art* 3:1, 1988.
2. Caldron PH, Calabrese LH, Clough JD, et al: A survey of musculoskeletal problems encountered in high-level musicians. *Med Probl Perform Art* 1:136, 1986.
3. Fry HJH: Incidence of overuse syndrome in the symphony orchestra. *Med Probl Perform Art* 1:51–55, 1986.
4. Fry HJH: Prevalence of overuse (injury) syndrome in Australian music schools. *Br J Industr Med* 44:35–40, 1987.
5. Fry HJH: Overuse syndrome of the upper limb in musicians. *Med J Aust* 144:182, 1986.

Playing-related Musculoskeletal Disorders in Musicians: A Systematic Review of Incidence and Prevalence
Zaza C (Univ of Western Ontario, London)
Can Med Assoc J 158:1019–1025, 1998
13–6

Background.—Performing arts medicine is a growing field. A systematic review of the literature on the incidence and prevalence of playing-related musculoskeletal disorders (PRMDs) in classical musicians was presented.

Methods.—Seven databases were searched to identify reports published between 1980 and 1996. Eighteen cross-sectional surveys and cohort studies were reviewed.

Findings.—The incidence of PRMD was estimated in only 1 study. Because of low response rates and other methodological problems, 10 of the 17 prevalence studies were not eligible for data combination. In the 7 eligible studies, PRMD point prevalences ranged from 39% to 87% in adults and from 34% to 62% in secondary school music students. The best PRMD prevalence estimates were derived from 3 studies that excluded mild symptoms. In these studies, PRMD prevalence ranged from 39% to 47% in adults and was 17% in secondary school music students.

Conclusions.—The prevalence of PRMD in adult classical musicians is apparently comparable with that of work-related musculoskeletal disorders in other occupational groups. Further research is needed.

▶ During the last 15–20 years, the medical literature on musical performance-related illness has gradually advanced. Zaza nicely reviews the literature on prevalence and incidence of such illnesses. Clearly, the studies of musical problems have many deficiencies. However, this area of medicine is still in its infancy and lacks dedicated researchers with adequate funding to pursue longitudinal studies. Despite the limitation of these studies, their conclusions are notable. Most importantly, these performance-related illnesses are quite common and greatly affect the act of making music. More published studies are needed to advance knowledge in this area and to raise awareness with hand practitioners.

K.A. Bengtson, M.D.

Determinants of Use of Outpatient Rehabilitation Services Following Upper Extremity Injury
McCarthy ML, Ewashko T, MacKenzie EJ (Johns Hopkins Univ, Baltimore, Md; Community Rehabilitation Program, Calgary, Alta)
J Hand Ther 11:32–38, 1998   13–7

Background.—Most injuries to the upper extremity occur in working-aged adults; about one third of industrial injuries affect the arm and hand. The experience at a statewide hand referral center was reviewed to assess factors associated with referral for rehabilitation services after severe upper-extremity injury.

Methods.—The analysis included 112 patients referred for isolated injuries to the upper extremity, distal to and including the elbow, over 9 months in 1990. The study was conducted at a hand-trauma referral center serving the entire state of Maryland. Seven months after injury, each patient was interviewed about using rehabilitation services. Patient characteristics examined included disability compensation and Abbreviated Injury Scale score. Information gathered on rehabilitation services included the use, setting, intensity, and frequency of outpatient therapy services. The patients were also asked about other health care services, such as rehospitalization, doctor visits, special equipment, or vocational services. Unmet need was assessed by asking patients whether they felt they received adequate outpatient and other services.

Findings.—The patients were predominantly white men who were working before their injury occurred. Twenty-two percent were uninsured. About half of the injuries were work-related. About one fifth of the patients received no therapy services after their injury. At 7 months' follow-up, the patients had made a mean of 29 therapy visits. Eighty-seven percent of patients started outpatient therapy within 1 month after hospital discharge. Only 16% of patients said they received vocational services. Nearly one third of patients said they would have liked to receive vocational services but did not, because of either barriers or lack of awareness.

Injury severity was the factor with the greatest effect on use of outpatient services. Other variables associated with a higher number of therapy visits included female sex, nonwhite race, having health insurance, and receiving disability insurance. The effect of disability compensation on therapy services increased as the severity of injury decreased. About one fourth of patients felt they had not received sufficient services. Factors associated with the perception of unmet need included nonwhite race and lack of insurance.

Conclusions.—For patients with upper-extremity injuries, use of outpatient rehabilitative therapy services varies significantly. The amount of services received increases with severity of injury, suggesting that the patients in greatest need of services are most likely to receive them. Other patient characteristics and resources affected use of outpatient services as well. Being on disability compensation increases services received, particularly among patients with less severe injuries.

▶ This article from the Raymond B. Curtis Hand Center of Union Memorial Hospital documents the use of outpatient rehabilitation services among patients who suffered a hand injury severe enough to warrant hospitalization.

If you can stick with a detailed report of patient demographics, you will find some statistical analysis to support the clinical observations that we all make each day as we treat the hand-injured patient: Patients who had insurance received twice as many treatments as those who did not; women received an average of 3 times more therapy than men; patients with the less severe injuries had the greatest complaints; the difference between the amount of therapy service received by patients with disability compensation and the amount received by those without was much greater when the injury was minor than when the injury was moderate to severe. The authors acknowledge that the results should be interpreted with caution because the sample was small, with significant variations in types of injuries, and because the data are based on patient recall. The authors do conclude, however, that the use of rehabilitation services following upper-extremity injury is influenced by injury severity, disability compensation, and insurance status.

There are few outcome studies in hand therapy that support or focus on the use of therapy after injury, and the information provided in this study needs to be updated. The study includes 9 months from 1990 to 1991. No doubt the single most important variable today would be the allowed number of patient visits, as approved by the insurance adjustor or managed care plan. Another important variable might be access to care for the indigent patient. Many for-profit large rehabilitation facilities formed by mergers and acquisitions dominate the market now and do not accept nonpaying patients.

R.B. Evans, O.T.R./L., C.H.T.

Vibrotactile Sense and Hand Symptoms in Blue Collar Workers in a Manufacturing Industry
Flodmark BT, Lundborg G (Svedala-Skuruphälsan AB, Sweden; Malmö Univ, Lund, Sweden)
Occup Environ Med 54:880–887, 1997   13–8

Introduction.—Workers exposed to vibration can experience impairment in nerve function, reflected in changes in nerve conduction and vibrotactile sense. A group of workers employed in rock-crushing plants took part in a study that tested a screening procedure for sensorineural symptoms to be used in the health care service.

Methods.—The setting of the study was a rural community in the south of Sweden. A total of 159 male workers were invited and 135 agreed to participate. Ninety-four men had previous or current vibration exposure, 22 were engaged in heavy manual work but had no vibration exposure, and 19 were young trainees. All participants completed a questionnaire designed to elicit information about exposure to vibration, smoking, medical history, and 9 subjective symptoms. The index and little fingers of both hands were examined for vibrotactile sense. Clinical examination included tests for median nerve function, ulnar nerve function, 2-point discrimination, and Allen's test for ulnar artery function.

Results.—A correlation was found between impairment in vibrotactile sense and impairment in grip force, cold sensitivity, and other sensorineural symptoms. In only those workers with the poorest vibrotactile sense were clinical findings such as Phalen's test and 2-point discrimination related. When workers were grouped according to the Stockholm workshop scale (sensorineural staging), an increased severity of sensorineural symptoms was reflected in an increased tendency for numbness in the hands and fingers, decreased grip strength, wrist and finger pain, and hand or arm tremors. Workers with decreased vibrotactile sense were more likely to have muscle and joint problems.

Conclusion.—Assessment of vibrotactile sense by tactilometry can be a useful tool for assessing vibration-induced neuromuscular symptoms and confirming worker complaints. Mean vibrotactile sense was similar in vibration-exposed and nonexposed groups, indicating that heavy manual labor without vibration may result in impairment.

▶ The author should have had a nonworking matched control cohort. The reader should understand that all parameters used in this study are subjective, and should also understand this is a surveillance study and, therefore, not valid to establish causation. There was no measurement of dose.

M.L. Kasdan, M.D.

Haemodynamic Changes in Ipsilateral and Contralateral Fingers Caused by Acute Exposures to Hand Transmitted Vibration
Bovenzi M, Griffin MJ (Univ of Trieste, Italy; Univ of Southampton, England)
Occup Environ Med 54:566–576, 1997

Background.—Those who use handheld vibrating tools at work can experience digital blanching or vibration-induced white finger as a result of vasospasm of digital vessels. The effects of exposure to different combinations of magnitudes and frequencies of vibration on finger blood flow (FBF), finger systolic pressure (FSP), and finger skin temperature (FST) were examined in both vibrated and nonvibrated fingers of normal volunteers. These results were compared to the assumptions used for occupational exposure in the current international standard ISO 5349.

Methods.—The study group consisted of 8 healthy volunteers aged 23–44 years. None of these men had occupational exposure to vibrating tools. The FST, FBF, and FSP were assessed in the fingers of both hands. With a static load of 10 N, the right hand was exposed for 30 minutes to each of these root mean squared (rms) acceleration magnitudes and frequencies of vertical vibration: 22 m/sec^{-2} at 31.5 Hz, 22 m/sec^{-2} at 125 Hz, and 87 m/sec^{-2} at 125 Hz. Measures of digital circulation and vasomotor tone were taken before vibration and static load exposure and at 0, 20, 40, and 60 minutes after the end of exposure.

Results.—Exposure to the static load alone did not cause any significant changes in FST, FBF, or any changes in vasomotor tone in either exposed or unexposed digits. Exposure to a vibration of 125 Hz and 22 m/sec^{-2} was associated with a greater decrease in FBF and vasomotor tone in both digits than exposure to a vibration of 31.5 Hz and 22 m/sec^{-2}. In the exposed finger, a vibration of 125 Hz and 87 m/sec^{-2} caused an immediate vasodilation, which was followed by a vasoconstriction during recovery. The nonexposed finger had a significant increase in vasomotor tone throughout the 60-minute recovery period.

Conclusions.—Exposure of healthy controls to hand-transmitted vibration causes changes in digital circulatory response, which depend on the magnitude and frequency of the applied vibration. Exposure to a vibration of 125 Hz and 87 m/sec^{-2} rms acceleration magnitudes produced immediate, transitory increases in blood flow in the exposed digit through a local mechanism. This was followed by a vasoconstriction in both the exposed and nonexposed digit, suggesting involvement of a central sympathetic reflex mechanism. Exposure to a vibration of 31.5 or 125 Hz with a lower acceleration magnitude caused an increase in vasomotor tone in both exposed and unexposed digits throughout the recovery period. The pattern of the responses of the digital vessels to acute vibration with various combinations of frequencies and accelerations does not support the occupational standards currently employed in ISO 5349. More research is needed to understand the effects of chronic occupational exposure to hand-transmitted vibration.

▶ This article demonstrates that digital circulation can be affected by both the frequency and magnitude of vibration. Although this manuscript demonstrates that the stimulation of vibration and amplitude impact can induce changes in vascular response, these data do not address long-term influences on microcirculation and are not appropriate to define vibration as a causal agent in secondary Raynaud's phenomenon. This information provides support of the inappropriateness of international standards based upon incomplete data.

L.A. Koman, M.D.

Comparison Between Single Injection Transthecal and Subcutaneous Digital Blocks
Low CK, Wong HP, Low YP (Tan Tock Seng Hosp, Singapore)
J Hand Surg [Br] 22B:582–584, 1997   13–10

Objective.—The single-injection transthecal digital block can anesthetize the entire digit. The single subcutaneous injection sometimes does not anesthetize the dorsal digital nerves. Anesthesia to the dorsum of the digit using transthecal single injection was compared with subcutaneous single injection by means of a randomized, double-blind study.

Methods.—A total of 142 patients (14 female) admitted for finger surgery were randomly allocated to receive (1) a single injection transthecal block using 3 mL of lignocaine and bupivacaine (n = 71, 86 digits) or (2) a single subcutaneous injection of the same mixture (n = 71, 80 digits). Surgery was performed by 2 physicians blinded to the technique used. Anesthesia was determined by the pin-prick test at 1 and 5 minutes and at 5-minute intervals for 30 minutes after injection. Complications during the 2 weeks after surgery were to be reported by the patients.

Results.—Anesthesia was achieved in 83 of 86 digits (97%) in group 1 and in 75 of 80 digits (94%) in group 2. No complications were reported for either technique.

Conclusion.—Both anesthesia techniques were equally effective. Although there were no differences in effectiveness, distribution, onset, or duration, the subcutaneous technique was easier to use.

▶ In spite of the potential advantage (1 needle-stick), the transthecal route of digital anesthetic administration has not been widely accepted. For me, the real disadvantage is the perception that transthecal injections are unpleasant, i.e., they hurt the patient if the injection is truly within the flexor sheath. The palm seems to be a more sensitive area than, for example, the dorsal skin of the web. A single subcutaneous injection to the mid-digital nerve would avoid the discomfort associated with distending the digital flexor sheath but still require inserting the needle through the sensitive palmar skin. This single-injection technique is perhaps preferred in an infant or uncooperative child, for whom any discomfort is maximum discomfort.

V.R. Hentz, M.D.

Functional Distal Interphalangeal Joint Splinting for Trigger Finger in Laborers: A Review and Cadaver Investigation
Rodgers JA, McCarthy JA, Tiedeman JJ (Univ of Nebraska, Omaha)
Orthopedics 21:305–310, 1998 13–11

Introduction.—There is ongoing debate about many aspects of stenosing tenosynovitis or trigger finger. Treatment has generally consisted of surgery, which carries substantial morbidity. Most reports of conservative treatment have focused on corticosteroid injections. This study evaluated the results of functional splinting of the distal interphalangeal (DIP) joint as a treatment for trigger finger.

Methods.—The study included 21 meat-packing workers with stenosing tenosynovitis. A total of 31 fingers were affected. Symptoms had been present for a mean of 5 months; each patient's work involved repetitive gripping of knives. The ring finger was affected in 42% of cases and the long finger in 32%. All patients were managed with full-time DIP joint splinting with Alumafoam taped to the dorsum of the digit, or with a Stax splint. If there was no improvement by 6 weeks, the patient was offered corticosteroid injection; if there was still no improvement 6 weeks later, surgical release was offered. The study definition of treatment success was complete resolution of symptoms, or painless clicking that did not interfere with function. In addition, cadaver studies were performed to evaluate the effects of DIP splinting on excursion of the flexor digitorum profundus tendon.

Results.—Treatment with functional DIP splinting was successful in 81% of fingers and 71% of patients. Corticosteroid injection was performed in 32% of successfully treated digits and 40% of successfully treated patients. The success rate of splinting alone was 55% of digits and 52% of patients. Most patients returned to modified duties. There were 4 recurrences, all of which responded to splinting or injection. The treatment-failure rate was 29% of digits and 19% of patients. Symptom duration was longer in the treatment-failure group, 12 vs. 5 months. The treatment-failure group were also more likely to have stage 3 vs. stage 2 triggering.

In the cadaver study, splinting decreased flexor digitorum profundus excursion by 4.2 mm with a dorsal Alumafoam splint and by 4.8 mm with a Stax splint.

Conclusions.—Functional splinting of the DIP joint appears to be a useful treatment for trigger finger. Cadaver studies suggest that DIP splinting may work by decreasing excursion of the flexor digitorum profundus tendon. The dorsal Alumafoam splint appears to be the most convenient and functional splint, and is well tolerated on the job.

▶ The authors present an easy and inexpensive treatment for the triggering digit in the manual laborer. A 1-joint dorsal splint allows adequate hand function while limiting power grip, which will decrease tendon-pulley pressures at A1. I have found that this splint is most effective with early triggers with uneven tendon movement, occasional locking, and full posterior interphalangeal (PIP) motion. Limiting profundus motion, even the 4–5 mm noted in the cadaver portion of this study, with the 1-joint splint may allow the 2 edematous tendons to glide differentially through the chiasm and A1 pulley areas, decreasing friction and accommodating volume discrepancies between tendon and pulley. Clinically, splinting the DIP joint appears to decrease tendon excursion enough that in some cases the digit will not trigger at the end arc of flexion.

Repetitive finger flexion movements, external forces against the A1 pulley area when working with tools, and associated carpal tunnel also need to be addressed in the treatment of triggering digits, by using a larger-handled tool, limiting forceful gripping, and wearing fingertip-free work gloves with a gel-perm interface through the palmar area. Carpal tunnel symptoms also need managment, when they exist.

With more advanced triggers, patients with loss of PIP joint flexion, or "compulsive grippers" (those patients who constantly move their digits in an effort to relieve symptoms), it is often necessary to fit the patient with a hand-based splint that blocks the metaphalangeal joints of the affected digits in extension and leaves the PIP joints free.[1] This decreases pressures at the A1 level by 500–700 mm Hg, because flexion into the distal palmar crease is disallowed,[2] and redirects flexor forces to the PIP level. All patients should sleep in a volar digital extension splint which positions the PIP and DIP joints in full extension to correct flexion contracture and to prevent painful nocturnal triggering. Splinting thumb triggers with a dorsal interphalangeal joint splint is also an effective treatment technique.

The authors have provided an excellent solution for conservative management of the triggering digit in the laborer. They have concluded that this technique works best when initiated in the earliest stages of inflammation.

R.B. Evans, O.T.R./L., C.H.T.

References

1. Evans RB, Hunter JM, Burkhalter WE: Conservative management of the trigger finger: A new approach. *J Hand Ther* 1:59–68, 1988.
2. Azar CA, Fleeggler EJ, Culver JE: Dynamic anatomy of the flexor pulley system of the fingers and thumb. Presented at the Second International Meeting for International Federation of Societies for Surgery of the Hand, Boston, October, 1983.

Percutaneous Treatment of Trigger Finger: 34 Fingers Followed 0.5–2 Years
Cihantimur B, Akin S, Özcan M (Uludag Univ, Bursa, Turkey)
Acta Orthop Scand 69:167–168, 1998

Background.—Stenosing tenosynovitis, a common clinical entity, results from a disproportion between a flexor tendon and its sheath. Initial manifestations are pain, swelling, and triggering of the affected digit during finger motion. The efficacy and safety of treatment with percutaneous release of the A1 pulley were investigated.

> *Technique.*—With the finger held firmly and hyperextended at the metacarpophalangeal joint, a 22-gauge needle is inserted into the flexor tendon. Hyperextension is essential because it causes the flexor tendon sheath to lie directly under the skin, permitting the digital neurovascular bundles to displace to either side. After the needle position is confirmed, the needle is withdrawn slightly until it stops moving with flexion of the fingertip, when the needle will be lying in the A1 pulley. A 16-gauge angiocath needle is inserted to the same depth along the previous needle track, and the A1 pulley is cut by moving the needle bevel longitudinally from proximal to distal. The surgeon feels a grating sensation as the needle tip cuts through the transverse fibers of the A1 pulley. When this sensation stops, the release is complete. The patient then flexes and extends the finger to confirm successful cutting.

Patients and Outcomes.—Thirty patients with 34 fingers affected by stenosing tenosynovitis were treated with this procedure. In all digits, complete release was achieved. No further treatments were required. All fingers regained full range of motion, with no triggering. Pain relief was complete in 32 digits and partial in 2 at the 6-week follow-up. All patients were satisfied with the results of the procedure. At the 2-month follow-up, 1 patient reported local swelling and induration in the long finger. No long-term complications occurred.

Conclusions.—The best treatment for short-term stenosing tenosynovitis is probably steroid injection. However, when this treatment is inadequate, percutaneous release of the A1 pulley with a needle appears to be the best approach.

▶ This technique can be useful but, in my opinion, not for the thumb. As with open release, percutaneous release should be a second-line treatment if injection fails. Patient selection is critical; the ideal patients are those with a visibly locking and unlocking proximal interphalangeal joint, in whom the result of percutaneous A1 release will be dramatically evident instantly. Workers in dirty environments who want to miss little work and to avoid an incision, and patients with trigger finger and an unrelated, overlying, asymptomatic Dupuytren's cord, which should not be irritated with an open release, are the ideal candidates. Having said this, I fear that percutaneous release is 1 of those procedures with a very steep learning curve. In light of the success, with minimal complications, of open release, this technique will probably not gain wide acceptance.

Technically, I do not agree that metacarpophalangeal joint hyperextension is "essential." Rather to avoid digital nerve injury, as well as serial longitudinal lacerations in the flexor tendons, it is imperative to stay in the midline over the A1 pulley with the needle cut, and not to quickly, repetitively cut the A1 pulley. I have performed this procedure in patients in the operating room, and in cadavers, followed by immediate open release to see what was cut, and have documented longitudinal lacerations in the superficialis and profundus tendons.

J.M. Failla, M.D.

Suggested Reading

Bell PM, Crumpton L: A fuzzy linguistic model for the prediction of carpal tunnel syndrome risks in an occupational environment. *Ergonomics* 40:790–799, 1997.
▶ This is a case control study. The surgery for carpal tunnel syndrome does not indicate that the diagnosis is correct. Certainly, because this is a case control study, causation cannot be implied or established. Personal attributes were not evaluated. The series is too small to provide predictability or preventability. It involves a cross-sectional study that may not be satisfactory for epidemiologic criteria.

M.L. Kasdan, M.D.

Hughes S, Gibbs J, Dunlop D, et al: Predictors of decline in manual performance in older adults. *J Am Geriatr Soc* 45:905–910, 1997.
▶ The authors study 485 people of 60 years of age or older. Many variables were considered, including physician measures of joint impairment. This study suggests that joint impairment may be an important factor for future functional limitation, and the authors conclude that the development and testing of interventions to maintain or restore upper extremity function are of high priority for an aging population such as exists in the United States and many other industrialized countries of the world.

V.R. Hentz, M.D.

Keir PJ, Bacj JM, Rempel DM: Fingertip loading and carpal tunnel pressure: Differences between a pinching and a pressing task. *J Ortho Res* 16:112–115, 1998.
▶ The repeated and sustained elevated carpal tunnel pressure has been considered as a potential cause of the carpal tunnel syndrome. In this study, the authors successfully measured the carpal tunnel pressure associated with the fingertip loading. In general, the pressure increased with the increase of the fingertip loading. In addition, the pressure was significantly higher in the pinch function than in pressing task. These findings were interesting and might have significant implications in clinic evaluation and ergonomic consideration. However, explanations of these findings are somewhat difficult based on the current understanding of the carpal tunnel anatomy and biomechanics. In the past, the tunnel pressures had been measured extensively by numerous investigators. It is important to recognize that, depending on the transducer used, there were 2 different

types of pressures measured: the contact pressure and the hydrodynamic pressure. The contact pressure mechanically applied to the median nerve is directly related to the amount of tendon tension and the angle in contact with the nerve. On the other hand, the hydrodynamic pressure in the tunnel is more related to the change of the volume and the pressure applied to the surrounding wall of the tunnel. In this study, the tunnel hydrodynamic pressure was measured. The increase of the pressure with the increase of the fingertip force and the differences in the pressure measurement between pinching and pressing are most likely due to the involvement of the intrinsic muscles of the thumb and the lumbrical muscles of the finger. More studies of the biomechanic interaction of intrinsic muscles to the tunnel pressure need to be considered in the future.

K.-N. An, M.D.

Keller K, Corbett J, Nichols D: Repetitive strain injury in computer keyboard users: Pathomechanics and treatment principles in individual and group intervention. *J Hand Ther* 11:9–26, 1998.
▶ This article is subtitled "Pathomechanics and treatment principles in individual and group intervention." The authors, a physical therapist, an occupational therapist, and a social worker, describe their concept of keyboard-related discomfort as a "kinetic-chain, multifactorial disorder" in which postural changes away from the ideal play a significant role. They describe approaching the problem from a multidisciplinarian standpoint with the goal of educating the individual and providing him or her the principles of self-management. I found this to be an interesting article, one that reinforced my bias that there may be little need for the physician and even less need for the surgeon in the treatment paradigm.

V.R. Hentz, M.D.

Nordstrom DL, Vierkant RA, DeStefano F, et al: Risk factors for carpal tunnel syndrome in a general population. *Occup Environ Med* 54:734–740, 1997.
▶ The authors have failed to establish a verified diagnosis of carpal tunnel syndrome and are accepting the ICD-9 code as confirmation of the diagnosis. This is not sound or valid methodology.

M.L. Kasdan, M.D.

Tanaka S, Wild DK, Cameron LL, et al: Association of occupational and non-occupational risk factors with the prevalence of self-reported carpal tunnel syndrome in a national survey of the working population. *Am J Ind Med* 32:550–556, 1997.
▶ This manuscript does not establish a valid diagnosis. It also lacks an evaluation of non-occupational hand use. Pain, numbness, and tingling in the hand may be completely unrelated to a median neuropathy.

M.L. Kasdan, M.D.

14 Microsurgery

The Flow-Through Free Flap in Replantation Surgery: A New Concept
Costa H, Cunha C, Conde A, et al (S João Hosp, Oporto, Portugal; Cannieburn Hosp, Glasgow, Scotland)
Eur J Plast Surg 20:181–185, 1997   14–1

Introduction.—With improvements in microsurgical instrumentation, replantation surgery has been successfully performed in many thousands of cases. The concept of 1-stage coverage and revascularization of traumatized limbs by a flow-through radial mid-forearm free flap was previously described by the principal author of this study and his colleagues. The present study reports the use of the flow-though flap concept in 2 hand replants (Fig 1).

> *Case Report.*—Man, 27, sustained a transmetacarpal amputation of his right hand in a traffic accident. All 4 fingers were amputated, together with metacarpal joints and different parts of the metacarpal bones. After bone fixation, surgeons re-established arterial flow through a basilic vein graft harvested from the right forearm. The graft was end-to-side anastomosed to the radial and metacarpal arteries. Because no dorsal veins were present for venous drainage, a free dermal flow-through venous flap was harvested from the contralateral forearm. Proximal and distal end-to-end venous anastomoses were then performed between dorsal and cephalic veins, and a split-skin graft was applied over the venous flap. The patient had an uneventful postoperative course and achieved a good range of motion after rehabilitation.

Discussion.—The flow-through free flap concept is the method of choice in cases of major trauma of the extremities, including total and subtotal amputations, when exposure of deep structures is present. Two types of free flaps allow clinical application of the concept in replantation surgery: (1) the flow-through free fasciocutaneous flap for arterial supply and venous drainage of the replant and (2) the flow-through free venous flap for venous drainage of the replant. The first achieves a 1-stage technique of soft tissue cover and distal revascularization. Advantages include reconstruction of the arterial defect by another artery, maintenance of the

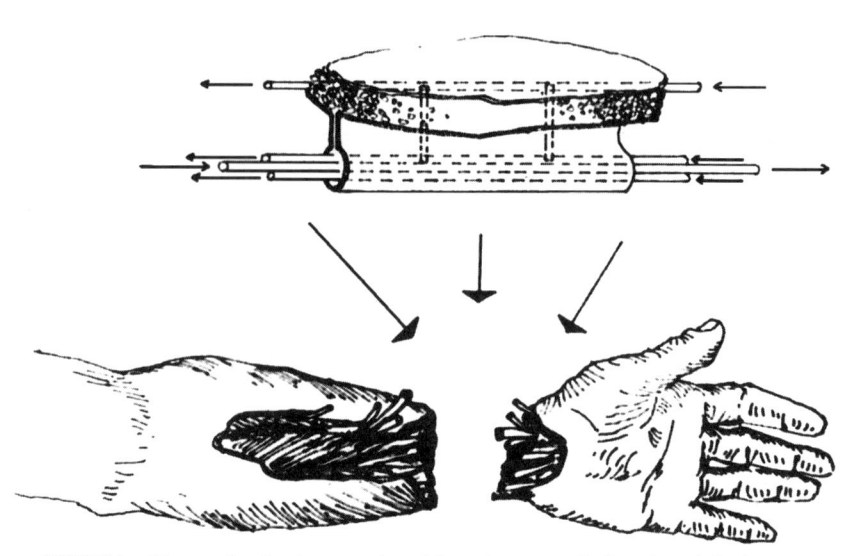

FIGURE 1.—Diagram showing the anatomic and dynamic concept of a flow-through fasciocutaneous free flap in replantation. (Courtesy of Costa H, Cunha A, Conde E, et al: The flow-through free flap in replantation surgery: A new concept. *Eur J Plast Surg* 20:181–185, 1997.)

collateral vessels in the traumatic defect by the flap tissue, and no major discrepancies in the microvascular anastomosis.

▶ The authors describe 2 patients undergoing hand replantation: in the first patient, a contralateral radial forearm free flap was used to restore arterial inflow as well as providing soft tissue coverage; in the second patient, a venous flow-through free flap was used to provide both venous outflow and soft-tissue coverage. This concept is not really new; the radial forearm flap, lateral arm flap and venous flaps have all been previously described for this purpose, but the paper serves to emphasize that a single free flap can sometimes provide 2 very useful functions in difficult situations where both arterial or venous continuity and soft tissue coverage are required.

N.F. Jones, M.D.

Toe-to-Hand Transfer for Traumatic Digital Amputations in Children and Adolescents
Wei F-C, El-Gammal TA, Chen H-C, et al (Chang Gung Mem College, Taipei, Taiwan, Republic of China)
Plast Reconstr Surg 100:605–609, 1997   14–2

Objective.—There are few reports in the literature about toe-to-hand transfer in children. Results of toe-to-hand transfer for traumatic digital amputations in children and adolescents before skeletal maturity, up to age 16 years, were evaluated. Three cases were discussed.

Methods.—Between July 1990 and August 1994, 45 toe transfers were performed in 28 children aged 3–16 years. Digits reconstructed included 13 thumbs, 12 index fingers, 14 middle fingers, and 6 ring fingers. Toes transplanted included 6 big toes, 24 second toes, 2 third toes, 4 combined second and third toes, 1 combined third and fourth toes, 1 vascularized second metatarsophalangeal joint, and 2 big toe pulps.

Results.—There was 1 failure of a second toe, 3 toes required reanastomosis for arterial insufficiency, and 2 digits had partial pulp loss. Patients were followed for an average of 3 years. Bony union was successful in all patients. Two-point discrimination was 6 mm while moving and 5 mm while static. Range of motion for the metaphalangeal, proximal interphalangeal, and distal interphalangeal joints of reconstructed fingers, and interphalangeal joint of the reconstructed thumbs averaged 69, 38, 13, and 15 degrees, respectively. Age did not affect outcome. None of the patients had a problem running or jumping. Transplanted digits grew normally.

Conclusions.—Toe transfer in children with traumatic digital amputations has a high success rate, requires fewer secondary procedures, and provides better sensory recovery than in adults.

▶ The authors present a series of toe transplants performed on children and adolescents. A wide variety of transplants were used, including 6 great toes, 24 second toes, 1 vascularized metatarsophalangeal joint, 2 third toes, and 5 toe combinations for a total of 45 transfers in 28 children. All original digit losses were traumatic.

One toe failed. Of the successful transplants, functional range of motion was achieved, and children had better sensation and fewer secondary procedures than adults undergoing similar procedures. The transplanted toes grew normally, and no long-term donor site morbidity occurred.

The authors' data add to a growing amount of information that toe transplantation in children is a reliable and functional reconstruction for traumatic and congenital abnormalities.[1,2]

W.C. Lineaweaver, M.D.

References

1. Canales F, Lineaweaver W, Furnas H, et al: Microvascular tissue transfer in pediatric patients: Analysis of 106 cases. *Br J Plast Surg* 44:423–427, 1991.
2. Shvedovchenko IV: Toe-to-hand transfers in children. *Ann Plast Surg* 31:251–254, 1993.

Distal Thumb Reconstruction With a Great Toe Partial-Nail Preserving Transfer Technique
Woo S-H, Seul J-H (Yeungnam Univ, Taegu, Korea)
Plast Reconstr Surg 101:114–122, 1998   14–3

Objective.—Using the big toe for thumb reconstruction poses a problem because of the size difference. Procedures developed to address this difference sometimes result in bone resorption, loss of the entire big toe or second toe, or complicated surgery. Transfer of a thumb-nail width of a toe nail, leaving a partial nail at the donor site, was described, and 2 cases were presented.

> *Technique.*—After the dorsal vein, the first dorsal metatarsal artery, the deep peroneal nerve, and both plantar digital nerves are dissected, a thumb-nail width of nail and skin flap from the big toe is attached to the distal phalangeal bone after performing an osteotomy or an arthrodesis with interosseous wiring. The remaining nail and medial skin flap was rotated 90 degrees and the donor site was closed. The flap was transferred, the circulation was restored. The dorsal vein, digital nerves, and deep peroneal nerve were reattached to the sutures of the thumb, and the deep peroneal nerve of the toe was sutured to the superficial radial nerve of the thumb. Patients were followed for at least 12 months.

Methods.—Between May 1993 and August 1996, 25 patients (4 female), aged 17–53 years, underwent distal thumb reconstruction, 16 of them immediately after injury.

Results.—The thumb-nail width had decreased an average of 1.8 mm in 9 patients at more than 24 months' follow-up. Pulp volumes of the transplanted and contralateral thumb were similar. Static 2-point discrimination averaged 8.5 mm. The average range of motion was 48 degrees. Key-pinch was 80% of normal in 18 thumbs with preservation of interphalangeal joint and 65% in 7 thumbs in which arthrodesis of the interphalangeal joint was performed.

Conclusion.—Distal thumb reconstruction with a thumb-nail width of the big toe toenail provides good aesthetic and functional results.

▶ The authors provide a technique of distal thumb reconstruction with preservation of the entire width of the toenail. In the cases presented, neither the reconstructed thumb nail nor the toe nail is perfect. One of the thumb nail margins is indistinct, and ingrowth may develop. The toenail is short and may be disposed to ingrowth and parrot-beak deformity. Long-term analysis of this technique will be necessary to confirm its value.

W.C. Lineaweaver, M.D.

Second Toe Plantar Flap for Partial Finger Reconstruction
Kimata Y, Mukouda M, Mizuo H, et al (Natl Cancer Ctr East, Chiba, Japan; Takeda Gen Hosp, Fukushima, Japan; Univ of Tokyo)
Plast Reconstr Surg 101:101–106, 1998   14–4

Objective.—Large finger defects require flap reconstruction. Donor site scarring is common, and postsurgical deformities can be a problem. Using a free neurovascular flap from the plantar surface of the second toe decreases postsurgical problems and complications and provides satisfactory functional and aesthetic results at donor and recipient sites. Two cases were discussed.

Full-Thickness Skin Graft Technique.—The full-thickness skin graft is harvested from the plantar skin up to the midlateral line of the second toe and is grafted to the defect. Another full-thickness skin graft is obtained from the inguinal crease and grafted to the donor site. Both are fixed with a tie-over fixation which is removed at day 5. Walking exercise is begun in 2 weeks.

Second Toe Plantar Flap Technique.—The second toe plantar flap must be 2–3 mm larger than the defect to relieve tension and uses the lateral or medial plantar digital artery of the injured finger or the first metatarsal artery if the digital artery is not satisfactory. The lateral or medial plantar digital nerve is used. The donor site dissection uses the standard tourniquet technique. After the incision is made, the plantar digital artery and digital nerve are ligated, the strip is elevated and dissected, with care being taken not to injure the plantar subcutaneous vein. The tourniquet is deflated, the flap is perfused for 20 minutes, and then the pedicle is divided for transfer. The donor site is closed. The recipient site is prepared and the flap is transferred as before.

Results.—Satisfactory results were obtained in 5 patients (2 females), aged 4–62 years, 2 with defects of the right ring finger and 1 each with a defect of the left ring finger, left index finger, and left middle finger. Three grafts survived and there were no rejections in 2 during a follow-up that ranged from 10 to 16 months. Among the surviving grafts, static 2-point discrimination ranged from 5 to 6. The advantage of this procedure is the aesthetic result at both donor and recipient sites. The disadvantages are the requirement for operations at 2 distant areas, a duration of surgery of 4 hours longer than for the local flap procedure, and a healing that takes 2–3 weeks.

Conclusion.—This 2-part procedure for partial finger reconstruction yields satisfactory aesthetic and functional results, particularly for significant pulp loss.

▶ This technique provides tailored, sensate full-thickness tissue to reconstruct small, critical areas such as tip pulps.

W.C. Lineaweaver, M.D.

Use of the Free Innervated Dorsalis Pedis Tendocutaneous Flap in Composite Hand Reconstruction

Cho BC, Lee JH, Weinzweig N, et al (Kyungpook Natl Univ, Taegu, Korea; Illinois Univ, Chicago)
Ann Plast Surg 40:268–276, 1998

14–5

Objective.—Reconstruction can be very difficult for patients with complete tissue loss of skin, tendon, or bone on the dorsum of the hand. These wounds are usually managed with a distant flap, with secondary tendon grafts or transfers. The dorsalis pedis composite flap has been used in various clinical situations, including composite hand injuries, as a free flap. An experience with the dorsalis pedis flap for management of composite loss of skin and tendons on the dorsum of the hand was presented.

Methods.—The experience included 7 patients with composite tissue loss of tendon and innervated skin on the dorsum of the hand. The extensor digitorum communis II and III were destroyed in 2 patients, the extensor digitorum communis II through V in 3, the extensor digitorum communis II in 1, and the extensor pollicis longus and extensor digitorum communis II in 1. The free dorsalis pedis flap included the extensor hallucis brevis if 1 tendon was needed, added the extensor digitorum longus II if 2 tendons were needed, and included the extensor digitorum longus II through IV if 4 tendons were needed. The exact tendon length needed was calculated with the interphalangeal and metacarpophalangeal joints in full extension and the wrist in 30 degrees of extension. The flaps ranged from 3 × 4 cm to 9.5 × 9 cm. After vascular anastomoses and tendon sutures were placed, the superficial peroneal nerve was coapted to a branch of the superficial radial nerve. Patients started active flexion and passive extension 1 week postoperatively.

Results.—The transferred flaps averaged 2-point discrimination of 25 mm. The average recovery rate for range of metacarpophalangeal joint motion was 91%. The color and texture of the transferred flaps matched the skin of the hand very well (Fig 1). One of 2 patients with skin loss over the donor area required repeat skin grafting.

Conclusion.—The dorsalis pedis free flap offers very good results in reconstruction of composite tissue defects of the dorsum of the hand. This flap provides up to 4 vascularized tendons, along with sensory nerve and bone. Other advantages include good skin matching, a 1-stage operation, faster healing, fewer adhesions, and early mobilization. Disadvantages

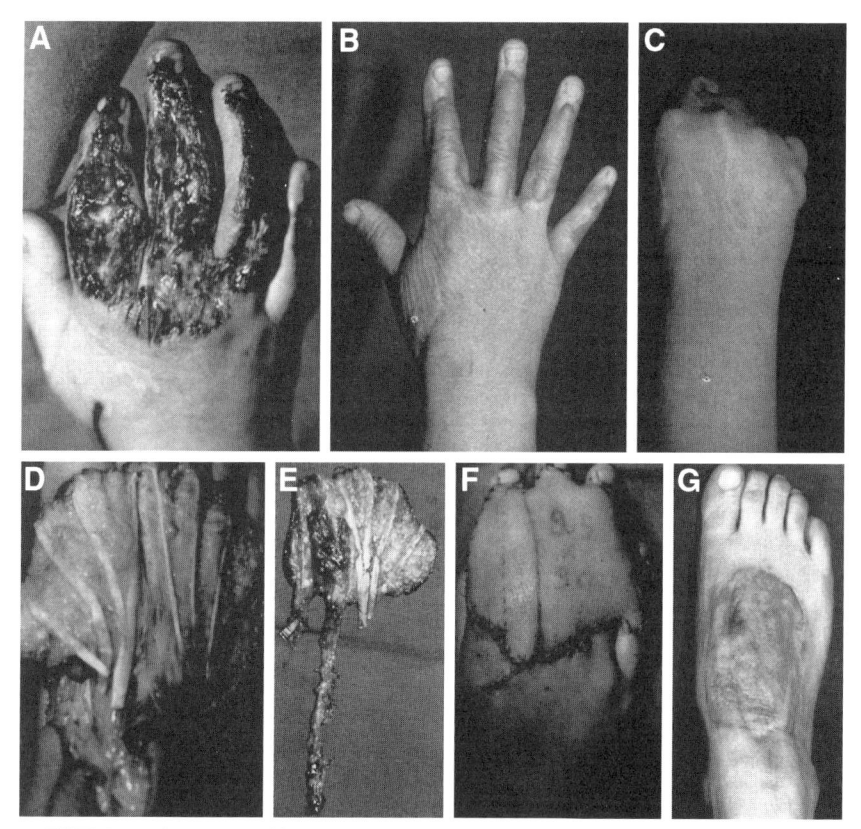

FIGURE 1.—**A**, a 42-year-old woman sustained a severe avulsion injury from an electric saw on the dorsum of her right hand. **B** and **C**, 2 years after separation of the individual fingers, the patient can flex and extend her fingers very effectively. **D** and **E**, harvesting of the 9 × 9.5-cm flap with 4 extensor digitorum longus tendons of the toe for transfer. **F**, immediate postoperative view. **G**, donor site 2 years after tendocutaneous flap was done. The patient has not experienced any functional problems. (Courtesy of Cho BC, Lee JH, Weinzweig N, et al: Use of the free innervated dorsalis pedis tendocutaneous flap in composite hand reconstruction. *Ann Plast Surg* 40:268–276, 1998.)

include variable anatomy of the first dorsal metatarsal artery, difficult dissection, limited skin flap size, and donor site morbidity.

▶ The authors describe a series of 7 patients with traumatic skin, soft-tissue tendon, and nerve substance loss on the dorsum of the hand. All patients had these complex soft-tissue defects reconstructed with a free, innervated dorsalis pedis tendocutaneous flap. This free flap consisted of a traditional dorsalis pedis flap with the inclusion of the superficial peroneal nerve as a vascularized nerve graft if nerve reconstruction was required. If reconstruction of a single extensor tendon was required, the extensor hallucis brevis was harvested with the flap as a vascularized tendon graft. If more than 1 tendon graft was required, extensor digitorum longus tendons were harvested as vascularized tendon grafts in the flap. All flaps were used to reconstruct extensor digitorum communis defects and, in 6 of the 7 patients, the superficial peroneal nerve was coapted to the superficial branch of the radial nerve to improve sensation on the dorsum of the hand.

At 1 week post surgery, the patients' extensor tendon injuries were managed with a passive extension/active flexion protocol. All flaps survived completely. The percentage of active range of motion for the 18 involved metacarpophalangeal joints was measured and ranged from 79 to 98% of normal. Donor site problems consisting of partial skin graft loss occurred in 2 of the 7 patients. One patient required a second skin graft.

The authors acknowledge drawbacks of using this flap, including variable anatomy of the first dorsal metatarsal artery, tedious dissection, limited flap size, and donor site morbidity. Nonetheless, I believe that this flap offers unique capabilities for reconstruction of the combined skin, soft-tissue, tendon, and nerve substance loss on the dorsum of the hand.

A.A. Smith, M.D.

Continuous Peripheral Nerve Block in Replantation and Revascularization
Taras JS, Behrman MJ (Thomas Jefferson Univ, Philadelphia)
J Reconstr Microsurg 14:17–21, 1998

Background.—The success of replantation after digital amputation depends on reestablishing the circulation and preventing thrombosis. One of the ways to limit thrombosis is to limit peripheral vasospasm, which can be achieved pharmacologically. These authors studied a continuous infusion of a local anesthetic both during and after digital replantation to determine its effectiveness in preventing neurogenically mediated vasospasm.

Methods.—The test group consisted of 55 patients who received a continuous infusion of 0.5% bupivacaine with 57 complete digital amputations and 26 subtotal amputations. The control group consisted of 10 patients who did not receive peripheral nerve blockade undergoing replantation and revascularization. With the patient under general anesthesia, a percutaneous catheter was placed between 4 cm and 8 cm proximal to the wrist crease and to the radial side of the palmaris longus tendon. A 5 ml bolus of 0.5% bupivacaine was infused before arterial repair began in the test patients; once arterial repair began, 3,000 units of heparin was infused at a rate of 1,000 units/hr for all patients. All patients were monitored in the hospital for up to a week after surgery. The test group continued to receive bupivacaine infusion at 2 mL/hr for 5 days postoperatively. All patients were given oral aspirin (325 mg twice daily) and chlorpromazine hydrochloride (25 mg three times daily) until discharge. Also, all patients were housed in a warm room (higher than 22°C) and hydration and heparin were maintained for at least 5 days. Dressings were changed as needed. Aspirin was prescribed for the first postoperative month.

Findings.—Of the 57 replanted digits, 53 survived (93%); of the 26 revascularized digits, 25 survived (96%). All 55 test patients reported decreased sensation in the distribution of the medial nerve while receiving bupivacaine; 12 also reported decreased sensation in the distribution of the ulnar nerve. After discontinuation of the infusion, however, all but 1 of the patients quickly recovered sensory function. The 1 patient with a delayed recovery of sensation (5 months) had had his thumb severed during an epileptic seizure. Patients in the test group used substantially less morphine for postoperative pain control than patients in the control group (15 mg vs. 56 mg, or 27%). There were no complications, including infection, hematoma, or compartment syndrome.

Conclusions.—Continuous peripheral nerve blockade with a percutaneous forearm catheter safely and effectively prevented vasospasm and thrombosis in patients undergoing digital replantation and revascularization.

▶ We do not routinely use continuous sympathetic blockade after replantation or revascularization. A long-acting axillary block, a warm room (80°F), and abstinence from vasoconstrictive substances are usually sufficient. Certainly, there are circumstances where additional measures are warranted, such as the need for a dressing change or inflow loss in the first few postoperative days. When inflow loss is detected, it is virtually impossible to clinically discriminate between occlusion secondary to vasospasm or thrombus. So, there is merit to the effort to continuously control vasospasm in the postoperative period. For this effort, the authors are to be commended. Unfortunately, this study fails to demonstrate conclusively that the described technique led to the laudable digital survival rate achieved. I think their effort deserves more attention, such as a randomized trial between those receiving continuous sympathetic blockade and those who do not. Digital temperatures could be measured using the contralateral digit as a control. Ratios within patients would then provide for a meaningful comparison between groups. The obvious potential complication with the technique described in this paper is compartment syndrome. The authors deny that this occurred, although they were monitoring a semianesthetized hand. The paucity of vascular and long-term neurologic compromise reported would suggest that their assessment is correct; however, final functional outcomes were not reported. I would suggest if continuous sympathetic blockade is done, an indwelling axillary catheter is conceptually safer. This method would also yield better coverage of the ulnar side of the hand.

S.M. Topper, M.D.

Acute Effects of Periarterial Sympathectomy on the Cutaneous Microcirculation
Pollock DC, Li Z, Rosencrance E, et al (Wake Forest Univ, Winston-Salem, NC)
J Orthop Res 15:408–413, 1997

Introduction.—A peripheral sympathectomy performed at the distal extremity offers an alternative to cervicothoracic sympathectomy in patients with vaso-occlusive disease. Although peripheral periarterial sympathectomy improves cutaneous perfusion and increases the nutritional component of peripheral blood flow, the mechanisms of its effects are not known. Using a rabbit ear model of digital microcirculation, investigators observed the acute effects of periarterial sympathectomy of the central artery of the ear on the thermoregulatory microcirculation.

Methods.—Experiments were performed on 19 male New Zealand White rabbits. A microscope system was used to record acute microvascular observations in 9 of the animals. Measurements were obtained before and after periarterial sympathectomy of the auricular artery at the base of the rabbit ear. Auricular temperatures were measured in 10 rabbits, 8 of which also underwent laser Doppler perfusion imaging.

Results.—Immediately after sympathectomy, the central auricular artery became dilated, with an increase of 50% to 100% over baseline diameter. The arterioles, arteriovenous anastomoses, and venules dilated to 165%, 156%, and 223%, respectively, at 30 minutes, and to 187%, 174%, and 204%, respectively, at 60 minutes, relative to baseline diameters. Laser Doppler perfusion imaging, a measure of cutaneous perfusion, had increased a mean of 8.9% at 120 minutes after sympathectomy. Although the core temperature of the rabbits did not change, ear temperatures rose a mean of 3°C at 120 minutes.

Conclusion.—A primary function of the rabbit ear is thermoregulation, a task also performed by human digits. The rabbit ear and the digits of the human hand are similar in morphology, function, and innervation. Findings in this rabbit ear model suggest that periarterial sympathectomy may improve the symptoms of vasospastic diseases of the hand by reducing the adrenergic tone of the distal microvasculature and improving overall microcirculatory blood flow.

▶ Peripheral sympathectomy has been considered as an alternative to destruction of the cervical sympathetic ganglia, or the next procedure to try if cervicothoracic sympathectomy has failed or its effect has been lost. The procedure is conceptually appealing. It "targets" the affected zone and avoids the risk of unpleasant side effects such as a Horner's sign. The experiments described in this study demonstrate that the effects of peripheral sympathectomy are of rapid onset and multilevel. The study provides additional experimental foundation favoring the choice of this procedure over stellate ganglionectomy.

V.R. Hentz, M.D.

Limited Microsurgical Arteriolysis for Complications of Digital Vasospasm
Tham S, Grossman JAI (New York Univ)
J Hand Surg [Br] 22B:359–361, 1997 14–8

Objective.—Patients with vasospasm are sometimes resistant to medical treatment. The results of limited microsurgical arteriolysis of the digital arteries for the treatment of patients with chronic digital ischemia associated with vasospasms refractory to medical management were presented.

Methods.—During a 3-year period, surgical microarteriolysis was performed on 22 digits of 6 patients with Raynaud's phenomenon, including 2 with scleroderma and 4 with CREST (*c*alcinosis cutis, *R*aynaud's phenomenon, *e*sophageal motility disorder, *s*clerodactyly, and *t*elangiectasia), and 1 with idiopathic vasospasm. There were chronic ulcers on 7 digits and dry gangrene on 1.

Technique.—Fingertip ulcers were debrided and heparin infused intravenously. A tourniquet was applied, and general anesthesia or axillary block was administered. The digital arteries were exposed, and the adventitia was stripped from the entire length. The incisions were closed and allowed to heal for a week before limited mobility was permitted.

Results.—Blood flow increased through the stripped artery unless the disease had progressed distally and proximally. After 12–36 months, pain and cold sensitivity had improved significantly in 19 digits. Three digits had residual pain on exposure to cold. Ulcers healed in an average of 27 days. There was stiffness in the joints of 2 digits, but no recurrence of symptoms.

Conclusions.—When medical intervention fails, adventitial stripping of affected arteries in patients with vasospasm is effective in reducing pain and cold sensitivity, and in promoting healing of ulcers.

▶ Digital sympathectomy diminishes symptoms and promotes wound (ulcer) healing in patients with refractory ulceration, cold intolerance, and Raynaud's phenomenon. This article supports reports on the value of adventitial stripping to maximize nutritional or total digital flow (or both).[1] Maximizing nutritional flow and reducing inappropriate arteriovenous shunting promotes tissue healing and decreases pain. Caution should be exercised in requiring a plethysmographic response to digital block as an inclusion criteria for peripheral sympathectomy. The ability of the digit to increase its total blood flow as demonstrated by plethysmography or temperature supports an excellent response to sympathectomy. However, because nutritional flow may be increased significantly without affecting total flow in patients with vasospastic and occlusive disease, the requirement to increase total flow after block will deny surgical relief in a segment of the population. Patients who require amputation for a necrotic fingertip secondary to vas-occlusive disease and secondary Raynaud's benefit from limited sympathectomy at the time of digital amputation. It is unfortunate that the authors have introduced "arteriolysis" as another synonym for "peripheral sympathectomy," or "digital sympathectomy."

L.A. Koman, M.D.

Reference

1. Koman LA, Smith BP, Pollock FE Jr, et al: The microcirculatory effects of peripheral sympathectomy. *J Hand Surg [Am]* 20A:709–717, 1995.

Suggested Reading

Adani R, Busa R, Castagnetti C, et al: Replantation of degloved skin of the hand. *Plast Reconstr Surg* 101:1544–1551, 1998.
▶ Degloving injuries such as ring avulsions present particular difficulties and difficult technical decisions. The majority of the part still remains and retains potentially good function. However, resurfacing the remaining tissues with skin grafts or burying the part in a pedicled flap are poor functional alternatives. The authors describe several technical steps that have allowed them to salvage skin degloved from fingers and hands. The most effective of these techniques included performing preliminary flow-through loops using long vein grafts and transfers of vessels from uninjured adjacent digits. The results shown, while not striking, are better than if the alternative sources of skin cover mentioned above were used. The authors suggest that if the degloved skin cannot be revascularized, then one should consider proceeding to amputation rather than using these other conventional techniques.

V.R. Hentz, M.D.

Bertelli JA, Paglieli A: The neurocutaneous flap based on the dorsal branches of the ulnar artery and nerve: A new flap for extensive reconstruction of the hand. *Plast Reconstr Surg* 101:1537–1543, 1998.
▶ The authors describe a retrograde modification of the dorsal ulnar island flap. The neurovascular axis is the dorsal sensory branch of the ulnar artery and the dorsal branch of the ulnar artery, also named the *descending branch* by Becker and Gilbert.[1] Bertelli and Paglieli describe their use of this flap in 5 patients with distally located defects on both the dorsal and palmer side of the hand. They suggest a modification that would permit transfer of a portion of the distal ulna for osteocutaneous reconstruction at the metacarpal or proximal phalangeal level.

V.R. Hentz, M.D.

Reference

1. Becker C, Gilbert A: The cubital flap [French]. *Ann Chir Main* 7:136–142, 1988.

Janezic TF, Arnez ZM, Šolinc M, et al: One hundred sixty-seven thumb replantations and revascularisations: Early microvascular results. *Microsurgery* 17:259–263, 1996.
▶ This is a very large series of thumb replantations and revascularizations performed over a 10-year period. The follow-up is relatively long-term. The

overall success rate was 66%, the most frequent cause of failure was venous thrombosis, and the most critical time was 4 days following replantation. After 7 days there were no microvascular complications. Key information included the finding that none of the failures occurring after the third day were successfully salvaged. This had bearing on how long patients need in-hospital monitoring.

V.R. Hentz, M.D.

Janezic TF, Arnez ZM, Šolinc M, et al: Functional results of 46 thumb replantations and revascularisations. *Microsurgery* 17:264–267, 1996.

▶ The authors analyzed the outcome of 46 thumb replantations. They studied various functional parameters and other parameters indicating patient satisfaction. Thumb replantations are functional. In spite of their functionality, patients are not happy if there has been little regard for the aesthetic aspects in addition to the functional considerations. The evolution is evident; first make it survive, next make it work, and finally, make it look good.

V.R. Hentz, M.D.

15 Vascular and Dystrophic Problems

Effective Treatment of Lymphedema of the Extremities
Ko DSC, Lerner R, Klose G, et al (Harvard Med School, Boston; Lerner Lymphedema Services, Boston)
Arch Surg 133:452–458, 1998   15–1

Introduction.—Most patients with chronic lymphedema of the extremities are advised to learn to live with the chronic swelling because of the lack of effective therapy. The Foeldi technique, or complete (or complex) decongestive physiotherapy (CDP), consists of skin care, eradication of infections, compression bandaging, and remedial exercises. The immediate and long-term volumetric reductions of upper and lower lymphedematous extremities were prospectively evaluated after a single course of CDP.

Methods.—Two hundred ninety-nine consecutive patients with lymphedema of the upper (2% primary, 98% secondary) or lower (61.3% primary, 38.7% secondary) extremities were treated with CDP for an average of 15.7 days. Patients underwent 2 phases of CDP. Phase 1 consisted of manual lymphatic massage, multilayered inelastic compression bandaging, remedial exercises, and meticulous skin care; self-care was the focus of phase 2, with use of daytime elastic sleeve or stocking compression, nocturnal wrapping, and continued exercises. Patients were evaluated for reduction of lymphedema at completion of phase 1 and at 6- and 12-month intervals during phase 2.

Results.—The average lymphedema reduction was 59.1% and 67.7%, respectively, after upper- and lower-extremity treatment. At an average follow-up of 9 months, the improvement was sustained in 86% of compliant patients at 90% of the initial reduction for upper and lower extremities. The 33% of patients who were noncompliant lost part of their initial reduction. The rate of infections decreased from 1.10 to 0.65 infections per patient year after a complete series of CDP treatments.

Conclusion.—Complete decongestive physiotherapy was highly effective in treating primary and secondary lymphedema. Initial volume reductions were maintained in most patients. Patients reported a significant recovery from their previous cosmetic and functional impairments and from the physical stigma they believed was frequently trivialized by the medical and payor communities.

▶ Decongestive physiotherapy, such as the Foeldi technique, is widely used in lymphedema clinics at major medical centers. These are intensive techniques that require 1–2 hours per day of therapist's time for 2–3 weeks. Most of the time is spent on manual lymph mobilization and decongestive massage. The amount of time commitment may limit the patient population that can use such treatments. The long-term at-home phase also requires considerable patient compliance with nighttime wrappings, daily exercises, and daytime compressive wraps. One wonders where the authors found such a highly compliant population (84% of upper extremity edema cases were termed "compliant") or how they were able to get reimbursement for this expensive protocol.

No head-to-head comparison is made between Foeldi's technique and the older and much simpler pump and wrap techniques. Clearly, Foeldi's technique is highly effective—according to this study and to experience at our institution. However, at our lymphedema center we reserve the Foeldi program for highly motivated patients who are able to commit to 3 weeks of daily therapy. We also find that fairly new pitting edema does not require the extensive manual decongestion and responds quite well to pumping and compressive garments with much less time, money, and effort. I would suspect that most upper extremity lymphedema seen in a hand surgeon's office would be acute or subacute in nature. Most of these patients with pitting edema would not need such intensive therapy as the Foeldi technique and would respond well to less expensive and intensive treatment.

K.A. Bengtson, M.D.

Sympathetic Vasoconstrictor Reflex Pattern in Patients With Complex Regional Pain Syndrome
Birklein F, Riedl B, Neundörfer B, et al (Friedrich-Alexander-Universität Erlangen, Germany)
Pain 75:93–100, 1998   15–2

Introduction.—Patients with complex regional pain syndrome (CRPS) also experience motor and sensory symptoms and autonomic disturbances. Peripheral sympathetic blockade has no uniform beneficial therapeutic effect, and the relationship between sympathetic dysfunction and disabling pain has not been determined. To examine whether sympathetic vasoconstrictor reflexes are altered in CRPS, different types of sympathetic vasoconstrictor reflexes were assessed in patients with untreated CRPS.

Methods.—Twenty patients and 21 healthy control subjects were included in the study. Patients were 12 women and 8 men with a mean age of 48.9 years. Nineteen had CRPS type I (previous noxious event without nerve lesion) and 1 had CRPS type II (noxious event with nerve lesion). The most common cause (10 patients) of CRPS was limb fracture. At the time of the study the mean duration of the disease was 8.5 weeks. The cutaneous blood flow of the affected and the contralateral limb was recorded during different maneuvers to produce vasoconstriction, including the veno-arteriolar reflex (VAR), inspiratory gasp (IG), cold pressor test (CP), and mental arithmetic (MA). Infrared thermography was used to record skin temperature immediately after assessment of the vasoconstrictor reflexes.

Results.—One affected leg and 19 affected arms were investigated. Although spontaneous pain was present in only 14 (70%) of 20 cases, 19 (95%) of 20 patients reported pain evoked by various mechanical and thermal stimuli. Seventeen (85%) of 20 patients had muscle weakness, 17 (85%) of 20 had edema, and 13 (65%) of 20 had trophic changes (hair or nails). Vasoconstriction caused by the provocation tests could be measured in 14 (70%) of 20 patients and 14 (70%) of 21 control subjects; these participants were included in the analysis. Sympathetic reflex vasoconstriction triggered by MA, which represents cortical-generated, moderate vasoconstrictor stimulus, was significantly reduced in affected limbs as compared with contralateral and control limbs (102.9% of prestimulus period vs. 85.0% and 84.8%, respectively). No differences in sympathetic vasoconstrictor reflexes were noted between affected limbs and contralateral and control limbs when VAR, IG, and CP were employed. Skin temperature did not differ between affected and unaffected limbs or between patients and control subjects.

Conclusion.—Sympathetic vasoconstrictor drive was found to be reduced in untreated CRPS, but no correlation was seen between pain and sympathetic dysfunction. The origin of vasoconstrictor reflex failure in CRPS has yet to be determined.

▶ The findings in this manuscript demonstrate the importance of peripheral thermoregulatory activity in the pathophysiology of complex regional pain. The importance of stress in evaluating diagnostic testing such as the VAR, the IG, the CP, and the MA is well supported. These data corroborate other studies and demonstrate that impairment of sympathetic vasoconstrictor activity after central vasoconstrictor stimulation is an important component of CRPS and supports the importance of physiologic staging. One third of the patients demonstrated vasodilatation; this explains, in part, individual variability seen in patients, and the variations observed in physiologic staging. In CRPS, the autonomic control of peripheral thermoregulation, vasomotor activity, and nutritional perfusion is controlled, in part, by adrenergic mechanisms and influences symptoms and function.

Treatment approaches based on pathophysiology and functional considerations provide clinical advantages and allow the practitioner to use medications in a specific and consistent fashion. The management of patients with abnormal vasoconstrictor tone should be directed at increasing nutritional perfusion and decreasing vasoconstriction by appropriate medications or interventions that modify alpha adrenergic control.

L.A. Koman, M.D.

Quantitative Evaluation of Sympathetic Nervous System Dysfunction in Patients With Reflex Sympathetic Dystrophy

Ide J, Yamaga M, Kitamura T, et al (Kumamoto Univ, Japan)
J Hand Surg [Br] 22B:102–106, 1997
15–3

Background.—The pathogenesis of reflex sympathetic dystrophy (RSD) is not known. To examine sympathetic nervous system dysfunction in patients with RSD, a noninvasive, quantitative laser Doppler method was developed to measure skin blood flow (SBF) at rest and the vasoconstrictor response.

Methods.—The study group consisted of 20 patients with RSD and 10 healthy controls. Patients were classified into Steinbrocker's stage 1 and 2. Nine patients were re-examined after successful treatment. A 2-channel laser Doppler flowmeter was used to assess SBF at rest and after the inspiratory gasp test. The skin vasoconstrictor response (SVR) to an inspiratory gasp was expressed as a percentage of the SBF. The ratio of the affected to unaffected extremity (A/U) was calculated for participants with RSD and the left/right (L/R) ratio was calculated for healthy controls.

Results.—In patients with stage 1 RSD, the A/U ratio of SBF was significantly higher than the L/R ratio of the healthy controls. The A/U of the SVR was the same for both groups. In patients with stage 2 RSD, the A/U ratio of SBF was significantly lower and the A/U ratio of SVR significantly higher than the L/R ratio of healthy controls. After treatment and recovery, all values became similar to those of healthy controls.

Conclusions.—Doppler measurement of SBF demonstrated that in patients with stage 1 RSD there was increased blood flow at rest and an unchanged vasoconstrictor response. In stage 2 RSD, blood flow at rest was decreased and the vasoconstriction response was increased. This implies that correct disease staging is necessary for proper treatment. Recovery from RSD was correlated with normalization of SBF and SVR. Quantitative analysis of sympathetic nervous system function appears to be useful in the diagnosis and management of RSD.

▶ This manuscript highlights the importance of physiologic staging in patients with complex regional pain syndrome (CRPS) or RSD. Recognizing the limitations of even the most sophisticated Doppler flowmeter, the combination of repeated measures over time with each patient serving as an internal control and a physiologic stress (inspiratory gas test) permits reproducible physiologic staging in CRPS. Laser Doppler flow analyzes both nutritional and thermoregulatory flow, but in isolation may fail to identify subtle changes in nutritional flow (a smaller and more superficial component of total flow). This manuscript helps explain "contradictory results" in the scientific literature secondary to inaccurate staging criteria and demonstrates the value of objective physiologic tests (resting SBF and SVR in defining clinical classifications or stages. In CRPS, the peripheral microcirculation follows 3 basic patterns: (1) increased total flow with decreased nutritional flow; (2) increased total flow with increased thermoregulatory flow and normal nutritional flow; and (3) decreased total flow with decreased nutritional flow. Thus, the presence of identical clinical pictures of pain and functional impairment in the presence of a hot swollen extremity and a cold atrophic extremity may be, in part, explained by the common finding of abnormal nutritional flow and segmental ischemia.

L.A. Koman, M.D.

Incidence and Characteristics of Patients With Hand Ischemia After a Hemodialysis Access Procedure
Morsy AH, Kulbaski M, Chen C, et al (Veterans Affairs Med Ctr, Decatur, Ga; Emory Univ, Atlanta, Ga)
J Surg Res 74:8–10, 1998

Background.—Ischemic complications associated with arteriovenous access in patients dependent on long-term hemodialysis can be devastating. The clinical characteristics of patients with chronic renal failure who develop hand ischemia in the limb with the dialysis angioaccess were investigated.

Methods and Findings.—Three hundred fifty-two patients with 409 upper extremity arteriovenous access sites were included in a retrospective review. Hand ischemia occurred in 4.3% of 299 hands with arteriovenous grafts and in 1.8% of 110 hands with direct forearm arteriovenous fistulas. Ischemic manifestations developed immediately after surgery in 6 patients, in the first week after surgery in 2, after 1 month in 4, and after 1 year in 1. Thirteen cases of ischemia were associated with the primary access procedure. Two followed graft thrombectomy and outflow dilation. Seven patients were midly symptomatic with dialysis-induced pain, coldness, or numbness. Eight patients experienced severe ischemic symptoms, including sensory loss in 3, severe intolerable pain with impalpable pulse in 3, and digital gangrene necessitation amputation in 2. Treatment was conservative in 3, by banding in 6, by ligation in 4, by embolization in 1, and by distal ligation and bypass surgery in 1. Hand ischemia developed in 10 patients with long-standing insulin-dependent diabetes, 12 with chronic hypertension, 14 with peripheral arterial disease, 8 with coronary artery disease, and 1 with systemic lupus erythematosis.

Conclusions.—Severe peripheral arterial diseases were common among these dialysis-dependent patients with hand ischemia and may be markers for risk after access surgery. Further prospective studies are needed to determine the major risk factors and way to prevent or reduce this complication.

▶ The problem here is a lack of alternatives. The authors suggest that if flow on 1 side is poor, to look contralaterally, and of course that is logical—but the problem may well be bilateral. Careful preoperative clinical examination, and Doppler, plethysmography and angiography, preoperatively, are all essential to avoid postoperative misadventures.

P.C. Amadio, M.D.

Pattern Recognition in Post-traumatic Cold Intolerance
Lithell M, Backman C, Nyström Å (Univ of Umeå, Sweden; Univ of Pittsburgh, Pa)
J Hand Surg [Br] 22B:783–787, 1997   15–5

Introduction.—Patients with a major injury to the hand are at high risk for the development of posttraumatic cold intolerance. Few studies have addressed the nature, cause and treatment of this condition, perhaps because it is difficult to define and to measure objectively. The subjective symptoms known as "posttraumatic cold intolerance" were retrospectively analyzed in a study of 40 patients.

Methods.—The study group was obtained from a review of hospital records. All patients were assumed to be at high risk for posttraumatic cold intolerance. Types of digital trauma included amputation, neurovascular laceration, or comminuted fracture requiring surgical reconstruction. All but 2 patients were men. The mean age of the group was 43.2 years, with a mean of 6.23 years since the injury. Patients were interviewed to determine the presence of cold intolerance and the degree of disability related to symptoms.

Results.—All 40 patients reported reduced tolerance to cold after the injury, and such intolerance often appeared within a few weeks. Wind-chill and humidity affected the degree of cold-related discomfort. Thus spring and autumn could be more troublesome than the drier, but colder winters of northern Sweden. Common symptoms were an unpleasant feeling of intense coldness, blanching or other discoloration of the fingers, pain, numbness, and stiffness. Many patients had abandoned certain leisure activities (24%) or changed jobs (18%) because of cold intolerance.

Conclusion.—The analysis of this group of patients with major injuries to the hand confirms the high incidence of posttraumatic cold intolerance. This problem can lead to disability among patients living in cold climates such as Sweden. Because the subjective expression of cold intolerance is quite varied, it is not possible to develop an adequate definition or assessment based on any single symptoms or group of symptoms.

Pseudo-Volkmann's Contracture Due to Tethering of Flexor Digitorum Profundus to Fractures of the Ulna in Children
Deeney VF, Kaye JJ, Geary SP, et al (Ochsner Clinic, New Orleans, La; Hosp for Sick Children, Toronto)
J Pediatr Orthop 18:437–440, 1998   15–6

Background.—Fractures of the radius and ulna in children may be complicated by compartment syndrome, which—if diagnosed late—may lead to Volkmann's ischemic contracture of the flexor muscles of the forearm. Even with extensive surgery to restore musculotendinous length, restoring normal function in these cases is usually not possible. An unusual

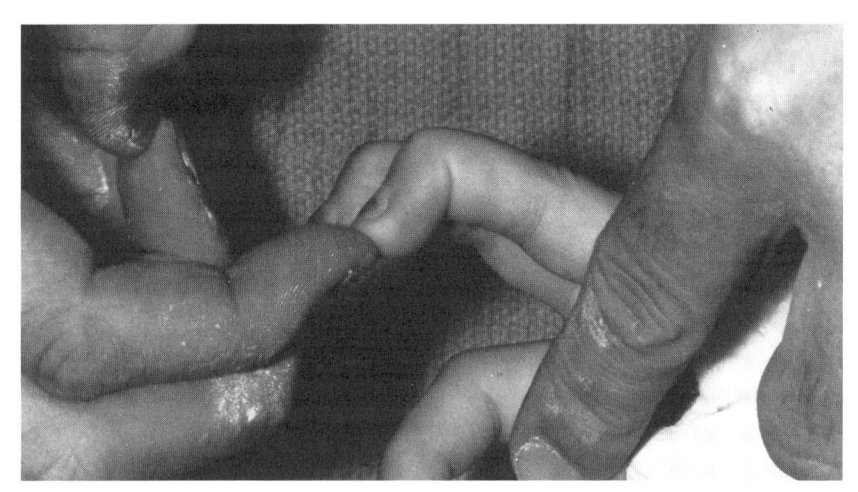

FIGURE 1, B.—Case 1, tenodesis of the flexor digitorum profundus tendons to the ring and long fingers, noted 2 days after the initial closed reduction. (Courtesy of Deeney VF, Kaye JJ, Geary SP, et al: Pseudo-Volkmann's contracture due to tethering of flexor digitorum profundus to fractures of the ulna in children. *J Pediatr Orthop* 18:437–440, 1998.)

complication of forearm fracture, pseudo-Volkmann's contracture caused by tethering of the flexor digitorum profundus, is reported.

Patients.—This complication was encountered in 7 children with forearm fractures. The patients were 6–14 years old at the time of the injury. The children were found to have partial tethering of the flexor digitorum profundus to the ulnar fracture, recognized 2 days to 16 years after injury. This complication caused inability to extend the joints of 2 or 3 fingers when the wrist was in neutral position, just as seen in Volkmann's ischemic contracture (Fig 1, B). However, there were no nerve palsies or undue pain after reduction.

Outcomes.—All patients were managed by untethering of the flexor digitorum profundus by manipulation or myotenolysis, which resulted in restoration of normal length, excursion, and function of the flexor digitorum profundus. There were no cases of forearm muscle wasting.

Conclusions.—Pseudo-Volkmann's contracture caused by tethering of the flexor digitorum profundus to an ulnar fracture is an unusual complication of forearm fracture in children. This complication can be detected by checking passive range of finger motion immediately after closed reduction of the fracture. Any muscle tethering can be released by remanipulation of the fracture. If necessary, surgical release can be performed through a small incision.

▶ This article is an excellent presentation of 7 children with entrapment of the flexor digitorum profundus at the site of ulna fractures, a relatively rare complication. The authors' inclusion of an individual with persistence of the contracture 16 years after injury suggests that not all of these cases resolve spontaneously. This article adds valuable information to the natural history of such entrapment phenomena, also reported by Jeffrey over 20 years ago.[1]

W.J. Shaughnessy, M.D.

Reference

1. Jeffery CC: Contracture of fingers due to fixation of the flexor profundus digitorum to the ulna. *Hand* 8:32–35, 1976.

Suggested Reading

Dowd PM, Goldsmith PC, Chopra S, et al: Cutaneous responses to endothelin-1 and histamine in patients with vibration white finger. *J Invest Dermatol* 110:127–131, 1998.

▶ The histamine flare and wheal response is well known to any medical student. Endothelin-1 produces a central area of pallor with a surrounding flare. In vibration white finger (VWF) both these responses are abnormal (smaller flares), whereas in normal people and in people exposed to vibration who do not have VWF both responses are preserved. In Raynaud's phenomenon the endothelin-1 response is abnormal while the histamine response is preserved. These tests are therefore useful in helping to distinguish VWF from Raynaud's phenomenon.

P.C. Amadio, M.D.

Stanec S, Tonković I, Stanec Z, et al: Treatment of upper limb nerve war injuries associated with vascular trauma. *Injury* 28:463–468, 1997.

▶ Each generation relearns the experience of the preceding generation. This series comes from the recent war in the former Yugoslavia. Functional outcome, when compared to civilian nerve and vascular trauma, was poor (poor or no recovery in 55% of cases) for all the usual reasons; 66% of the injuries were in proximal locations, nerve repair was delayed, usually with nerve grafts placed in injured and scarred tissues, and polytrauma predominated. However, the results are clearly better than those experienced in World War II, when few grafts were used.

V.R. Hentz, M.D.

16 Research

Gene Expression of Transforming Growth Factor Beta-1 in Rabbit Zone II Flexor Tendon Wound Healing: Evidence for Dual Mechanisms of Repair

Chang J, Most D, Stelnicki E, et al (Stanford Univ, Calif)
Plast Reconstr Surg 100:937–944, 1997   16–1

Background.—Pathologic scar formation is a complication that adversely affects function in patients who have undergone flexor tendon repair in the hand. Both intrinsic and extrinsic processes may contribute to repair, but the biology of hand flexor tendon wound healing has not been defined. Transforming growth factor–β, a cytokine with numerous biological activities related to wound healing, activates an aggressive inflammatory response in the local wound environment. Investigators used in situ hybridization and immunohistochemical techniques to examine the role of transforming growth factor–β1 gene expression in a rabbit flexor tendon wound-healing model.

Methods.—Experiments were performed in adult New Zealand White rabbits. Forty forepaws underwent complete transection and repair of the middle digit flexor digitorum profundus tendon in zone II. The rabbits were sacrificed at 1, 3, 7, 14, 28, and 56 days postoperatively and the tendons harvested for determination of the expression patterns of transforming growth factor–β1.

Results.—In contrast to control, unwounded rabbit flexor tendons, the transected and repaired flexor tendons showed a significantly elevated number of cells expressing transforming growth factor–β1 messenger RNA (mRNA) from resident tenocytes concentrated at the anastomosis and surrounding epitenon. The increased signal for transforming growth factor–β1 was also seen in the infiltrating fibroblasts and inflammatory cells from the tendon sheath. The tendon sheath was several times more cellular than the underlying tendon at all times after repair (1–56 days). Immunohistochemical studies showed active expression and secretion of transforming growth factor–β1 throughout the wound.

Conclusion.—Previous studies have implicated several growth factors in tendon wound healing. In this rabbit flexor tendon model, transforming growth factor–β1 mRNA upregulation was detected in wound tendon tissue by postoperative day 1. This upregulation was observed in wounded specimens from both the tendon parenchyma and the sheath. Early modulation of transforming growth factor–β1 may be a means of controlling the formation of adhesion, thereby improving functional outcome after hand flexor tendon repair.

▶ It is clear by now that advances in surgical techniques offer little in the way of improvements in the outcome of flexor tendon repair. On the other hand, altering the molecular environment at the wound site or altering the molecular processes of the organism itself offer the possibility of near-infinite variety in ways to affect outcome. Understanding the mechanisms that determine the sequential upregulation or downregulation of cytokines is only the initial step in this goal.

V.R. Hentz, M.D.

Suture Methods for Flexor Tendon Repair: A Biomechanical Analysis During the First Six Weeks Following Repair
Winters SC, Seiler JG III, Woo SL-Y, et al (Washington Univ, St Louis; Univ of Pittsburgh, Pa)
Ann Chir Main 16:229–234, 1997   16–2

Objective.—Although primary tendon repair is the treatment of choice for complete severing of the flexor tendon, poor outcome—usually resulting from adhesion formation—is not rare. Early active motion rehabilitation can improve outcome. The strength and gliding function of several different repair methods during the first 6 weeks after repair were compared, and their abilities to predict stress of early active digital motion were assessed in the dog.

Technique.—The transected flexor tendons of the second and fifth digits of the forepaw were repaired using either the Tajima, Tsuge, Savage, Kessler, double loop locking suture, or 8-strand method; 4-0 braided dacron sutures were used, in the case of the 8-strand method, 4-0 Supramid. With the latter method, the needle was extended from the repair site exiting 1 cm from the cut edge. Proceeding counterclockwise, the needle was inserted distal to the exit point. The next suture paralleled the first. The same method was used on the dorsal side and then on the palmar half. Tension on the double-stranded suture permitted apposition of the tendon ends.

Methods.—The techniques were compared in vitro using 64 fresh frozen digits from adult mongrel dogs and in vivo using 24 dogs. The dogs participated in passive mobilization of the wrists and digits 10 minutes each day, beginning on day 1 after surgery. Twelve dogs were sacrificed at 3 and then at 6 weeks. Digits were disarticulated, the metacarpal bone was removed, and gliding function and uniaxial tensile testing were done. Nonsevered tendons were used as controls.

Results.—In the in vitro experiment, the 8-strand and Tajima methods had the highest rotation values, and, along with the Savage method, yielded results similar to those for controls. Gliding functions for these 3 methods was significantly higher than for the Tsuge and Kessler methods. The 8-strand method had the highest tensile load before rupture (69 N). In the in vivo experiment, the Kessler method had the highest failure rate. Gliding function, joint rotation, and excursion of tendons repaired by the Tajima, Savage, and 8-strand methods were similar at 3 and 6 weeks but significantly less than for controls. The 8-strand method yielded repairs that were significantly stronger at 3 and 6 weeks (52.6 N and 70.9 N, respectively) than the Tajima and Savage repairs.

Conclusion.—Early active motion after tendon repair using the 8-strand method yields improved strength and functional results.

▶ Early active flexion after flexor tendon repair is being touted as an improvement over rehabilitation protocols centered about early passive motion or active entension protocols introduced by Kleinert. To reduce the risk of gap formation or rupture at the repair site, new suture techniques continue to be introduced. The authors describe an 8-strand technique, 2 more than the Savage technique. Previous studies confirm that strength of repair is proportional to the numbers of strands crossing the repair site. Recent work by Hotokezaka and Manske[1] and by Shaieb and Singer[2] suggest that there is a trade-off between the technical difficulty of multiple pass techniques and the added strength afforded by these techniques.

V.R. Hentz, M.D.

References

1. Hotokezaka S, Manske PR: Differences between locking loops and grasping loops: Effects on 2-strand core suture. *J Hand Surg [Am]* 22A:995–1003, 1997.
2. Shaieb M, Singer D: Tensile strengths of various suture techniques. *J Hand Surg [Br]* 22B:764–767, 1997.

Tensile Strengths of Various Suture Techniques
Shaieb MD, Singer DI (Univ of Hawaii, Honolulu)
J Hand Surg [Br] 22B:764–767, 1997.   16–3

Introduction.—The ideal suture for flexor tendon repair would be simple, allow early active motion, prevent gap formation and the development of adhesions, and avoid constriction of blood vessels and increased bulk. Using an animal model, 2 new suture techniques—a Double and Triple (modified) Kessler—were compared for strength with the Savage, Indiana, and modified Kessler techniques.

Methods.—In the 2-part study, 28 fresh New Zealand White rabbit Achilles' tendons and 14 fresh New Zealand White rabbit flexor digitorum longus (FDL) tendons were harvested and tested within 4 hours. All repairs were performed with core sutures of 4/0 Ethibond without an epitenon suture. The comparison of suture techniques was an in vitro biomechanical study of the forces required for 2 mm of gap formation and ultimate tensile strength.

Results.—In the test with rabbit Achilles' tendons, all failures occurred at the repair site. All methods were statistically different for gap formation and ultimate strength. The Double Kessler was almost twice as strong as the modified Kessler, and the Savage technique was strongest—even when compared with the Triple Kessler, another 6-stranded suture technique. In FDL tendons, the Double Kessler and Indiana techniques were similar in ultimate strength, but the Double Kessler was significantly stronger for gap formation. The Indiana technique's horizontal mattress suture allowed earlier gap formation by pulling out of the tendon early and at low forces.

Conclusions.—Although the Savage is the strongest suture, it can be technically difficult, time-consuming, and bulky. The Savage is almost twice as strong as the Double Kessler, and the Double Kessler almost twice as strong as the modified Kessler. The Savage technique is also stronger than another 6-stranded technique, the Triple Kessler, perhaps because the former uses only 1 knot and the latter 3 knots. Among 4-stranded techniques, the Double Kessler is stronger than the Indiana.

▶ The tensile strengths of suture techniques were studied for their biomechanical properties in vitro using rabbit Achilles' and FDL tendons. No epitendinous sutures were used. The study found that the Double Kessler was almost twice as strong as the modified Kessler, and the Savage was almost twice as strong as the Double Kessler.

Forces were recorded at the formation of a 2-mm gap; this is an important result of the study that should be stressed. In ascending order, 2-mm gaps formed, at low values, first in the modified Kessler, followed by the Double Kessler, Triple Kessler, and Savage. The authors acknowledge that the strongest suture that forms a 2-mm gap at the highest biomechanical value (in newtons) is the Savage, but this is technically difficult and time-consuming, and tends to increase the manipulation of the tendon.

Two 4-stranded techniques were also compared in this animal model—the Indiana and Double Kessler—but the ultimate strength was not significantly different.

This study tested at only a very early time frame—that is, 4 hours after tendon repair. The ultimate test of the tensile strength of these repairs should be tested in animal models first, with longer follow-up to 6–12 weeks after repair. Data from such investigation may provide a rationale for suggestions as to the tensile strength and gap formation that may be most advantageous for clinical practice.

M.A. Badalamente, Ph.D.

Anatomical Study of Flexor Digitorum Profundus Tendon Replacement by Flexor Superficialis Tendon Transfer [French]
Zuber Ch, Della Santa DR, Gajisin S (Hôpitaux Universitaires, Genève)
Ann Chir Main 16:235–244, 1997   16–4

Introduction.—The functional results of surgical repair of flexor tendon lesions are disappointing, especially when a secondary repair is needed. Tendon transfers for restoration of thumb flexion yield consistently good results. An anatomical study of superficial flexor tendons was described.

Findings.—The hands of 3 fresh cadavers were dissected to examine the length of superficial flexor tendons before advancement on the same finger to replace the deep flexor or their transfer to adjacent long fingers in the event of destruction of both flexor tendons. Excluding the superficial flexor of the fifth digit, the other 3 superficial flexors may be used for advancement or transfer, either alone or associated with proximal elongation according to Rouhier's technique.

Conclusions.—The superficial flexor of one finger may be used for advancement or transfer, with the exception of the little finger. This approach may be an optional deep flexor repair technique to the free graft and vascularized graft, particularly when direct repair is not possible.

▶ This anatomical study demonstrates that the superficialis of one finger can be transferred to another finger to substitute for loss of flexor profundus function in the same way that it can be used for flexor pollicis longus reconstruction. One philosophical problem with this study is that direct flexor tendon repair restores anatomy without disturbing an adjacent finger. This type of repair using a tendon transfer also carries the risk of adherence in the flexor sheath and rupture at the distal junction, so that it may not have a great advantage over direct repair. However, this may be an option if direct repair is impossible as in flexor profundus avulsion with retraction to the palm or loss of tendon substance.

J.M. Failla, M.D.

Mechanical Stress In Vitro Induces Increased Expression of MMPs 2 and 9 in Excised Dupuytren's Disease Tissue
Tarlton JF, Meagher P, Brown RA, et al (Univ of Bristol, England; Univ College, London; Univ of Westminster, London)
J Hand Surg [Br] 23B:297–302, 1998   16–5

Background.—Although collagen fibers are typically inextensible, in vivo stretching of fingers with severe Dupuytren's contractures nevertheless stretches the collagen fibers and reduces resistance. Thus the properties of the collagen must somehow change in these tissues, perhaps because of the mechanical stimulus or possibly owing to an inflammatory cell response. It hypothesized that the mechanical force of stretching would increase levels of degradative proteases such as matrix metalloproteinases

2 and 9 (MMPs 2 and 9) in these tissues, leading to depolymerization and thus weakened collagen fibers. The hypothesis was tested on Dupuytren's tissue samples in vitro.

Methods.—Tissue was sampled during fasciectomy from 21 patients (mean age, 62 years) who had Dupuytren's disease for 9 months to 30 years. Tissues were examined in vitro to avoid the influx of inflammatory cells and thus ensure that the results were caused by only biomechanical stress. A continuous elongation technique was mimicked by using a customized tensiometer that delivered defined creep loading to tissue strips at stresses of 0.25, 0.5, and 0.75 MPa. MMP-2 and MMP-9 enzymes in stretched and in control samples were extracted by gelatin substrate zymography.

Findings.—All 112 tissue specimens expressed proMMP-2, and all but 1 expressed MMP-2. Of 112 specimens 58 (52%) expressed proMMP-9, and 5 (4%) expressed MMP-9. ProMMP-2 levels were significantly higher at a load of 0.75 MPa than at a load of 0.25 MPa. MMP-2 levels were also higher at the 0.75 MPa load than in control tissues. MMP-9 levels were significantly higher at a load of 0.75 MPa than at 0.25 MPa, although MMP-9 expression varied throughout the experiment. To ensure there was no selection bias, pairs of stretched and control tissue samples were analyzed. Paired analysis confirmed that stretched specimens had lower levels of MMP-2 and MMP-9 than would be expected based on levels in controls.

Conclusions.—The constant exertion of tension on excised Dupuytren's disease tissue increased levels of the degradative MMP-2 and -9 and thus weakened the collagen fibers by depolymerization. This weakening allowed the collagen fibers to stretch, which accounts for the success of continuous elongation techniques. Furthermore, these events occurred in vitro, in the absence of inflammatory cell mediation.

▶ The question arises whether gradual mechanical elongation stretches tissue by mechanical disruption, by inducing remodelling, or both. This article shows evidence of the remodelling mechanism, although the differences between the control and experimental tissue was only significant at the highest load level applied. Further, this data shows that the Dupuytren's nodule tissue tested had baseline degradative enzyme levels lower than normal, suggesting perhaps some sort of inhibition of normal processes. All this is good evidence in favor of elongation as a part of a biological approach to the management of Dupuytren's disease.

P.C. Amadio, M.D.

Changes in Interstitial Pressure and Cross-Sectional Area of the Cubital Tunnel and of the Ulnar Nerve With Flexion of the Elbow: An Experimental Study in Human Cadavera

Gelberman RH, Yamaguchi K, Hollstien SB, et al (Washington Univ, St Louis)
J Bone Joint Surg Am 80-A:492–501, 1998   16–6

Introduction.—The exact mechanism of compression of the ulnar nerve within the cubital tunnel has not been completely defined. Twenty specimens from human cadavers were assessed to determine the relationship between the ulnar nerve and the cubital tunnel during elbow flexion.

Methods.—In positions of incremental flexion, elbows underwent magnetic resonance imaging. Cross-sectional images were made at 3 anatomical regions of the cubital tunnel: medial epicondyle, deep to the cubital tunnel aponeurosis, and deep to the flexor carpi ulnaris muscle. The cross-sectional areas of the cubital tunnel and the ulnar nerve were estimated and compared for varying positions of ulnar flexion. Ultrasonographic imaging was used to measure interstitial pressures within the cubital tunnel and 4 cm proximal to it, at 10-degree increments from 0 to 130 degrees of elbow flexion.

Results.—The mean cross-sectional area of the 3 regions of the cubital tunnel were reduced by 30, 39, and 41 degrees, respectively, as the elbow was moved from full extension to 135 degrees of flexion; the mean area of the ulnar nerve was reduced by 33, 50, and 34 degrees, respectively. Changes in all 3 cubital tunnel regions were significant, with the greatest changes observed in the region beneath the aponeurosis of the cubital tunnel with the elbow in 135-degree flexion. The mean intraneural pressure within the cubital tunnel was significantly greater than the mean extraneural pressure with the elbow in 90, 100, 110, and 130 degrees of flexion. The mean intraneural pressure was 45 degrees greater than the mean extraneural pressure. The mean intraneural pressure 4 cm proximal to the cubital tunnel was significantly greater than the mean extraneural pressure with elbow flexion of 120 degrees or greater. Within the cubital tunnel and proximal to it, intraneural pressure increased at smaller angles of flexion than did extraneural pressure. After surgical release of the aponeurotic roof of the cubital tunnel, there were no significant differences in intraneural pressure at the level of the cubital tunnel or 4 cm proximally.

Conclusion.—The cubital tunnel is a morphologically dynamic region. The cubital tunnel and the ulnar nerve change as much as 50% with elbow flexion and extension. There is no evidence of direct, focal compression of the ulnar nerve when it is flattened during elbow flexion. These morphological findings parallel those of measurements of interstitial pressure, which demonstrated an initial rise in intraneural pressure without a corresponding increase in extraneural pressure. Traction on the ulnar nerve is a primary cause of increased intraneural pressure during flexion of the elbow.

▶ The conservative management of cubital tunnel syndrome is predicated on teaching patients to avoid unnecessary elbow flexion and direct pressure over the ulnar nerve in the cubital tunnel. Patients are advised to modify their activities with such maneuvers as the use of headsets or speaker phones; they are told to sleep with their arms by their sides and to hold the steering wheel a little farther in front of them. These recommendations are based on our understanding that elbow flexion increases pressure to the ulnar nerve and also increases tension on the ulnar nerve as suggested in the early work by Pechan and Julis.[1] This elegant study by Gelberman et al adds to our understanding of the cause of cubital tunnel syndrome and emphasizes that certain positions and postures will, indeed, affect neural function. Thus, an awareness of these various positions should be emphasized to our patients in order that they might make alterations in their work, nonwork, and sleep postures to prevent such problems as cubital tunnel syndrome.[2]

S.E. Mackinnon, M.D., F.R.C.S.C.

References

1. Pechan J, Julia I: The pressure measurement in the ulnar nerve: A contribution to the pathophysiology of the cubital tunnel syndrome. *J Biomechanics* 8:75–79, 1975.
2. Mackinnon SE, Novak C: Clinical commentary: Pathogenesis of cumulative trauma disorder. *J Hand Surg [Am]* 19A:873–883, 1994.

Variables Affecting Axonal Regeneration Following End-to-Side Neurorrhaphy
Al-Qattan MM, Al-Thunyan A (King Saud Univ, Riyadh, Saudi Arabia)
Br J Plast Surg 51:238–242, 1998   16–7

Introduction.—The concept that end-to-end nerve coaptation can encourage collateral sprouting has recently been reintroduced; findings conflict. Described are some of the variables affecting axonal regeneration after end-to-side repair in the rat sciatic nerve model.

Findings.—Two experiments were performed.

Experiment 1.—Twenty Sprague-Dawley rats were divided into 2 groups of 10 animals each to evaluate the rate of axonal regeneration after end-to-side neurorrhaphy with nerve grafts and to compare epineurial vs. perineurial sutures. In group A, the nerve graft was sutured to the epineurium. In group B rats, it was sutured to the perineurium. Nerve grafts underwent histologic and electron microscopic examination 50 days after repair. The nerve grafts in group A had no evidence of nerve-regenerating axons, compared with 50% for the nerve grafts in group B. Between-group differences were significant. Electron microscopy revealed that the repair process after end-to-side neurorrhaphy was structurally similar to axonal regeneration after end-to-end neurorrhaphy.

Experiment 2.—The feasibility of inducing collateral sprouting by means of silicone tubes sutured in an end-to-side fashion to the epineurium or perineurium of intact rat sciatic nerves was assessed in 2 groups of 10 rats each. The site of silicone tube attachment was exposed at 50-day follow-up, and the tube was meticulously removed. The silicone tube contained soft tissue, which was firmly attached to the side of the nerve. This attached soft tissue segment had no histologic or electron microscopic evidence of any nerve regeneration.

Conclusion.—Axonal regeneration after end-to-side nerve coaptation is significantly more likely to occur when the nerve graft is sutured to the parent nerve with perineurial rather than epineurial sutures. Failure to establish collateral sprouting within the attached soft tissue segment may be explained by the absence of Schwann cells in the transplanted silicone tubes.

▶ We are all familiar with end-to-side vessel repair. However, in spite of the fact that the concept of an end-to-side nerve repair was introduced a century ago, the concept has only recently been revisited with several experimental studies. There is agreement that sensory axons will sprout de novo from an intact nerve into the distal stump of a second nerve sutured end-to-side to the perineurium of the intact donor nerve. In a clinical situation in which limited sensory axonal regeneration would be superior to no sensory recovery and traditional alternatives for reinnervation are not available, consideration of an end-to-side nerve repair to recover some sensibility is indicated. This has been used in head and neck reconstruction in which the lateral antebrachial cutaneous nerve of the radial forearm flap is sutured end-to-side to the lingual nerve to provide limited sensory reinnervation of this intraoral flap. The concept of collateral sprouting of sensory axons is observed after the harvest of sensory nerves for nerve graft procedures. Over subsequent months to years large areas of sensory deficit gradually decrease in size, in keeping with collateral sensory sprouting from adjacent uninjured sensory nerves. By contrast, the ability of motor axons to collaterally sprout in an end-to-side repair remains controversial. In our laboratory, when retrograde tracing studies were performed, there was little to no tracking back to the motor neuron pool.[1] By contrast, the few axons that had sprouted into the distal end-to-side nerve were traced back by retrograde labeling to the dorsal root ganglion. Motor recovery noted in other experimental studies is possibly related to contamination of motor axon sprouting from the divided proximal end of the recipient nerve, not the normal donor nerve. Although there has been a scant number of clinical reports on the use of end-to-side repair for motor recovery, I remain skeptical of this technique for motor recovery in the clinical situation. Further experimental studies are needed.

S.E. Mackinnon, M.D., F.R.C.S.C.

Reference

1. Tarasidis G, Watanabe O, Mackinnon SE, et al: End-to-side neurorrhaphy resulting in limited sensory axonal regeneration in a rat model. *Ann Otol Rhinol Laryngol* 106:506–512, 1997.

End-to-Side Neurorrhaphy: A Histologic and Morphometric Study of Axonal Sprouting Into an End-to-Side Nerve Graft

Noah EM, Williams A, Jorgenson C, et al (Internatl Inst for Reconstructive Surgery and Microsurgical Research Ctr, Norfolk, Va)
J Reconstr Microsurg 13:99–106, 1997
16–8

Objective.—Although nerve repairs have been effected by borrowing axons from adjacent nerves, quantitative morphological proof of how this occurs is lacking. To shed light on this situation, factors that can enhance or inhibit lateral sprouting were identified in the rat.

Technique.—The peroneal nerve was severed where it joins the sciatic nerve in 20 Sprague-Dawley rats. The connective tissue sheaths of the posterior tibial nerve were allowed to remain intact in group 1. The epineurium was removed in group 2, and the peroneal nerve was sutured end-to-side to the posterior tibial nerve. In group 3, the epineurium and perineurium were removed at the site of nerve coaptation. In group 4, one third of the cross-sectional neural area was excised and the peroneal nerve was coapted and sutured end-to-end to the prepared site. After 30 days, nerve specimens were harvested and examined by light and electron microscopy, and quantitative morphometry was performed.

Results.—Axonal regeneration was apparent in all groups. Morphometry revealed spare regeneration in group 1, with infrequent Schwann cells and degeneration and demyelination. In group 2, specimens were densely packed with Schwann cells and endoneural connective tissue. Group 3 revealed clusters of myelinated axons embedded in Schwann cells, myelin formation, and pronounced vascularization. Group 4 also had a substantial increase in the number of axons, with a significantly smaller diameter and a significantly smaller myelin area than those found in the other groups. Groups 1 and 2 had statistically similar results. Groups 3 and 4 had statistically similar results but significantly more axons than groups 1 and 2.

Conclusion.—Axon regeneration was significantly higher in groups in which the perineurium was incised and end-to-end neurorrhaphy was performed.

▶ The jury is still "out" on this issue. What do we know for certain? . . . that nerves are easily stimulated to grow, regenerate, and sprout. There must be many chemical signals and appropriate receptors active. Among the most important known source of these agents is the Schwann cell. Any perineural injury leads to significant demyelination/remyelination, all under the influence of Schwann cells, and to retrograde transport of neuroactive triggers. To an axon bud, 1 chemical target may be as attractive as another. The ultimate clinical significance of these findings remains to be determined.

V.R. Hentz, M.D.

A New Type of "Bioartificial" Nerve Graft for Bridging Extended Defects in Nerves
Lundborg G, Dahlin L, Kanje M, et al (Lund Univ, Malmö, Sweden)
J Hand Surg [Br] 22B:299–303, 1997   16–9

Introduction.—Silicone tubes offer an alternative to the use of autologous nerve grafts or frozen muscle to promote axonal growth over segmental defects in peripheral nerves. In the rat sciatic nerve model, however, a silicone tube usually fails to support axonal growth in defects greater than 10 mm. A new artificial nerve graft composed of polyamide filaments placed inside silicon tubes was tested for its ability to bridge an extended gap.

Methods.—Sciatic nerve defects of 15 mm were created in 20 female Wistar rats. In all animals the defect was bridged by a 19-mm silicone tube with an inner diameter of 1.8 mm. Nerve ends were pulled 2 mm into each opening and secured by two 9/0 Ethilon stitches. Eight polyamide filaments (15 mm in length and 250 µm in diameter) were placed inside the silicone tube in 12 rats (filament group); 8 rats served as controls. All tubes were filled with saline and the wound was sutured. Four weeks later, a pinch reflex test was performed distal to the tube. The rats were then killed and the nerve segments prepared for routine histology and immunocytochemistry.

Results.—The pinch test gave a clear response in all rats in the filament group, but no response was observed in any of the controls. A well-developed, rounded structure with the appearance of smooth connective tissue was organized around the filaments in the filament group. The tube contained only fluid in 6 controls; tubes in the 2 remaining controls contained a minute threadlike structure that bridged the defect. Histology indicated axonal growth along the whole length of the tube in the filament group, and there was positive staining for neurofilaments in the distal nerve segment.

Conclusion.—Synthetic filaments have the potential to promote axonal growth across greater distances in extended nerve defects. Success with bioartificial nerve grafts may help to limit or avoid the need to sacrifice healthy nerves in patients requiring autologous nerve transplantation.

▶ Any technique that will enhance regeneration across a silicone tubing that is 12–15 mm in length is an important advance. Although *bioabsorbable* conduits will allow nerve regeneration to 3 cm, gaps much greater than 1 cm in length bridged with a *silicone* conduit will not support axonal regeneration. Although this study involved only 12 experimental animals, and no histomorphometry was done to quantitate the degree of neural regeneration, the fact that there was any regeneration across this conduit is exciting information and suggests that the future management of the short nerve gap will include nerve conduits of some sort as an option for reconstruction.

S.E. Mackinnon, M.D., F.R.C.S.C.

Forearm Muscle Oxygenation Decreases With Low Levels of Voluntary Contraction

Murthy G, Kahan NJ, Hargens AR, et al (Univ of California, Berkeley; Sports and Occupation Med Associates, Cupertino; Natl Aeronautics and Space Administration Ames Research Ctr, Moffett Field, Calif; et al)
J Orthop Res 15:507–511, 1997   16–10

Background.—Although the causes of muscle fatigue and pain resulting from repetitive motion of the hand and arm are unclear, many contributing factors have been identified. Among these are impaired blood flow and local hypoxemia or ischemia. Near infra-red spectroscopy, a noninvasive technique that directly measures relative changes in tissue oxygenation, was evaluated for its ability to detect changes in tissue oxygenation at low levels of isometric contraction in the extensor carpi radialis brevis muscle. This technique has been validated for human skeletal muscle, but has not been used to study tissue oxygenation at low levels of muscle contraction.

Methods.—Study participants were 7 men and 2 women with a mean age of 34, good health, and no history of upper extremity musculoskeletal disorders. They were seated with the right arm abducted to 45 degrees, elbow flexed to 85 degrees, forearm pronated 45%, and wrist and forearm supported on an arm rest. Baseline measurements were obtained with the muscle relaxed. A near infrared spectroscopy probe was used to measure altered tissue oxygenation after application of 4 different loads proximal to the metacarpophalangeal joint so that participants isometrically contracted the extensor carpi radialis brevis at 5%, 10%, 15%, and 50% of the maximum voluntary contraction for 1 minute each.

Results.—At each level of contraction, tissue oxygenation usually increased to above baseline levels within 10 seconds after the onset of contraction, then declined below baseline levels, reached a plateau 10–40 seconds into the contraction, and remained at the reduced level until the end of the 60-second contraction period. Mean tissue oxygenation levels at 10%, 15%, and 50% of the maximum voluntary contraction were all significantly lower than the baseline value. At 5% maximum voluntary contraction level, tissue oxygenation did not differ significantly from baseline and it recovered to 100% of baseline value within 3 minutes. The perceived exertion at each level of contraction showed a linear increase with decreasing tissue oxygenation.

Conclusion.—Tissue oxygenation significantly decreases during brief, low levels of static muscle contraction. Near infra-red spectroscopy can be used to detect this deoxygenation at low levels of forearm muscle contraction.

▶ This is an interesting article. Unfortunately, it lacks adequate controls, and has too narrow a scope and too small a series to draw any conclusions. However, it is an interesting pilot study that merits further investigation.

M.L. Kasdan, M.D.

Adhesion Receptors and Cytokine Profiles in Controlled Tourniquet Ischaemia in the Upper Extremity
Germann G, Drücke D, Steinau HU (BG-Univ Hosp "Bergmannsheil", Bochum, Germany)
J Hand Surg [Br] 22B:778–782, 1997   16–11

Purpose.—Cytokine-mediated adhesion mechanisms are intimately involved in ischemia-reperfusion mechanisms. Studies of organ transplantation have shown this relationship clearly, but it has not been studied in patients undergoing upper extremity surgery. This study used controlled tourniquet ischemia of the upper extremity, in surgical patients and volunteers, to study changes in adhesion receptors and cytokines in ischemia and reperfusion.

Methods.—The study included 8 patients undergoing elective hand surgery and 2 normal controls. All were studied during tourniquet ischemia of the upper arm, with a maximum pressure of 250 mm Hg. For up to 30 minutes after reperfusion was restored, blood samples were taken for measurement of the adhesion molecules (CD11/CD18); the cytokines tumor necrosis factor (TNF)-α and interleukin (IL)-1; CD4+ and CD8+ lymphocytes; and polymorphonuclear neutrophils.

Results.—Ischemia time averaged 67 minutes, and was unrelated to levels of adhesion molecules. Leukocyte counts did not change significantly, nor did the counts and ratio of CD4+/CD8+ cells. TNF-α did not increase significantly after reperfusion. However, 2 patients with ischemia times of 67 and 147 minutes had outstanding peaks in their levels of adhesion molecules and a sharp rise in TNF-α.

Conclusions.—Even brief periods of ischemia during upper extremity surgery are associated with detectable changes in the immune system. Ischemia stimulates adhesion molecules and cytokines, which are involved in the early pathophysiology of reperfusion. The adhesion molecule and cytokine patterns noted in humans are comparable to those noted in previous animal studies. The data support the concept that receptor-blocking agents may be useful in reducing the effects of prolonged ischemia in severe hand injury, compartment syndrome, or free-flap revisions.

▶ This is a preliminary study investigating the potential contribution of adhesion molecules (CD11/CD18), certain cytokines (TNF-α and IL-1, CD4+ and CD8+) lymphocytes and PMNs to adverse effects after ischemia in the human upper extremity.

Mean tourniquet time was 67 minutes at 250 mm Hg. Eight patients having Dupuytren's or tendon surgery and two control subjects were studied. Blood samples were taken at 0, 1, 2, 5 and 30 minutes after perfusion was restored.

Results indicate no significant correlation between levels of adhesion molecules and duration of ischemia time, no alteration in CD4+/CD8+ counts, and no significant difference in TNF-α and IL-1. Outlier values in 2 patients were recorded as sharp increases in TNF-α with 67 and 147 minutes of ischemia.

Although this study has not shown any significant changes in the parameters of various molecules that may be important to the pathophysiology of tissue damage after ischemia reperfusion, the study used clinical standards for upper extremity surgery known to be safe. The value of this study may be that it will serve as a useful model to study the serious adverse effects of severe hand injuries, such as replantation surgery. The agents under investigation in this study have been shown to have potential in animal models for mediating adverse tissue events after ischemia reperfusion.

The ultimate contribution of these agents to the pathophysiology of reperfusion injury will await future study which investigates more severe upper extremity injuries.

M.A. Badalamente, Ph.D.

Suggested Reading

Pohl D, Bass LS, Stewart R, et al: Effect of optical temperature feedback control on patency in laser-soldered microvascular anastomosis. *J Reconstr Microsurg* 14:23–29, 1998.

▶ Although interrupted sutures remain the gold standard for microsurgical vascular repair, the search continues for a more efficient and less technique-dependent method. In this study, 2 different laser methods were compared with freehand sutures in a rat model. Long-term patency of the freehand technique was 96%. The freehand laser technique was faster but produced a lower patency rate (71%). A modification of the laser technique, which provided optical feedback (an infrared thermometer) of weld temperature, resulted in a significant improvement in laser patency of 88%. As control of laser technology improves, it may be possible to use these techniques clinically. However, the risks of rupture and aneurysm formation continue to relegate laser-assisted vascular anastomosis to the experimental laboratory.

P.C. Amadio, M.D.

Van Turnhout AA, Hage JJ, De Groot PJ, et al: Lack of difference in sensibility between the dominant and nondominant hands as tested with Semmes-Weinstein monofilaments. *J Hand Surg [Br]* 22B:768–771, 1997.

▶ A previous study showed equal or better sensibility in the pulp of the non-dominant vs. the dominant index finger. These authors tested multiple sites in 50 healthy volunteers and found no difference between these palmar sites in 51%, better sensibility in the all the non-dominant sites in 34%, and better sensibility in the dominant hand in 15%.

V.R. Hentz, M.D.

Subject Index

A

Acutrak cannulated screw
  fixation for scaphoid, comparison with other screws during application of cyclical bending loads, 163
Adduction
  contractures of thumb, release procedures for, and anatomy of adductor pollicis muscle, 2
Adductor
  pollicis muscle, anatomy of, 2
Adhesion
  receptors in controlled tourniquet ischemia in upper extremity, 299
Adolescents
  carpal tunnel syndrome in, with no history trauma, 130
  digit amputation in, traumatic, toe-to-hand transfer for, 266
Aesthesiometer
  Semmes-Weinstein pressure, effect of wrist position on testing light touch sensation with, 41
Algodystrophy
  after fracture of distal radius, predictive criteria of outcome after 1 year, 184
Allodynia
  touch, after endoscopic or open carpal tunnel release, 119
Allograft
  osteoarticular, in reconstruction of distal radius after excision of skeletal tumor, 227
Alumafoam splint
  dorsal, for trigger finger, 259
Amputation
  digital, traumatic, toe-to-hand transfer for, in children and adolescents, 266
  fingertip, eponychial flap for, 67
Amyotrophic
  lateral sclerosis and carpal tunnel syndrome, 131
Anastomosis
  microvascular, laser-soldered, effect of optical temperature feedback control on patency in (in rat), 300
Anatomical
  basis of vascularized pronator quadratus pedicled bone graft, 24
  classification of sites of compression of palmar cutaneous branch of median nerve, 5

factors predisposing to focal dystonia in musician's hand, 201
investigation of distal tract of interosseous membrane, 191
study
  of flexor digitorum profundus tendon replacement by flexor superficialis tendon transfer, 291
  of interosseous flap, 62
  of interosseous nerve, posterior, and radial tunnel syndrome, 128
  of venous drainage of radial forearm and anterior tibial reverse flow flaps, 12
Anatomy, 1
  of adductor pollicis muscle, 2
  detailed, of palmar cutaneous nerves, 8
  of interosseous nerve, posterior, in relation to fixation of radial head, 11
  of palmar ligamentous structures of carpal canal, 3
Anchor
  Mitek mini, in gamekeeper's thumb, 56
Anesthesia, 27
  regional, IV, vs. general, for outpatient hand surgery, pharmacoeconomics of, 38
  techniques, comparison of three, for reduction of distal radius fractures, 40
Anesthetic
  digit, completely, once-twice test for evaluation of, 41
Anomalies
  congenital, Ilizarov distraction-lengthening in, 242
Antiinflammatory
  drugs, nonsteroidal, for piper's palsy, 203
AO classification
  of Colles' fractures, 168
  of radius fractures, distal, 167
Aponeurosis
  palmar, mechanical properties of, and Dupuytren's contracture, 235
Arteriolysis
  limited microsurgical, for complications of digital vasospasm, 275
Artery(ies)
  carpal, palmar, vascularized bone graft from, for scaphoid nonunion, 144
  digital, reverse island flap, clinical experience with, 64
  interosseous
    anterior, experience with, 25

301

flap (see Flap, interosseous)
periarterial sympathectomy, acute effects on cutaneous microcirculation (in rabbit), 274
radial, perforators, proximal, island fasciocutaneous flap based on, for resurfacing of burned cubital fossa, 70
ulnar
 dorsal branch, neurocutaneous flap based on, 276
 flap, dorsal, use in hand and wrist tissue cover, 59
Arthritis, 207
 osteoarthritis (see Osteoarthritis)
 posttraumatic
  thumb carpometacarpal joint, de la Caffinière replacement for, long-term follow-up, 210–211
  trapeziometacarpal joint replacements for, cemented and non-cemented, 213
 rheumatoid
  carpometacarpal joint, thumb, de la Caffinière replacement for, long-term follow-up, 210
  early stage, bone scintigraphy in, 223
  hand joints in, destruction and reconstruction of, 224
  synovectomy of elbow and radial head excision in, 225
  trapeziometacarpal joint replacements for, cemented and non-cemented, 213
  wrist, does wrist fusion cause destruction of first carpometacarpal joint in? 222
  wrist, evolution of surgical indications in treatment of, 218, 224
  wrist, synovectomy for, arthroscopic, long-term follow-up, 217
Arthrodesis
 wrist, limited, for scapholunate advanced collapse, 162
Arthrography
 conventional vs. magnetic resonance, in diagnosis of gamekeeper thumb, 34
 magnetic resonance, vs. MRI in diagnosis of gamekeeper thumb, 34
 of triangular fibrocartilage complex lesion in distal forearm fractures of children, 187
 vs. MRI in diagnosis of triangular fibrocartilage injuries, 31
 wrist, after acute trauma to distal radius, 169

Arthroplasty
 scaphoid costo-osteochondral replacement, proximal, 140
 wrist, total, review of last 30 years, 219
Arthroscopy
 -assisted reduction of intraarticular fractures of distal radius, 178
 elbow, interosseous nerve injury after, 98
 in evaluation and treatment of thumb carpometacarpal joints, 208
 of intraarticular lesions in distal fractures of radius, in young adults, 179
 synovectomy of rheumatoid wrist by, long-term follow-up, 217
 of trapeziometacarpal joint, portals for, 209
 wrist
  after carpal injuries, 133
  in management of triangular fibrocartilage complex tears, 194
Articular
 fracture of phalanx, external traction for, 57
Aspiration
 simple, or with injection of corticosteroid and/or hyaluronidase for carpal and digital ganglions, 232
 of wrist ganglia, 238
Ataxia
 cerebellar, late onset, and carpal tunnel syndrome, 131
Avulsion
 brachial plexus
  C5-C6 or C5-C6-C7, ulnar nerve fascicle transfer onto biceps muscle nerve in, 199
  complete, elbow extension in reconstruction of prehension with reinnervated free muscle transfer after, 200
 fracture, metacarpophalangeal joint, 47
Axial
 loading induces rotation of proximal carpal row bone around unique screw-displacement axes, 166
Axon
 regeneration after end-to-side neurorrhaphy (in rat), 294
 sprouting into end-to-side nerve graft, histologic and morphometric study of (in rat), 296

B

Bagpipers
  focal dystonia in, 203
Bandage
  elastic, in treatment of ring and little metacarpal neck fractures, 47
Bandaging
  compression, for lymphedema of extremities, 279
Biaxial total wrist arthroplasty prosthesis, 219, 221
Biceps
  muscle nerve, ulnar nerve fascicle transfer onto, in C5-C6 or C5-C6-C7 avulsion of brachial plexus, 199
"Bioartificial" nerve graft
  for bridging extended defects in nerve, new type of (in rat), 297
Biomechanical
  analysis
    of limited intercarpal fusion for Kienböck's disease, 155
    of suture repair methods for flexor tendon repair (in dog), 288
Biomechanics, 1
Block
  digital, single injection transthecal vs. subcutaneous, 258
  hematoma, with sedation, for reduction of distal radius fractures, 40
  nerve, continuous peripheral, in replantation and revascularization, 272
Blood
  supply of lumbrical muscles, 2
Blue collar workers
  in manufacturing industry, vibrotactile sense and hand symptoms in, 256
Body
  mass index, effect on prevalence of median mononeuropathy at wrist, 107
Bone
  carpal
    motion relative to radius, 3-D analysis of, 165
    proximal row, rotation around unique screw-displacement axis, axial loading induces, 166
  graft (see Graft, bone)
  loss, segmental, isolated forearm nonunion with, surgical treatment of, 50
  nerves implanted in, prevention of neuroma formation in (in rat), 93

scintigraphy in early stage lupus erythematosus and rheumatoid arthritis, 223
substitute for enchondroma, 238
tumors, juxta-articular giant cell, vascularized bone grafts for, 230
Botulinum
  toxin
    in piper's palsy, 203
    in writer's cramp, 251
Brace
  functional, for ring and little metacarpal neck fractures, 47
Brachial plexus
  avulsion
    C5-C6 or C5-C6-C7, ulnar nerve fascicle transfer onto biceps muscle nerve in, 199
    complete, elbow extension in reconstruction of prehension with reinnervated free muscle transfer after, 200
  lesions, traumatic, role of neurophysiological investigation in, 29
Brunelli procedure
  modified, for scapholunate instability, early results, 149
Bruner approach
  modified, to proximal interphalangeal joint denervation, 207
Bupivacaine
  nerve block, continuous peripheral, in replantation and revascularization, 272
Burn(s)
  cubital fossa, resurfacing for, island fasciocutaneous flap based on proximal perforators of radial artery for, 70

C

Camptodactyly
  Ilizarov distraction-lengthening in, 242
Care
  skin, for lymphedema of extremities, 279
Carpal
  (See also Wrist)
  artery, palmar, vascularized bone graft from, for scaphoid nonunion, 144
  bone
    motion relative to radius, 3-D analysis of, 165
    proximal row, rotation around unique screw-displacement axis, axial loading induces, 166

canal
- ligamentous structures of, palmar, anatomical study of, 3
- morphologic changes after open carpal tunnel release, effect of transverse carpal ligament on, 17
- compression test, value in diagnosis of carpal tunnel syndrome, 100
- dislocations, perilunate, lunotriquetral lesions and their sequelae in, 152
- fracture-dislocations, perilunate, lunotriquetral lesions and their sequelae in, 152
- fractures in children, 166
- impaction, ulnar, ulnar shortening osteotomy for, 153
- injuries, wrist arthroscopy after, 133
- instability, ulnar, ulnar shortening osteotomy for, 153
- intercarpal fusion, limited, for Kienböck's disease, biomechanical analysis of, 155
- kinematics (see Kinematics, carpal)
- ligament, transverse
  - effect on flexor tendon excursion after open carpal tunnel release, 17
  - lengthening vs. simple division, in carpal tunnel syndrome, 116
  - stability, study of, 134
- tunnel (see below)
- ulnocarpal stress test in diagnosis of ulnar-sided wrist pain, 146

Carpal tunnel
- MRI of, median nerve compression detected by, 104
- pressure
  - effects of static fingertip loading on, 249
  - fingertip loading and, 262
- release
  - endoscopic, review of, 114
  - endoscopic, touch allodynia after, 119
  - open, effect of transverse carpal ligament on flexor tendon excursion, morphologic changes of carpal canal, and pinch and grip strength after, 17
  - open, touch allodynia after, 119
  - open, wound tenderness after, effect of vascularized hypothenar fat pad on, 121
  - pillar pain after, 120
  - return to work after, predictors of, 118
  - safe, via limited palmar incision, 122
- syndrome
  - in amyotrophic lateral sclerosis and late onset cerebellar ataxia, 131
  - carpal ligament lengthening vs. simple division of ligament in, 116
  - in children and adolescents with no history of trauma, 130
  - diagnosis, value of carpal compression test in, 100
  - electrodiagnostic studies in, predictive value of, 263
  - exercises for, nerve and tendon gliding, 110
  - forearm velocity in, 131
  - MRI of, dynamic, 41
  - in mucopolysaccharidoses and mucolipidoses, 109
  - with normal electrodiagnostic study, 113
  - outcome instrument in, self-administered, 130
  - provocative test for, new, 99
  - after reduction of intraarticular fractures of distal radius, arthroscopically-assisted, 179
  - release (see Carpal tunnel, release above)
  - risk factors for, 263
  - risk factors for, occupational and personal, in industrial workers, 264
  - risks in occupational environment, linguistic model for prediction of, 262
  - self-reported, in working population, prevalence of, association with occupational and non-occupational risk factors, 264
  - sensory function after median nerve decompression in, 115
  - test battery for, sensory and psychomotor functional, in confirmed cases and normal subjects, 101
  - test battery for, sensory and psychomotor functional, in industrial subjects, 103
  - ultrasound treatment for, 111
  - vitamin B_6 related to, in industrial workers, 106

Carpectomy
- proximal row
  - case reviews, 159
  - palmar, 160

Carpometacarpal joint
- thumb
  - arthroscopic evaluation and treatment of, 208
  - destruction caused by wrist fusion in rheumatoid arthritis, 222
  - replacements, de la Caffinière, long-term follow-up, 210

Cast
  plaster-of-Paris, for ring and little metacarpal neck fractures, 47
Castle
  flap in treatment of skin retraction in severe stiffness of hand and fingers, 63
Cell
  giant cell tumors of bone, vascularized bone graft for, 230
Cellulitis
  Escherichia coli, upper limb, in immunocompromised patients, 69
Cemented
  replacement of trapeziometacarpal joint, 213
  trapeziometacarpal prosthesis, radiological course of, 214
Centralization
  for radial club hand, long-term follow-up, 239
Cerebellar
  ataxia, late onset, and carpal tunnel syndrome, 131
Cerebral
  palsy, surgery of spastic hand in, 204
Cheiralgia
  paresthetica, case reports, 127
Children
  brachial plexus lesions in, traumatic, role of neurophysiological investigation in, 29
  carpal tunnel syndrome in
    with mucopolysaccharidoses and mucolipidoses, 109
    with no history trauma, 130
  digit amputation in, traumatic, toe-to-hand transfer for, 266
  digital tip replacement in, composite graft, 68
  elbow ossification centers in, sequential development, 245
  fingertip injuries in, crush, late diagnosis and treatment of, 71
  fracture in
    carpal, 166
    forearm, distal, epidemiology, 171
    forearm, distal, role of radiographs in follow up, 49
    forearm, distal, triangular fibrocartilage complex lesion in, 187
  median nerve repair in, primary epineural, 89
  physis injuries in, distal radius, corrective osteotomies after, 182
  pseudo-Volkmann's contracture due to tethering of flexor digitorum profundus to fractures of ulna in, 284
  scar contracture in, recurrent digital, proximal phalangeal island flap for, 70
  tendon sheath of snapping digits in, operative and histopathological study, 245
Chondral
  lesions in distal fractures of radius, in young adults, 179
Chow technique of endoscopic tunnel release
  review of, 114
Cigarette
  smoking and cold intolerance after peripheral nerve injuries, 96
Club
  hand, radial
    Ilizarov distraction-lengthening in, 242
    operative correction, long-term follow-up, 239
Cold
  intolerance
    after peripheral nerve injury, 95
    posttraumatic, pattern recognition in, 284
Colles' fracture (*see* Fracture, Colles')
Compression
  bandaging for lymphedema of extremities, 279
  carpal, test, value in diagnosis of carpal tunnel syndrome, 100
  median nerve (*see* Median nerve, compression)
  neuropathy, 99
Computer
  keyboard users, repetitive strain injury in, pathomechanics and treatment, 263
Conduits
  ePTFE, reconstruction of upper extremity peripheral nerve injuries with, 87
Congenital
  anomalies, Ilizarov distraction-lengthening in, 242
  problems, 239
Contraction
  voluntary, low levels, forearm muscle oxygenation decreases with, 298
Contracture
  adduction, of thumb, release procedures for, and anatomy of adductor pollicis muscle, 2

Dupuytren's
  fasciotomy for, percutaneous, 237
  pathogenesis, mechanical properties of palmar aponeurosis in, 235
joint
  interphalangeal, proximal, correction of, multiplanar distracter in, 45
  moderate, after controlled active motion after primary flexor tendon repair, 73
  pseudo-Volkmann's, due to tethering of flexor digitorum profundus to fractures of ulna, in children, 284
  scar, digital, recurrent, proximal phalangeal island flap for, in children, 70
Coonrad-Morrey semiconstrained elbow prosthesis
  for osteoarthrosis, posttraumatic, 225
Coronoid
  reconstruction for chronic dislocation of elbow, 55
Corpuscles
  pacinian, in hand
    distribution of, 7
    painful hyperplasia and hypertrophy of, 97
Cortical
  dysfunction associated with writer's cramp not reversed by botulinum toxin, 251
Corticosteroid
  injection
    with aspiration for carpal and digital ganglions, 232
    for ganglia of wrist, 238
    local, with splinting, for ulnar neuropathy at elbow, 125
Cost
  of continuous passive motion after rigid fixation of isolated unicondylar fractures of proximal phalanx, 44
Costo-osteochondral
  replacement arthroplasty, proximal scaphoid, 140
Cramp
  writer's, botulinum toxin does not reverse cortical dysfunction associated with, 251
CREST
  digital vasospasm in, complications of, limited microsurgical arteriolysis for, 275
Crush injuries
  of fingertip, late diagnosis and treatment, in children, 71

Cubital
  fossa, burned, resurfacing of, island fasciocutaneous flap based on proximal perforators of radial artery for, 70
  tunnel
    interstitial pressure and cross-sectional area changes with flexion of elbow, 293
    syndrome, long-term results of modified King's method for, 131
Cumulative trauma disorders
  reliability of Postural and Repetitive risk-factors Index in, 247
Cutaneous
  (See also Skin)
  branch
    dorsal, of ulnar nerve, 24
    palmar, of median nerve, anatomical classification of sites of compression of, 5
  microcirculation, acute effects of periarterial sympathectomy on (in rabbit), 274
  nerves, palmar, detailed anatomy of, 8
  responses to endothelin-1 and histamine in vibration white finger, 286
Cytokine
  profiles in controlled tourniquet ischemia in upper extremity, 299

D

de la Caffinière
  prosthesis, trapeziometacarpal joint, 213
    radiological course of, 214
  thumb carpometacarpal replacements, long-term follow-up, 210
Decompression
  median nerve, in carpal tunnel syndrome, sensory function after, 115
Decongestive
  physiotherapy, complete, for lymphedema of extremities, 279
Deformity
  mallet, of finger, 5-year follow-up of conservative treatment, 83
Degloved skin
  of hand, replantation of, 276
Delta frame
  for intraarticular fractures of distal radius, 173
Denervation
  interphalangeal joint, proximal, 207
  radiocarpal joint, follow-up study, 161

Subject Index / 307

Diagnosis, 27
Digit
  (*See also* Finger; Thumb; Toe)
  amputation, traumatic, toe-to-hand transfer for, in children and adolescents, 266
  completely anesthetic, once-twice test for evaluation of, 41
  ganglia, simple aspiration or aspiration and injection of corticosteroid and/or hyaluronidase for, 232
  replantation (*see* Replantation)
  snapping, tendon sheath of, operative and histopathological study, in children, 245
  vasospasm, complications of, limited microsurgical arteriolysis for, 275
Digital
  artery island flap, reverse, clinical experience with, 64
  blocks, single injection transthecal *vs.* subcutaneous, 258
  scar contracture, recurrent, proximal phalangeal island flap for, in children, 70
  tip (*see* Fingertip)
Disability
  elbow, validity of observer-based aggregate scoring systems as descriptors of, 27
Dislocation
  elbow, chronic, coronoid reconstruction for, 55
  fracture-dislocation, perilunate carpal, lunotriquetral lesions and their sequelae in, 152
  interphalangeal joint, dorsal, neglected, "S" Quattro turbo in management of, 56
  perilunate
    carpal, lunotriquetral lesions and their sequelae in, 152
    transscaphoid, management of, 148
  radioulnar joint, distal
    chronic palmar, Sauvé-Kapandji procedure for, 193
    ulnar styloid malunion with, 187
  trapeziometacarpal, recent closed, pinning for, 56
Distracter
  multiplanar, in correction of proximal interphalangeal joint contracture, 45
Distraction
  Ilizarov distraction-lengthening in congenital anomalies, 242

Doppler
  flowmeter, laser, in quantitative evaluation of sympathetic nervous system dysfunction in reflex sympathetic dystrophy, 282
  ultrasound, color, of tendon and muscle movements, 1
Dorsalis
  pedis tendocutaneous flap, free innervated, in composite hand reconstruction, 270
Drainage
  venous, of radial forearm and anterior tibial reverse flow flaps, 12
Drugs
  antiinflammatory, nonsteroidal, for piper's palsy, 203
Dupuytren's contracture
  fasciotomy for, percutaneous, 237
  pathogenesis, mechanical properties of palmar aponeurosis in, 235
Dupuytren's disease
  primary, severe, skeletal traction for, 233
  recurrent, myofibroblasts in, 238
  tissue, excised, mechanical stress in vitro induces increased expression of MMPs 2 and 9 in, 291
Durkan's test
  of carpal compression in diagnosis of carpal tunnel syndrome, 100
Dysplasia
  radial, correction of, five different incisions for, 240
Dystonia
  focal
    in musician's hand, anatomical factors predisposing to, 201
    in pipers, 203
Dystrophic
  problems, 279
Dystrophy
  reflex sympathetic, sympathetic nervous system dysfunction, quantitative evaluation of, 282

E

Economic
  repercussions, indirect, of radiography *vs.* MRI in diagnosis of occult scaphoid fractures, 143
Elastic
  bandage in treatment of ring and little metacarpal neck fractures, 47
Elbow
  arthroscopy, interosseous nerve injury after, 98

dislocation, chronic, coronoid reconstruction for, 55
extension in reconstruction of prehension with reinnervated free muscle transfer after complete brachial plexus avulsion, 200
flexion, changes in interstitial pressure and cross-sectional area of cubital tunnel and ulnar nerve with, 293
function, validity of observer-based aggregate scoring systems as descriptors of, 27
mobilization, immediate active, after operative treatment of posttraumatic proximal radioulnar synostosis, 53
ossification centers, sequential development, in children, 245
pain, validity of observer-based aggregate scoring systems as descriptors of, 27
replacement, semiconstrained total, for posttraumatic osteoarthrosis, 225
synovectomy and radial head excision in rheumatoid arthritis, 225
ulnar neuropathy at (see Ulnar, neuropathy at elbow)
Elderly
  forearm fracture in, distal, epidemiology, 171
  manual performance decline in, predictors of, 263
Electrodiagnostic
  study
    in carpal tunnel syndrome, predictive value of, 263
    normal, carpal tunnel syndrome with, 113
Electromyography
  surface, of wrist extensors, effect of wrist orthosis use during functional activities on, 20
Electrophysiological
  evaluation of splinting and local steroid injection for ulnar neuropathy at elbow, 125
Enchondroma
  bone substitute for, 238
Endoscopic
  carpal tunnel release
    review of, 114
    touch allodynia after, 229
Endothelin-1
  cutaneous responses to, in vibration white finger, 286
Entrapment
  nerve
    distal, after nerve repair, 98
    radial, superficial branch, case reports, 127
Epicondylitis
  lateral, chronic, etiology, and sarcomere length in wrist extensor muscles, 24
Epineural
  repair of median nerve, primary, in children, 89
Eponychial
  flap, 67
Escherichia coli
  cellulitis, upper limb, in immunocompromised patients, 69
Evaluation, 27
Excision
  radial head, and elbow synovectomy in rheumatoid arthritis, 225
  of skeletal tumor of distal radius, reconstruction with osteoarticular allograft after, 227
  ulna, combined with radial Z-plasty for correction of radial dysplasia, 240
Exercises
  nerve and tendon gliding, for carpal tunnel syndrome, 110
  remedial, for lymphedema of extremities, 279
Extension
  elbow, in reconstruction of prehension with reinnervated free muscle transfer after complete brachial plexus avulsion, 200
  moments, wrist, effect of muscle architecture and moment arms on, 13
  torque, isometric wrist, reliability using LIDO WorkSET for late follow-up of postoperative wrist patients, 138
Extensor(s)
  muscles, wrist, sarcomere length in, 24
  tendon
    injuries, early active mobilization for, 78
    rupture, repeated, due to fluoroquinolones, 84
    tenorrhaphy, simplified functional splinting after, 80
  wrist
    effect of radial shortening on muscle length and moment arms of, 16
    electromyography of, surface, effect of wrist orthosis use during functional activities on, 20
Extremity
  lymphedema, treatment of, 279
  upper
    anomalies of, congenital, Ilizarov distraction-lengthening in, 242

Subject Index / 309

cellulitis, *Escherichia coli,* in immunocompromised patients, 69
cumulative trauma disorders in, reliability of Postural and Repetitive Risk-Factors Index in, 247
injuries, in music students, instrument-specific rates of, 252
injuries, outpatient rehabilitation after, determinants of use of, 254
nerve injuries, associated with vascular trauma, treatment of, 286
nerve injuries, peripheral, reconstruction with ePTFE conduits, 87
neuroprosthesis, implanted, follow-up, 197
reconstruction with reverse flaps, 71
surgery, fluoroscopy in, operative, 28
tourniquet ischemia in, controlled, adhesion receptors and cytokine profiles in, 299
work-related disorders of, prevalence in printing factory, 248

F

Factory
  printing, prevalence of work-related upper limb disorders in, 248
Falls
  forearm fractures due to, distal, 171
Fascicle
  ulnar nerve, transfer onto biceps muscle nerve in C5-C6 or C5-C6-C7 avulsion of brachial plexus, 199
Fasciocutaneous
  flap, island, based on proximal perforators of distal radial artery for resurfacing of burned cubital fossa, 70
Fasciotomy
  percutaneous, for Dupuytren's contracture, 237
Fat
  pad, vascularized hypothenar, effect on wound tenderness after open carpal tunnel release, 121
Fibrocartilage
  triangular (*see* Triangular fibrocartilage)
Finger
  (*See also* Digit)
  deformity, mallet, 5-year follow-up of conservative treatment, 83
  flexion
    sign for ulnar neuropathy, 41
    strength, isokinetic, measurement of, 23
  ipsilateral and contralateral, hemodynamic changes due to acute exposures to hand transmitted vibration, 257
  little, fracture of metacarpal neck of, treatment, 46
  nail transfer, evolution of, 68
  reconstruction, partial, second toe plantar flap for, 269
  ring, fracture of metacarpal neck of, treatment, 46
  splints for piper's palsy, 203
  stiffness, severe, castle flap in treatment of skin retraction in, 63
  trigger
    percutaneous treatment of, long-term follow-up, 261
    splinting for, functional distal interphalangeal joint, in laborers, 259
  tumors of, glomus, MRI of, 238
  vibration white, cutaneous responses to endothelin-1 and histamine in, 286
Fingertip
  amputation, eponychial flap for, 67
  injuries, crush, late diagnosis and treatment, in children, 71
  loading
    carpal tunnel pressure and, 262
    static, effects on carpal tunnel pressure, 249
  reconstruction, reverse digital artery island flap for, 64
  replacement, composite graft, in children, 68
  values, normal, for Weinstein Enhanced Sensory Test, 36
Fixation
  device, external, skeletal traction with, for Kienböck's disease, 157
  external
    metaphyseal, for intraarticular fractures of distal radius, 173
    vs. percutaneous pinning for unstable Colles' fracture, 172
  internal
    after bone grafting, intercalary, in isolated forearm nonunion with segmental bone loss, 50
    of radius fracture, distal, displaced intraarticular, 177
    of radial head, anatomy of posterior interosseous nerve related to, 11
  screw
    Herbert, of transscaphoid perilunate dislocations, 148
    lag, of isolated unicondylar fractures of proximal phalanx, 43

scaphoid, comparison during
    application of cyclical bending
    loads, 163
staple, customized, in hand and wrist
    surgery, 139
wire, of metacarpophalangeal joint
    fracture, avulsion, 48
Flap
  bilobed, in correction of radial
      dysplasia, 240
  castle, in treatment of skin retraction in
      severe stiffness of hand and fingers,
      63
  digital artery island, reverse, clinical
      experience with, 64
  dorsalis pedis tendocutaneous, free
      innervated, in composite hand
      reconstruction, 270
  eponychial, 67
  fasciocutaneous, island, based on
      proximal perforators of distal
      radial artery for resurfacing of
      burned cubital fossa, 70
  forearm, radial reverse flow, venous
      drainage of, 12
  free, flow-through, in replantation
      surgery, 265
  interosseous
      anatomical study of, 62
      free, posterior, types of, 61
      posteroanterior, concept of, 62
  neurocutaneous, based on dorsal
      branches of ulnar artery and nerve,
      276
  phalangeal
      dorsal middle, mid-term results, 66
      proximal, island flap, for recurrent
          digital scar contracture, in children,
          70
  plantar, second toe, for partial finger
      reconstruction, 269
  reverse, upper limb reconstruction with,
      71
  tibial, anterior, reverse flow, venous
      drainage of, 12
  ulnar artery, dorsal, use in hand and
      wrist tissue cover, 59
Flexion
  elbow, changes in interstitial pressure
      and cross-sectional area of cubital
      tunnel and ulnar nerve with, 293
  finger, sign, for ulnar neuropathy, 41
  mobilization, active and passive, range
      of excursion of flexor tendons in
      zone V after, 76
  moments, wrist, effect of muscle
      architecture and moment arms on,
      13

strength, isokinetic finger, measurement
    of, 23
wrist (*see* Wrist, flexion)
Flexor(s)
  digitorum profundus tendon
      replacement by flexor superficialis
      tendon transfer, anatomical study
      of, 291
  tethering to fractures of ulna causing
      pseudo-Volkmann's contracture, in
      children, 284
  superficialis tendon transfer, flexor
      digitorum profundus tendon
      replacement by, anatomical study
      of, 291
  tendon
      excursion after open carpal tunnel
          release, effect of transverse carpal
          ligament on, 17
      excursion in zone V, range of, after
          active *vs.* passive flexion
          mobilization regimes, 76
      profundus, double-armed reinsertion
          suture of, with immediate active
          mobilization, 74
      repair, primary, controlled active
          motion after, 73
      repair, suture methods for (in dog),
          288
      rupture, two-stage treatment of, 84
      wound healing, zone II, gene
          expression of transforming growth
          factor beta-1 in (in rabbit), 287
  wrist, effect of radial shortening on
      muscle length and moment arms of,
      16
Flowmeter
  laser Doppler, in quantitative evaluation
      of sympathetic nervous system
      dysfunction in reflex sympathetic
      dystrophy, 282
Fluoroquinolones
  extensor tendon rupture to due,
      repeated, 84
Fluoroscopy
  operative, in hand and upper limb
      surgery, 28
Foeldi technique
  for lymphedema of extremities, 279
Forearm
  flaps, radial reverse flow, venous
      drainage of, 12
  fracture (*see* Fracture, forearm)
  mobilization, immediate active, after
      operative treatment of
      posttraumatic proximal radioulnar
      synostosis, 53

muscle oxygenation decreases with low levels of voluntary contraction, 298
nonunion, isolated, with segmental bone loss, surgical treatment of, 50
radioulnar load-sharing in, 21
velocity in carpal tunnel syndrome, 131
Fossa
  cubital, burned, resurfacing of, island fasciocutaneous flap based on proximal perforators of radial artery for, 70
Fracture
  carpal, in children, 166
  Colles'
    (See also Fracture, radius, distal below)
    classifications of, AO and Frykman's, 168
    Older type 1 and 2, immobilization for, 3 vs. 5 weeks, 181
    ulnar styloid affection in, predictive value of, 187
    unstable, external fixation vs. percutaneous pinning for, 172
  -dislocation, perilunate carpal, lunotriquetral lesions and their sequelae in, 152
  forearm, distal
    epidemiology, 171
    follow up, role of radiographs in, in children, 49
    triangular fibrocartilage complex lesion in, in children, 187
  metacarpal neck, ring and little, treatment of, 46
  metacarpophalangeal joint, 58
    avulsion type, 47
  phalanx
    articular, external traction for, 57
    base, middle, classification, management, and long-term results, 58
    proximal, isolated unicondylar fracture, treatment approach for, 43
  radius, distal
    (See also Fracture, Colles' above)
    algodystrophy after, predictive criteria of outcome after 1 year, 184
    classifications of, simplified Frykman and AO, 167
    fusion after, radioscapholunate, long-term results, 183
    intraarticular, displaced, 177
    intraarticular, fixation for, metaphyseal external, 173
    intraarticular, reduction of, arthroscopically-assisted, 178
    intraarticular lesions in, in young adults, 179
    physiotherapy after, 186
    pinning for, Kapandji's or Py's, 174
    reduction of, comparison of three anesthetic techniques for, 40
  scaphoid
    diagnosis, combining clinical signs improves, 32
    occult, radiography vs. MRI in diagnosis, 143
Frame
  delta, for intraarticular fractures of distal radius, 173
Frykman classification
  of Colles' fracture, 168
  simplified, of distal radius fractures, 167
Functional
  activities, use of wrist orthosis during, effect on surface electromyography of wrist extensors, 20
Fusion
  intercarpal, limited, for Kienböck's disease, biomechanical analysis of, 155
  radioscapholunate, after distal radius fracture, long-term results, 183
  wrist, does it cause destruction of first carpometacarpal joint in rheumatoid arthritis? 222

G

Gamekeeper thumb
  diagnosis, MR arthrography vs. conventional arthrography and MRI in, 34
  Mitek mini anchor in, 56
Ganglia
  digital, simple aspiration or aspiration and injection of corticosteroid and/or hyaluronidase for, 232
  wrist
    aspiration vs. steroid filtration in, 238
    simple aspiration or aspiration and injection of corticosteroid and/or hyaluronidase for, 232
Gene
  expression of transforming growth factor beta-1 in zone II flexor tendon wound healing (in rabbit), 287
Giant cell
  tumors of bone, vascularized bone graft for, 230
Glomus
  tumors of finger, MRI of, 238

Graft
    allograft, osteoarticular, in
        reconstruction of distal radius after
        excision of skeletal tumor, 227
    bone
        intercalary, in isolated forearm
            nonunion with segmental bone loss,
            50
        pronator quadratus pedicled,
            anatomical basis of, 24
        vascularized, for bone tumors, juxta-
            articular giant cell, 230
        vascularized, for scaphoid nonunion,
            166
        vascularized, from palmar carpal
            artery for scaphoid nonunion, 144
        composite, for replacement of digital
            tips, in children, 68
    nerve
        "bioartificial," new type, for bridging
            extended defects in nerves (in rat),
            297
        end-to-side, axonal sprouting into,
            histologic and morphometric study
            (in rat), 296
        olecranon, in coronoid reconstruction
            for chronic dislocation of elbow, 55
Grip
    strength after open carpal tunnel
        release, effect of transverse carpal
        ligament on, 17
Growth
    transforming growth factor beta-1 gene
        expression in zone II flexor tendon
        wound healing (in rabbit), 287

H

Hand
    club, radial
        Ilizarov distraction-lengthening in,
        242
        operative correction, long-term
        follow-up, 239
    corpuscles in, pacinian
        distribution of, 7
        painful hyperplasia and hypertrophy
        of, 97
    injuries, mutilating, "Tic-Tac-Toe"
        classification system for, 35
    ischemia after hemodialysis access
        procedure, incidence and
        characteristics of patients with, 283
    joints in rheumatoid arthritis,
        destruction and reconstruction of,
        224
    musician's, focal dystonia in,
        anatomical factors predisposing to,
        201
    neuromas, painful, treatment by
        relocation into pronator quadratus
        muscle, 91
    reconstruction, composite, free
        innervated dorsal pedis
        tendocutaneous flap in, 270
    sensibility between dominant and
        nondominant, lack of difference as
        tested with Semmes-Weinstein
        monofilaments, 37, 300
    skin, degloved, replantation of, 276
    spastic, in cerebral palsy, surgery of,
        204
    stiffness, severe, castle flap in treatment
        of skin retraction in, 63
    surgery
        fluoroscopy in, operative, 28
        outpatient, pharmacoeconomics of IV
            regional vs. general anesthesia for,
            38
        staple fixation in, customized, 139
    symptom pattern associated with
        objective evidence of median nerve
        compression, 108
    symptoms and vibrotactile sense in blue
        collar workers in manufacturing
        industry, 256
    tissue cover, use of dorsal ulnar artery
        flap in, 59
    toe-to-hand transfer for traumatic
        digital amputations in children and
        adolescents, 266
    transmitted vibration exposures, acute,
        causing hemodynamic changes in
        ipsilateral and contralateral fingers,
        257
Healing
    wound, zone II flexor tendon, gene
        expression of transforming growth
        factor beta-1 in (in rabbit), 287
Hematoma
    block with sedation for reduction of
        distal radius fractures, 40
    subchondral, with distal fractures of
        radius in young adults, 180
Hemodialysis
    access procedure, hand ischemia after,
        incidence and characteristics of
        patients with, 283
Hemodynamic
    changes in ipsilateral and contralateral
        fingers due to acute exposures to
        hand transmitted vibration, 257
Herbert screw
    fixation

of metacarpophalangeal joint fracture, avulsion, 48
of osteotomy of radial styloid for scapholunate collapse and radiostyloid pain syndrome, 158
of perilunate dislocations, transscaphoid, 148
for scaphoid, comparison with other screws during application of cyclical bending loads, 163
removal from scaphoid, useful technique for, 166
Herbert-Whipple screw
fixation for scaphoid, comparison with other screws during application of cyclical bending loads, 163
Histamine
cutaneous responses to, in vibration white finger, 286
Histologic
study of axonal sprouting into end-to-side nerve graft (in rat), 296
Histopathological
study of tendon sheath of snapping digit, in children, 245
Hueston flap
dorsal, in treatment of skin retraction in severe stiffness of hands and fingers, 63
Hyaluronidase
injection with aspiration for carpal and digital ganglions, 232
Hyperplasia
painful, of pacinian corpuscles in hand, 97
Hypertrophy
painful, of pacinian corpuscles in hand, 97
Hypothenar
fat pad, vascularized, effect on wound tenderness after open carpal tunnel release, 121

I

Ilizarov distraction-lengthening
in congenital anomalies, 242
Imaging
magnetic resonance (see Magnetic resonance imaging)
Immobilization
for anterior interosseous nerve syndrome, 129
for Colles' fracture, Older type 1 and 2, immobilization for, 3 vs. 5 weeks, 181

Immunocompromised patients
cellulitis in, upper limb *Escherichia coli*, 69
Implanted neuroprosthesis
upper extremity, follow-up, 197
Incision(s)
five different, for correction of radial dysplasia, 240
palmar, limited, safe carpal tunnel release via, 122
Industrial workers
active, vitamin B_6 status related to median nerve function and carpal tunnel syndrome in, 106
carpal tunnel syndrome in
risk factors for, occupational and personal, 264
sensory and psychomotor functional test battery for, 103
Industry
manufacturing, vibrotactile sense and hand symptoms in blue collar workers in, 256
Injury(ies)
(*See also* Trauma)
crush, of fingertip, late diagnosis and treatment, in children, 71
extremity, upper
in music students, instrument-specific rates of, 252
outpatient rehabilitation after, determinants of use of, 254
hand, mutilating, "Tic-Tac-Toe" classification system for, 35
nerve
interosseous, after elbow arthroscopy, 98
peripheral, cold intolerance after, 95
peripheral, reconstruction with ePTFE conduits, 87
vascular trauma associated with, treatment of, 286
physis, distal radius, corrective osteotomies after, in children, 182
repetitive strain, in computer keyboard users, pathomechanics and treatment, 263
tendon, extensor, early active mobilization for, 78
triangular fibrocartilage, arthrography vs. MRI in diagnosis, 31
Innervated
dorsalis pedis tendocutaneous flap, free, in composite hand reconstruction, 270
Instrument
-specific rates of upper extremity injuries in music students, 252

Intercalary
  bone graft in isolated forearm nonunion with segmental bone loss, 50
Intercarpal
  fusion, limited, for Kienböck's disease, biomechanical analysis of, 155
Interobserver
  agreement of simplified Frykman and AO classifications of distal radius fractures, 167
Interosseous
  artery, anterior, experience with, 25
  flap (see Flap, interosseous)
  membrane, effect on distal radioulnar joint, 191
  nerve
    anterior, injury after elbow arthroscopy, 98
    anterior, palsy, case reviews, 96
    anterior, syndrome, literature review and case reports, 129
    posterior, anatomy of, in relation to fixation of radial head, 11
    posterior, and radial tunnel syndrome, 128
    posterior, palsy, traumatic, clinical features and management of, 94
Interphalangeal joint
  dislocation, dorsal, neglected, "S" Quattro turbo in management of, 56
  distal, functional splinting for trigger finger in laborers, 259
  proximal
    contracture, correction of, multiplanar distracter in, 45
    denervation, 207
Interstitial
  pressure changes of cubital tunnel and ulnar nerve with flexion of elbow, 293
Intraarticular
  fractures of distal radius (see Fracture, radius, distal, intraarticular)
  lesions in distal fractures of radius, in young adults, 179
Intraobserver
  agreement of simplified Frykman and AO classifications of distal radius fractures, 167
Ischemia
  hand, after hemodialysis access procedure, incidence and characteristics of patients with, 283
  tourniquet, controlled, in upper extremity, adhesion receptors and cytokine profiles in, 299

Isokinetic
  finger flexion strength, measurement of, 23
Isometric
  wrist extension torque reliability using LIDO WorkSET for late follow-up of postoperative wrist patients, 138

J

Jebsen test
  after centralization for radial club hand, 239
Joint(s)
  carpometacarpal, thumb
    arthroscopic evaluation and treatment of, 208
    replacements, de la Caffinière, long-term follow-up, 210
  contracture, moderate, after controlled active motion after primary flexor tendon repair, 73
  hand, in rheumatoid arthritis, destruction and reconstruction of, 224
  interphalangeal (see Interphalangeal joint)
  laxity, effect on periscaphoid carpal kinematics, 136
  metacarpophalangeal (see Metacarpophalangeal, joint)
  radiocarpal, denervation, follow-up study, 161
  radioulnar (see Radioulnar, joint)
  trapeziometacarpal (see Trapeziometacarpal joint)
Juxta-articular
  giant cell tumors of bone, vascularized bone graft for, 230

K

Kapandji's pinning
  for radial fractures, distal, 174
Kessler suture
  Double, tensile strength of (in rabbit), 289
  modified, for primary flexor tendon repair, controlled active motion after, 73
  Triple, tensile strength of (in rabbit), 289
Keyboard
  users, computer, repetitive strain injury in, pathomechanics and treatment, 263
Kienböck's disease
  carpectomy for, proximal row, 159

palmar, 160
fusion for, limited intercarpal,
  biomechanical analysis of, 155
skeletal traction for, 156
Kinematics
  carpal
    normal, 165
    periscaphoid, effect of joint laxity on, 136
    during wrist flexion in vivo, load dependence in, 25
King's method
  modified, for cubital tunnel syndrome, long-term results, 131
Kirschner wire(s)
  in arthroscopically-assisted reduction of intraarticular fractures of distal radius, 178
  fixation of osteotomy of radial styloid for scapholunate collapse and radiostyloid pain syndrome, 158
  pinning, percutaneous, *vs.* external fixation for unstable Colles' fracture, 172

L

Laborers
  trigger finger in, functional distal interphalangeal joint splinting for, 259
Laceration
  median nerve, acute transectional, primary epineural repair of, in children, 89
Lag
  screw fixation of isolated unicondylar fractures of proximal phalanx, 43
Laser
  Doppler flowmeter in quantitative evaluation of sympathetic nervous system dysfunction in reflex sympathetic dystrophy, 282
  -soldered microvascular anastomosis, effect of optical temperature feedback control on patency in (in rat), 300
Ledoux prosthesis
  trapeziometacarpal joint, 213
  radiological course of, 214
Lengthening
  Ilizarov distraction-lengthening in congenital anomalies, 242
  ligament, transverse carpal, *vs.* simple division, in carpal tunnel syndrome, 116

LIDO WorkSET
  reliability of isometric wrist extension torque using, for late follow-up of postoperative wrist patients, 138
Ligament
  carpal, transverse
    effect on flexor tendon excursion after open carpal tunnel release, 17
    lengthening *vs.* simple division, in carpal tunnel syndrome, 116
  lesions in distal fractures of radius in young adults, 179–180
  reconstruction, trapeziectomy with, 212
  scapholunate
    disruption, chronic, isolated scaphotrapeziotrapezoid osteoarthritis as radiographic marker of, 151
    tears with distal fractures of radius in young adults, 180
Ligamentous
  repair of perilunate dislocations, transscaphoid, 148
  structures, palmar, of carpal canal, anatomical study of, 3
Light
  touch sensation testing with Semmes-Weinstein pressure aesthesiometer, effect of wrist position on, 41
Limb (*see* Extremity)
Linguistic
  model, for prediction of carpal tunnel syndrome risks in occupational environment, 262
Load
  dependence in carpal kinematics during wrist flexion in vivo, 25
  -sharing, radioulnar, in forearm, 21
Loading
  axial, induces rotation of proximal carpal row bone around unique screw-displacement axes, 166
  fingertip
    carpal tunnel pressure and, 262
    static, effects on carpal tunnel pressure, 249
Loads
  bending, cyclical, comparison of fixation screws for scaphoid during application of, 163
Lumbrical
  muscles, blood supply of, 2
Lunate
  scapholunate instability, Brunelli procedure for, modified, early results, 149

Lunotriquetral
  lesions and their sequelae in perilunate carpal dislocations and fracture-dislocations, 152
Lupus
  erythematosus, systemic, early stage, bone scintigraphy in, 223
Luxation (*see* Dislocation)
Lymphedema
  of extremities, treatment of, 279

M

Magnetic resonance arthrography
  vs. MRI in diagnosis of gamekeeper thumb, 34
Magnetic resonance imaging
  of carpal tunnel, median nerve compression detected by, 104
  dynamic, of carpal tunnel syndrome, 41
  of glomus tumors of finger, 238
  high-resolution, of triangular fibrocartilage complex, 189
  sagittal, in assessment of dorsal or ventral intercalated segmental instability configurations of wrist, 42
  vs. arthrography, magnetic resonance, in diagnosis of gamekeeper thumb, 34
  vs. arthrography in diagnosis of triangular fibrocartilage injuries, 31
  vs. radiography in diagnosis of occult scaphoid fractures, 143
Mallet deformity
  of finger, 5-year follow-up of conservative treatment, 83
Malunion
  ulnar styloid, with dislocation of distal radioulnar joint, 187
Manual
  performance decline in older adults, predictors of, 263
Manufacturing
  industry, vibrotactile sense and hand symptoms in blue collar workers in, 256
Matrix metalloproteinases 2 and 9
  increased expression in excised Dupuytren's disease tissue induced by mechanical stress in vitro, 291
MCPP
  profile analysis, role in treatment of triphalangeal thumbs, 243
Mechanical
  stress in vitro induces increased expression of MMPs 2 and 9 in excised Dupuytren's disease tissue, 291

Median mononeuropathy
  at wrist, effect of body mass index and work activity on, 107
Median nerve
  compression
    hand symptom pattern associated with objective evidence of, 108
    on MRI of carpal tunnel, 104
    at palmar cutaneous branch, anatomical classification of sites of, 5
    with wrist flexion as provocative test for carpal tunnel syndrome, 99
  decompression in carpal tunnel syndrome, sensory function after, 115
  function in industrial workers, relation to vitamin B_6 status, 106
  palmar cutaneous branch, anatomical classification of sites of compression of, 5
  reconstruction with ePTFE conduits, 87
  repair
    epineural, primary, in children, 89
    function recovery after, rationale for evaluation, 37
Medicine
  physical and occupational, 247
Menisci
  of metacarpophalangeal joint of thumb, 22
Metacarpal
  first, osteotomy, for trapeziometacarpal osteoarthritis, 215
  neck, ring and little, treatment of fractures of, 46
Metacarpophalangeal
  joint
    fracture, 58
    fracture, avulsion, 47
    thumb, menisci and synovial folds of, 22
  pattern profile analysis, role in treatment of triphalangeal thumbs, 243
Metalloproteinases
  2 and 9, matrix, increased expression in excised Dupuytren's disease tissue induced by mechanical stress in vitro, 291
Metaphyseal
  external fixation for intraarticular fractures of distal radius, 173
Microcirculation
  cutaneous, acute effects of periarterial sympathectomy on (in rabbit), 274

Microsurgery, 265
Microsurgical
  arteriolysis, limited, for complications of digital vasospasm, 275
Microvascular
  anastomosis, laser-soldered, effect of optical temperature feedback control on patency in (in rat), 300
  results, early, after thumb replantations and revascularizations, 276
Mitek mini anchor
  in gamekeeper's thumb, 56
MMPs 2 and 9
  expression in excised Dupuytren's disease tissue increased by mechanical stress in vitro, 291
Moberg "pick up" test
  after centralization for radial club hand, 239
Mobilization
  active
    early, for extensor tendon injuries, 78
    flexion, range of excursion of flexor tendons in zone V after, 76
    immediate, after profundus flexor tendon repair with double-armed reinsertion suture, 74
    immediate, of elbow and forearm after operative treatment of posttraumatic proximal radioulnar synostosis, 53
  passive flexion, range of excursion of flexor tendons in zone V after, 76
  wrist, early, after Herbert screw fixation and ligamentous repair of transscaphoid perilunate dislocations, 148
Model
  linguistic, for prediction of carpal tunnel syndrome risks in occupational environment, 262
Moment
  arms
    effect on wrist flexion–extension moments, 13
    of wrist flexors and extensors, effect of radial shortening on, 16
Monofilaments
  Semmes-Weinstein, lack of difference in sensibility between dominant and nondominant hands as tested with, 37, 300
Mononeuropathy
  median, at wrist, effect of body mass index and work activity on, 107
Morphologic
  changes of carpal canal after open carpal tunnel release, effect of transverse carpal ligament on, 17
Morphometric
  study of axonal sprouting into end-to-side nerve graft (in rat), 296
Motion
  active, controlled, after flexor tendon repair, primary, 73
  passive, continuous, after lag screw fixation of isolated unicondylar fractures of proximal phalanx, 43
Motor
  function recovery after nerve repair, rationale for evaluation, 37
Movements
  tendon and muscle, color Doppler analysis of, 1
MRI (see Magnetic resonance imaging)
Mucolipidoses
  carpal tunnel syndrome in, 109
Mucopolysaccharidoses
  carpal tunnel syndrome in, 109
Muscle(s)
  adductor pollicis, anatomy of, 2
  architecture, effect on wrist flexion–extension moments, 13
  biceps muscle nerve, ulnar nerve fascicle transfer onto, in C5-C6 or C5-C6-C7 avulsion of brachial plexus, 199
  extensor, wrist
    electromyography of, surface, effect of wrist orthosis use during functional activities on, 20
    sarcomere length in, 24
  length of wrist flexors and extensors, effect of radial shortening on, 16
  lumbrical, blood supply of, 2
  movements, color Doppler analysis of, 1
  oxygenation, forearm, decrease with low levels of voluntary contraction, 298
  pronator quadratus, relocation into, treatment of painful neuromas of hand and wrist by, 91
  relaxants for piper's palsy, 203
  transfer, reinnervated free, after complete brachial plexus avulsion, elbow extension in reconstruction of prehension with, 200
Musculoskeletal
  disorders in musicians, playing-related, incidence and prevalence of, 253
Music
  students, instrument-specific rates of upper extremity injuries in, 252

Musicians
  hands of, focal dystonia in, anatomical factors predisposing to, 201
  musculoskeletal disorders in, playing-related, incidence and prevalence of, 253
Mutilating
  injuries of hand, "Tic-Tac-Toe" classification system for, 35
MWPIII total wrist arthroplasty prosthesis, 219, 222
Myofibroblasts
  in Dupuytren's disease, recurrent, 238

N

Nail
  great toe partial-nail preserving transfer for thumb reconstruction, 268
  transfer, evolution of, 68
Near infra-red spectroscopy
  for forearm muscle oxygenation decrease with low levels of voluntary contraction, 298
Nerve(s)
  biceps muscle, ulnar nerve fascicle transfer onto, in C5-C6 or C5-C6-C7 avulsion of brachial plexus, 199
  block, continuous peripheral, in replantation and vascularization, 272
  cutaneous, palmar, detailed anatomy of, 8
  defects, extended, bridging with new type of "bioartificial" nerve graft (in rat), 297
  distal, entrapment after nerve repair, 98
  gliding exercises for carpal tunnel syndrome, 110
  graft
    "bioartificial," new type, for bridging extended defects in nerves (in rat), 297
    end-to-side, axonal sprouting into, histologic and morphometric study (in rat), 296
  implanted in bone, prevention of neuroma formation in (in rat), 93
  injuries associated with vascular trauma, treatment of, 286
  interosseous (see Interosseous, nerve)
  median (see Median nerve)
  peripheral, injuries
    cold intolerance after, 95
    reconstruction with ePTFE conduits, 87
  radial, superficial branch, entrapment of, case reports, 127
  reconstruction, 87
  relocation into pronator quadratus muscle for painful neuromas of hand and wrist, 91
  repair
    nerve entrapment after, distal, 98
    recovery of sensory and motor function after, rationale for evaluation, 37
  resection for posttraumatic neuralgia, pain relief after, 89
  trauma, 87
  ulnar (see Ulnar, nerve)
Nervous
  system, sympathetic, dysfunction in reflex sympathetic dystrophy, quantitative evaluation of, 282
Neuralgia
  posttraumatic, pain relief after nerve resection for, 89
Neurocutaneous
  flap based on dorsal branches of ulnar artery and nerve, 276
Neurolysis
  for interosseous nerve palsy, posterior traumatic, 95
Neuroma
  formation in nerves implanted in bone, prevention of (in rat), 93
  painful, of hand and wrist, treatment by relocation into pronator quadratus muscle, 91
Neuromuscular
  disorders, 197
Neuropathy
  compression, 99
  ulnar (see Ulnar, neuropathy)
Neurophysiological
  investigation, role in traumatic brachial plexus lesions, 29
Neuroprosthesis
  implanted upper extremity, follow-up, 197
Neurorrhaphy
  end-to-side (in rat)
    axonal regeneration after, 294
    axonal sprouting into graft after, histologic and morphometric study of, 296
Nonunion
  forearm, isolated, with segmental bone loss, surgical treatment of, 50
  scaphoid, vascularized bone graft for, 166
  from palmar carpal artery, 144
Norwich regime
  for extensor tendon injuries, 78

O

Obstetric
  brachial plexopathy, neurophysiologic investigation of, 30
Occupational
  environment, carpal tunnel syndrome risks in, linguistic model for prediction of, 262
  medicine, 247
  risk factors for carpal tunnel syndrome association with prevalence of self-reported carpal tunnel syndrome in working population, 264
  in industrial workers, 264
Olecranon
  graft in coronoid reconstruction for chronic dislocation of elbow, 55
Once-twice test
  for evaluation of completely anesthetic digit, 41
Optical
  temperature feedback control, effect on patency in laser-soldered microvascular anastomosis (in rat), 300
Orthosis
  wrist, use during functional activities, effect on surface electromyography of wrist extensors, 20
Ossification
  centers, elbow, sequential development, in children, 245
Osteoarthritis
  carpometacarpal joint, thumb, de la Caffinière replacement for, long-term follow-up, 210
  scapholunate, advanced collapse-type, proximal row carpectomy through palmar approach for, 160
  scaphotrapeziotrapezoid, isolated, as radiographic marker of chronic scapholunate ligament disruption, 151
  trapeziometacarpal joint
    osteotomy for, first metacarpal, 215
    replacements for, cemented and non-cemented, 213
Osteoarthrosis
  posttraumatic, semiconstrained total elbow replacement for, 225
Osteoarticular
  allograft reconstruction of distal radius after excision of skeletal tumor, 227
Osteotomy
  corrective, after injuries of distal radial physis, in children, 182
  metacarpal, first, for trapeziometacarpal osteoarthritis, 215
  radial styloid, for scapholunate collapse and radiostyloid pain syndrome, 158
  ulnar shortening, for ulnar carpal instability and ulnar carpal impaction, 153
Outcome
  instrument, self-administered, in carpal tunnel syndrome, 130
Outpatient
  rehabilitation services, determinants of use after upper extremity injury, 254
Oxygenation
  forearm muscle, decrease with low levels of voluntary contraction, 298

P

Pacinian
  corpuscles in hand
    distribution of, 7
    painful hyperplasia and hypertrophy of, 97
Pain
  elbow, validity of observer-based aggregate scoring systems as descriptors of, 27
  pillar, after carpal tunnel release, 120
  relief after nerve resection for posttraumatic neuralgia, 89
  after surgery for ulnar neuropathy at elbow, 126
  syndrome
    complex regional, sympathetic vasoconstrictor reflex pattern in, 280
    radiostyloid, and scapholunate collapse, radial styloid osteotomy for, 158
  wrist, ulnar-sided, ulnocarpal stress test in diagnosis of, 146
Painful
  hyperplasia and hypertrophy of pacinian corpuscles in hand, 97
  neuromas of hand and wrist, treatment by relocation into pronator quadratus muscle, 91
Palmar
  aponeurosis, mechanical properties of, and Dupuytren's contracture, 235
  carpal artery, vascularized bone graft from, for scaphoid nonunion, 144
  carpectomy, proximal row, 160

cutaneous branch of median nerve,
    anatomical classification of sites of
    compression of, 5
cutaneous nerves, detailed anatomy of,
    8
incision, limited, safe carpal tunnel
    release via, 122
ligamentous structures of carpal canal,
    anatomical study of, 3
radioulnar dislocation, chronic distal,
    Sauvé-Kapandji procedure for, 193
Palsy
  cerebral, surgery of spastic hand in, 204
  interosseous nerve
    anterior, case reviews, 96
    posterior, traumatic, clinical features
      and management of, 94
  piper's, study of, 203
Paraplegics
  rotator cuff repairs in, 205
Percutaneous
  fasciotomy for Dupuytren's contracture,
    237
  pinning *vs.* external fixation for
    unstable Colles' fracture, 172
  treatment of trigger finger, long-term
    follow-up, 261
Perfusion
  study, radiographic, of venous drainage
    of radial forearm and anterior
    tibial reverse flow flaps, 12
Periarterial
  sympathectomy, acute effects on
    cutaneous microcirculation (in
    rabbit), 274
Perilunate
  dislocations
    carpal, lunotriquetral lesions and
      their sequelae in, 152
    transscaphoid, management of, 148
  fracture-dislocations, carpal,
    lunotriquetral lesions and their
    sequelae in, 152
Peripheral nerve
  block, continuous, in replantation and
    revascularization, 272
  injury
    cold intolerance after, 95
    reconstruction with ePTFE conduits,
      87
Periscaphoid
  carpal kinematics, effect of joint laxity
    on, 136
PET
  for effect of botulinum toxin on cortical
    dysfunction associated with writer's
    cramp, 251

Pfeiffer syndrome
  hand in, 245
Phalanx
  fracture (*see* Fracture, phalanx)
  middle, flap, dorsal, mid-term results,
    66
  proximal
    flap, island, for recurrent digital scar
      contracture, in children, 70
    fracture, isolated unicondylar,
      treatment approach for, 43
Pharmacoeconomics
  of anesthesia, IV regional *vs.* general,
    for outpatient hand surgery, 38
Phylogeny
  of wrist, 25
Physical
  medicine, 247
  therapy (*see* Physiotherapy)
Physiotherapy
  for anterior interosseous nerve
    syndrome, 129
  complete decongestive, for lymphedema
    of extremities, 279
  after fractures of distal radius, 186
  after operative treatment of
    posttraumatic proximal radioulnar
    synostosis, 53
Physis
  distal radial, injuries, corrective
    osteotomies after, in children, 182
Pillar
  pain after carpal tunnel release, 120
Pinch
  strength after open carpal tunnel
    release, effect of transverse carpal
    ligament on, 17
Pinning
  closed, for recent, closed
    trapeziometacarpal luxation, 56
  Kapandji's, for distal radius fracture,
    174
  percutaneous, *vs.* external fixation for
    unstable Colles' fracture, 172
  Py's, for distal radius fracture, 174
Piperacillin
  in cellulitis, *Escherichia coli* upper limb,
    in immunocompromised patient, 70
Piper's palsy
  study of, 203
Plantar
  flap, second toe, for partial finger
    reconstruction, 269
Plaster-of-Paris
  for metacarpal neck fractures, ring and
    little, 47

Playing
 -related musculoskeletal disorders in musicians, incidence and prevalence of, 253
Poland's syndrome
 syndactyly due to, 241
Polytetrafluoroethylene
 expanded, conduits of, reconstruction of upper extremity peripheral nerve injuries with, 87
Portals
 for arthroscopy of trapeziometacarpal joint, 209
Positron emission tomography
 for effect of botulinum toxin on cortical dysfunction associated with writer's cramp, 251
Postoperative
 wrist patients, reliability of isometric wrist extension torque using LIDO WorkSET for late follow-up of, 138
Postural and Repetitive Risk-Factors Index reliability in cumulative trauma disorders, 247
Prehension
 reconstruction with reinnervated free muscle transfer after complete brachial plexus avulsion, elbow extension in, 200
Preiser's disease
 carpectomy for, proximal row, 159
Pressure
 aesthesiometer, Semmes-Weinstein, effect of wrist position on testing light touch sensation with, 41
Printing
 factory, prevalence of work-related upper limb disorders in, 248
Profundus
 flexor tendon, double-armed reinsertion suture of, with immediate active mobilization, 74
Pronator
 quadratus muscle, relocation into, treatment of painful neuromas of hand and wrist by, 91
 quadratus pedicled bone graft, vascularized, anatomical basis of, 24
Prosthesis
 de la Caffinière, for thumb carpometacarpal joint, long-term follow-up, 210
 elbow, semiconstrained total, for posttraumatic osteoarthrosis, 225
 neuroprosthesis, implanted upper extremity, follow-up, 197
 trapeziometacarpal joint, cemented and uncemented, 213
 radiological course of, 214
Pseudoarthritis
 scaphoid, proximal row carpectomy through palmar approach for, 160
Pseudoarthrosis
 carpectomy for, proximal row, 159
Pseudo-Volkmann's contracture
 tethering of flexor digitorum profundus to fractures of ulna causing, in children, 284
Psychomotor
 /sensory functional test battery for carpal tunnel syndrome
   in confirmed cases and normal subjects, 101
   in industrial subjects, 103
PTFE
 expanded, conduits of, reconstruction of upper extremity peripheral nerve injuries with, 87
Py's pinning
 for radial fractures, distal, 174

Q

Quattro turbo
 "S", in management of neglected dorsal interphalangeal dislocations, 56

R

Radial
 artery perforators, proximal, island fasciocutaneous flap based on, for resurfacing of burned cubital fossa, 70
 club hand
   Ilizarov distraction-lengthening in, 242
   operative correction, long-term follow-up, 239
 dysplasia, correction of, five different incisions for, 240
 flaps, forearm, reverse flow, venous drainage of, 12
 nerve, superficial branch, entrapment of, case reports, 127
 styloid osteotomy for scapholunate collapse and radiostyloid pain syndrome, 158
 tunnel syndrome and posterior interosseous nerve, 128
Radiocarpal
 joint denervation, follow-up study, 161

Radiographic
  marker of chronic scapholunate ligament disruption, isolated scaphotrapeziotrapezoid osteoarthritis as, 151
  perfusion study of venous drainage of radial forearm and anterior tibial reverse flow flaps, 12
  role during follow up of distal forearm fractures, in children, 49
  vs. MRI in diagnosis of occult scaphoid fractures, 143
Radiological
  course of cemented and uncemented trapeziometacarpal prostheses, 214
Radioscapholunate
  fusion after distal radius fracture, long-term results, 183
Radiostyloid
  pain syndrome and scapholunate collapse, radial styloid osteotomy for, 158
Radioulnar
  joint, distal, 187
    dislocation, chronic palmar, Sauvé-Kapandji procedure for, 193
    dislocation, ulnar styloid malunion with, 187
    effect of interosseous membrane on, 191
  load-sharing in forearm, 21
  synostosis, posttraumatic proximal, operative treatment of, 53
Radius
  carpal bone motion relative to, 3-D analysis of, 165
  distal, 167
    physis, injuries of, corrective osteotomies after, in children, 182
    trauma to, acute, wrist arthrography after, 169
    tumor of, skeletal, reconstruction with osteoarticular allograft after excision of, 227
  fracture (see Fracture, radius)
  head
    excision and elbow synovectomy in rheumatoid arthritis, 225
    fixation of, anatomy of posterior interosseous nerve related to, 11
  shortening, effect on muscle length and moment arms of wrist flexors and extensors, 16
Raynaud's phenomenon
  digital vasospasm in, complications of, limited microsurgical arteriolysis for, 275

Reconstruction
  coronoid, for chronic dislocation of elbow, 55
  finger, partial, second toe plantar flap for, 269
  fingertip, reverse digital artery island flap for, 64
  hand, composite, free innervated dorsal pedis tendocutaneous flap in, 270
  of hand joints in rheumatoid arthritis, 224
  ligament, trapeziectomy with, 212
  limb, upper, with reverse flaps, 71
  nail, 68
  nerve, 87
    peripheral, upper extremity, with ePTFE conduits, 87
  of prehension with reinnervated free muscle transfer after complete brachial plexus avulsion, elbow extension in, 200
  radius, distal, with osteoarticular allograft after excision of skeletal tumor, 227
  skeletal, 43
  soft tissue, 59
  tendon, 73
  thumb, distal, with great toe partial-nail preserving technique, 268
Reduction
  arthroscopically-assisted, of intraarticular fractures of distal radius, 178
  open, for distal radius fracture, displaced intraarticular, 177
  of radius fractures, distal, comparison of three anesthetic techniques for, 40
Reflex
  sympathetic dystrophy, sympathetic nervous system dysfunction in, quantitative evaluation of, 282
  sympathetic vasoconstrictor, pattern in complex regional pain syndrome, 280
Regeneration
  axonal, after end-to-side neurorrhaphy (in rat), 294
Rehabilitation
  services, outpatient, determinants of use after upper extremity injury, 254
Reinnervated
  free muscle transfer after complete brachial plexus avulsion, elbow extension in reconstruction of prehension with, 200

Repetitive strain injury
  in computer keyboard users,
      pathomechanics and treatment, 263
Replantation
  of degloved skin of hand, 276
  nerve block in, continuous peripheral,
      272
  surgery, flow-through free flap in, 265
  thumb, results
    functional, 277
    microvascular, early, 276
Research, 287
Resurfacing
  cubital fossa, burned, island
      fasciocutaneous flap based on
      proximal perforations of radial
      artery for, 70
Retraction
  skin, in severe stiffness of hand and
      fingers, castle flap in treatment of,
      63
Return to work
  after carpal tunnel release, predictors of,
      118
Revascularization
  nerve block in, continuous peripheral,
      272
  thumb, results
    functional, 277
    microvascular, early, 276
Rheumatoid
  arthritis (see Arthritis, rheumatoid)
Rod
  silicon, in two-stage treatment of flexor
      tendon ruptures, complications of,
      84
Rotator
  cuff repairs in paraplegics, 205
Rupture
  ligament, scapholunate, with distal
      fractures of radius in young adults,
      180
  tendon
    extensor, repeated, due to
        fluoroquinolones, 84
    flexor, after controlled active motion
        after primary flexor tendon repair,
        73
    flexor, two-stage treatment of, 84
  triangular fibrocartilage complex
    MRI of, high-resolution, 189
    wrist arthroscopy in management of,
        194

S

"S" Quattro turbo
  in management of neglected
      dorsointerphalangeal dislocations,
      56
Sarcomere
  length in wrist extensor muscles, 24
Sauvé-Kapandji's procedure
  modification of, 194
  for radioulnar dislocation, chronic
      palmar distal, 193
Scaphocapitate
  fusion for Kienböck's disease,
      biomechanical analysis of, 155
Scaphoid
  costo-osteochondral replacement
      arthroplasty, proximal, 140
  fracture
    diagnosis, combining clinical signs
        improves, 32
    occult, radiography *vs.* MRI in
        diagnosis, 143
  Herbert screw removal from, useful
      technique, 166
  nonunion, vascularized bone graft for,
      166
  from palmar carpal artery, 144
  pseudoarthritis, proximal row
      carpectomy through palmar
      approach for, 160
  screws for, fixation, comparison during
      application of cyclical bending
      loads, 163
  transscaphoid perilunate dislocations,
      management of, 148
Scapholunate
  collapse
    advanced, arthrodesis for, limited
        wrist for, 162
    advanced, carpectomy for, proximal
        row, 159
    radiostyloid pain syndrome and,
        radial styloid osteotomy for, 158
  instability, Brunelli procedure for,
      modified, early results, 149
  ligament
    disruption, chronic, isolated
        scaphotrapeziotrapezoid
        osteoarthritis as radiographic
        marker of, 151
    tears with distal fractures of radius in
        young adults, 180
  osteoarthritis, advanced collapse-type,
      proximal row carpectomy through
      palmar approach for, 160

Scaphotrapeziotrapezoid
  osteoarthritis, isolated, as radiographic marker of chronic scapholunate ligament disruption, 151
Scaphotrapeziotrapezoidal
  fusion for Kienböck's disease, biomechanical analysis of, 155
Scar
  contracture, digital, recurrent, proximal phalangeal island flap for, in children, 70
Scintigraphy
  bone, in early stage lupus erythematosus and rheumatoid arthritis, 223
Scleroderma
  digital vasospasm in, complications of, limited microsurgical arteriolysis for, 275
Sclerosis
  amyotrophic lateral, and carpal tunnel syndrome, 131
Scoring
  systems, observer-based aggregate, validity as descriptors of elbow pain, function, and disability, 27
Screw
  -displacement axes, unique, axial loading induces rotation of proximal carpal row bone around, 166
  fixation for scaphoid, comparison during application of cyclical bending loads, 163
  Herbert (see Herbert screw)
  lag, in fixation of isolated unicondylar fractures of proximal phalanx, 43
Sedation
  hematoma block with, for reduction of distal radius fractures, 40
Semmes-Weinstein monofilaments
  lack of difference in sensibility between dominant and nondominant hands as tested with, 37, 300
Semmes-Weinstein pressure aesthesiometer
  effect of wrist position on testing light touch sensation using, 41
Sensation
  light touch, testing with Semmes-Weinstein pressure aesthesiometer, effect of wrist position on, 41
Sensibility
  lack of difference between dominant and non-dominant hands, as tested with Semmes-Weinstein monofilaments, 37, 300
Sensory
function
  after median nerve decompression in carpal tunnel syndrome, 115
  recovery after nerve repair, rationale for evaluation, 37
  /psychomotor functional test battery for carpal tunnel syndrome
    in confirmed cases and normal subjects, 101
    in industrial subjects, 103
  Weinstein Enhanced Sensory Test, normal digit tip values for, 36
Shortening
  osteotomy, ulnar, for ulnar carpal instability and ulnar carpal impaction, 153
  radius, effect on muscle length and moment arms of wrist flexors and extensors, 16
Silicon
  rod in two-stage treatment of flexor tendon ruptures, complications of, 84
Skeletal
  musculoskeletal disorders in musicians, playing-related, incidence and prevalence of, 253
  reconstruction, 43
  traction
    for Dupuytren's disease, severe primary, 233
    for Kienböck's disease, 156
  trauma, 43
  tumor of distal radius, reconstruction with osteoarticular allograft after excision of, 227
Skin
  (See also Cutaneous)
  care for lymphedema of extremities, 279
  hand, degloved, replantation of, 276
  retraction in severe stiffness of hand and fingers, castle flap in treatment of, 63
Smoking
  cold intolerance after peripheral nerve injuries and, 96
Snapping digit
  tendon sheath of, operative and histopathological study, in children, 245
Soft tissue
  cover, hand and wrist, use of dorsal ulnar artery flap in, 59
  reconstruction, 59
  trauma, 59
Spastic hand
  in cerebral palsy, surgery of, 204

Subject Index / 325

Spectroscopy
  near infra-red, for forearm muscle oxygenation decrease with low levels of voluntary contraction, 298
Spinal
  cord injured patients, rotator cuff repairs in, 205
Splint
  finger, for piper's palsy, 203
  thermoplastic, for mallet deformity of finger, 5-year follow-up, 83
Splinting
  alone or with local steroid injection for ulnar neuropathy at elbow, 125
  functional
    of interphalangeal joint, distal, for trigger finger in laborers, 259
    simplified, after extensor tenorrhaphy, 80
Staple
  fixation, customized, in hand and wrist surgery, 139
Stax splint
  dorsal, for trigger finger, 259
Steroid (see Corticosteroid)
Stiffness
  severe, of hand and fingers, castle flap in treatment of skin retraction in, 63
Strain
  injury, repetitive, in computer keyboard users, pathomechanics and treatment, 263
Strength
  finger flexion, isokinetic, measurement of, 23
  pinch and grip, after open carpal tunnel release, effect of transverse carpal ligament on, 17
  tensile, of various suture techniques (in rabbit), 289
Stress
  mechanical, in vitro, induces increased expression of MMPs 2 and 9 in excised Dupuytren's disease tissue, 291
  test, ulnocarpal, in diagnosis of ulnar-sided wrist pain, 146
Students
  music, instrument-specific rates of upper extremity injuries in, 252
Styloid
  radial, osteotomy, for scapholunate collapse and radiostyloid pain syndrome, 158
  ulnar
    affection in Colles' fractures, predictive value of, 187

  malunion with dislocation of distal radioulnar joint malunion with dislocation of distal radioulnar joint, 187
Subchondral
  hematomas with distal fractures of radius in young adults, 180
Subcutaneous
  vs. transthecal digital blocks, single injection, 258
Surgery
  hand (see Hand, surgery)
  limb, upper, operative fluoroscopy in, 28
  replantation, flow-through free flap in, 265
  wrist, customized staple fixation in, 139
Suture
  high-strength, primary flexor tendon repair with, controlled active motion after, 73
  methods for flexor tendon repair (in dog), 288
  pull-out, for avulsion fracture of metacarpophalangeal joint, 48
  reinsertion, double-armed, of profundus flexor tendon, with immediate active mobilization, 74
  techniques, tensile strengths of (in rabbit), 289
Symbrachydactyly
  Ilizarov distraction-lengthening in, 242
Sympathectomy
  periarterial, acute effects on cutaneous microcirculation (in rabbit), 274
Sympathetic
  dystrophy, reflex, sympathetic nervous system dysfunction in, quantitative evaluation of, 282
  nervous system dysfunction in reflex sympathetic dystrophy, quantitative evaluation of, 282
  vasoconstrictor reflex pattern in complete regional pain syndrome, 280
Syndactyly
  comparison of patients with different types of, 241
Synostosis
  radioulnar, posttraumatic proximal, operative treatment of, 53
Synovectomy
  arthroscopic, of rheumatoid wrist, long-term follow-up, 217
  of elbow and radial head excision in rheumatoid arthritis, 225

Synovial
  folds of metacarpophalangeal joint of thumb, 22

T

Tear (see Rupture)
TEC apparatus
  for skeletal traction in severe primary Dupuytren's disease, 234
Temperature
  optical, feedback control, effect on patency in laser-soldered microvascular anastomosis (in rat), 300
Tendocutaneous
  flap, free innervated dorsalis pedis, in complete hand reconstruction, 270
Tendon
  extensor
    injuries, early active mobilization for, 78
    rupture, repeated, due to fluoroquinolones, 84
  flexor (see under Flexor)
  gliding exercises for carpal tunnel syndrome, 110
  interposition, trapeziectomy with, 212
  movements, color Doppler analysis of, 1
  reconstruction, 73
  sheath of snapping digit in children, operative and histopathological study, 245
  transfer for interosseous nerve palsy, posterior traumatic, 95
  trauma, 73
Tenorrhaphy
  extensor, simplified functional splinting after, 80
Tensile
  strengths of various suture techniques (in rabbit), 289
Tethering
  of flexor digitorum profundus to fractures of ulna causing pseudo-Volkmann's contracture, in children, 284
Tetraplegic patient
  neuroprosthesis for, implanted upper extremity, follow-up, 197
Thermoplastic
  splint for mallet deformity of finger, 5-year follow-up, 83
Thumb
  (See also Digit)
  contractures, adduction, release procedures for, and anatomy of adductor pollicis muscle, 2
  distal, reconstruction with great toe partial-nail preserving transfer technique, 268
  gamekeeper
    diagnosis, MR arthrography vs. conventional arthrography and MRI in, 34
    Mitek mini anchor in, 56
  joint
    carpometacarpal (see Carpometacarpal joint, thumb)
    metacarpophalangeal, menisci and synovial folds of, 22
  replantation results
    functional, 277
    microvascular, early, 276
  revascularization results
    functional, 277
    microvascular, early, 276
  triphalangeal, role of metacarpophalangeal pattern profile analysis in treatment of, 243
Tibial
  flaps, anterior, reverse flow, venous drainage of, 12
"Tic-Tac-Toe"
  classification system for mutilating injuries of hand, 35
Tissue
  Dupuytren's disease, excised, mechanical stress in vitro induces increased expression of MMPs 2 and 9 in, 291
  soft (see Soft tissue)
Tobramycin
  in cellulitis, Escherichia coli upper limb, in immunocompromised patient, 70
Toe
  (See also Digit)
  great toe partial-nail preserving transfer technique for distal thumb reconstruction, 268
  second, plantar flap, for partial finger reconstruction, 269
  -to-hand transfer for traumatic digital amputations in children and adolescents, 266
Tomography
  positron emission, for effect of botulinum toxin on cortical dysfunction associated with writer's cramp, 251
Touch
  allodynia after endoscopic or open carpal tunnel release, 119
  sensation, light, testing with Semmes-Weinstein pressure aesthesiometer, effect of wrist position on, 41

Subject Index / 327

Tourniquet
  ischemia, controlled, in upper extremity, adhesion receptors and cytokine profiles in, 299
Toxin
  botulinum
    in piper's palsy, 203
    in writer's cramp, 251
Traction
  external, for articular fractures of phalanges, 57
  skeletal
    for Dupuytren's disease, severe primary, 233
    for Kienböck's disease, 156
Transfer
  great toe partial-nail preserving, for distal thumb reconstruction, 268
  muscle, reinnervated free, after complete brachial plexus avulsion, elbow extension in reconstruction of prehension with, 200
  nail, evolution of, 68
  tendon
    flexor superficialis, flexor digitorum profundus replacement by, anatomical study of, 291
    for interosseous nerve palsy, posterior traumatic, 95
  toe-to-hand, for traumatic digital amputations in children and adolescents, 266
  ulnar nerve fascicle, onto biceps muscle nerve in C5-C6 or C5-C6-C7 avulsion of brachial plexus, 199
Transforming growth factor
  beta-1 gene expression in zone II flexor tendon wound healing (in rabbit), 287
Transscaphoid
  perilunate dislocations, management of, 148
Transthecal
  vs. subcutaneous digital blocks, single injection, 258
Trapeziectomy
  alone, with tendon interposition or with ligament reconstruction? 212
Trapeziometacarpal joint
  arthroscopy, portals for, 209
  dislocation, recent closed, pinning for, 56
  osteoarthritis, first metacarpal osteotomy for, 215
  replacements, cemented and uncemented, 213
  radiological course of, 214

Trauma
  (See also Injury)
  amputation due to, digital, toe-to-hand transfer for, in children and adolescents, 266
  arthritis after
    thumb carpometacarpal joint, de la Caffinière replacement for, long-term follow-up, 210–211
    trapeziometacarpal joint replacements for, cemented and non-cemented, 213
  brachial plexus lesions due to, role of neurophysiological investigation in, 29
  carpal, wrist arthroscopy after, 133
  cold intolerance after, pattern recognition in, 284
  disorders, cumulative, reliability of Postural and Repetitive Risk-Factors Index in, 247
  interosseous nerve palsy after, posterior, clinical features and management of, 94
  nerve, 87
  neuralgia after, pain relief after nerve resection for, 89
  osteoarthrosis after, semiconstrained total elbow replacement for, 225
  radioulnar synostosis due to, proximal, operative treatment of, 53
  radius, acute distal wrist arthrography after, 169
  skeletal, 43
  soft tissue, 59
  tendon, 73
  vascular, treatment of nerve injuries associated with, 286
Triamcinolone
  injection
    aspiration and, for carpal and digital ganglions, 233
    local, with splinting, for ulnar neuropathy at elbow, 125
Triangular fibrocartilage
  complex
    injuries with distal fractures of radius in young adults, 180
    lesion in distal forearm fractures of children, 187
    MRI of, high-resolution, 189
    tears, wrist arthroscopy in management of, 194
  injuries, arthrography vs. MRI in diagnosis, 31
Trigger finger
  percutaneous treatment of, long-term follow-up, 261

splinting for, functional distal
  interphalangeal joint, in laborers,
  259
Trihexyphenidyl
  for piper's palsy, 203
Triphalangeal
  thumbs, role of metacarpophalangeal
    pattern profile analysis in treatment
    of, 243
Trispherical total wrist arthroplasty
  prosthesis, 219, 220
Tumor(s), 227
  bone, juxta-articular giant cell,
    vascularized bone grafts for, 230
  glomus, of finger, MRI of, 238
  skeletal, of distal radius, reconstruction
    with osteoarticular allograft after
    excision of, 227
Turbo
  "S" Quattro, in management of
    neglected dorsal interphalangeal
    dislocations, 56

U

Ulna
  excision combined with radial Z-plasty
    for radial dysplasia, 240
  fracture, tethering of flexor digitorum
    to, causing pseudo-Volkmann's
    contracture, 284
  radioulnar load-sharing in forearm, 21
Ulnar
  artery
    dorsal branch, neurocutaneous flap
      based on, 276
    flap, dorsal, use in hand and wrist
      tissue cover, 59
  carpal impaction, ulnar shortening
    osteotomy for, 153
  carpal instability, ulnar shortening
    osteotomy for, 153
  centralization of hand on, for radial
    club hand, long-term follow-up,
    239
  nerve
    conduction studies, three, for ulnar
      neuropathy at elbow, 123
    cutaneous branch of, dorsal, 24
    dorsal branch, neurocutaneous flap
      based on, 276
    fascicle transfer onto biceps muscle
      nerve in C5-C6 or C5-C6-C7
      avulsion of brachial plexus, 199
    interstitial pressure and
      cross-sectional area changes with
      flexion of elbow, 293

  reconstruction with ePTFE conduits,
    87
  repair, function recovery after,
    rationale for evaluation, 37
  neuropathy
    at elbow, splinting and local steroid
      injection for, 125
    at elbow, surgery for, pain after, 126
    at elbow, ulnar nerve conduction
      studies for, three, 123
    finger flexion sign for, 41
  osteotomy, shortening, for ulnar carpal
    instability and ulnar carpal
    impaction, 153
  -sided wrist pain, ulnocarpal stress test
    in diagnosis of, 146
  styloid
    affection in Colles' fractures,
      predictive value of, 187
    malunion with dislocation of distal
      radioulnar joint, 187
Ulnocarpal
  stress test in diagnosis of ulnar-sided
    wrist pain, 146
Ultrasound
  Doppler, color, of tendon and muscle
    movements, 1
  treatment for carpal tunnel syndrome,
    111
Universal Compression screw
  fixation for scaphoid, comparison with
    other screws during application of
    cyclical bending loads, 163

V

Vascular
  microvascular anastomosis,
    laser-soldered, effect of optical
    temperature feedback control on
    patency in (in rat), 300
  microvascular results, early, after thumb
    replantations and
    revascularizations, 276
  problems, 279
  trauma, treatment of nerve injuries
    associated with, 286
Vascularized
  graft, bone
    for bone tumors, juxta-articular giant
      cell, 230
    from palmar carpal artery for
      scaphoid nonunion, 144
    pronator quadratus pedicled,
      anatomical basis of, 24
    for scaphoid nonunion, 166

hypothenar fat pad, effect on wound tenderness after open carpal tunnel release, 121
Vasoconstrictor
  reflex pattern, sympathetic, in complex regional pain syndrome, 280
Vasospasm
  digital, complications of, limited microsurgical arteriolysis for, 275
Vein
  drainage of radial forearm and anterior tibial reverse flow flaps, 12
Verona apparatus
  for skeletal traction in severe primary Dupuytren's disease, 234
Vibration
  hand transmitted, acute exposure causing hemodynamic changes in ipsilateral and contralateral fingers, 257
  white finger, cutaneous responses to endothelin-1 and histamine in, 286
Vibrotactile
  sense and hand symptoms in blue collar workers in manufacturing industry, 256
Vitamin
  B_6 status, relation to median nerve function and carpal tunnel syndrome in industrial workers, 106

W

Wartenberg's syndrome
  case reports, 127
Weinstein Enhanced Sensory Test
  normal digit tip values for, 36
Whipple technique
  for rheumatoid wrist, long-term follow-up, 217
White
  finger, vibration, cutaneous responses to endothelin-1 and histamine in, 286
Wire
  fixation of metacarpophalangeal joint fracture, avulsion, 48
  Kirschner (*see* Kirschner wire)
Wisconsin test battery
  for carpal tunnel syndrome
    in confirmed cases and normal subjects, 101
    in industrial subjects, 103
Work
  activity, effect on prevalence of median mononeuropathy at wrist, 107
  -related upper limb disorders, prevalence in printing factory, 248
  return to, after carpal tunnel release, predictors of, 118
Workers
  blue collar, in manufacturing industry, vibrotactile sense and hand symptoms in, 256
  industrial (*see* Industrial workers)
Wound
  healing, zone II flexor tendon, gene expression of transforming growth factor beta-1 in (in rabbit), 287
  tenderness after open carpal tunnel release, effect of vascularized hypothenar fat pad on, 121
Wrist, 133
  (*See also* Carpal)
  arthritis, rheumatoid (*see* Arthritis, rheumatoid, wrist)
  arthrodesis, limited, for scapholunate advanced collapse, 162
  arthrography after acute trauma to distal radius, 169
  arthroplasty, total, review of last 30 years, 219
  arthroscopy
    after carpal injuries, 133
    in management of triangular fibrocartilage complex tears, 194
  configurations, dorsal or ventral intercalated segmental instability, sagittal MRI in assessment of, 42
  extension
    moments, effect of muscle architecture and moment arms on, 13
    torque, reliability using LIDO WorkSET for late follow-up of postoperative wrist patients, 138
  extensor(s)
    effect of radial shortening on muscle length and moment arms of, 16
    electromyography of, surface, effect of wrist orthosis use during functional activities on, 20
    muscles, sarcomere length in, 24
  flexion
    in vivo, load dependence in carpal kinematics during, 25
    median nerve compression and, as provocative test for carpal tunnel syndrome, 99
    moments, effect of muscle architecture and moment arms on, 13
  flexors, effect of radial shortening on muscle length and moment arms of, 16

fusion, does it cause destruction of first
carpometacarpal joint in
rheumatoid arthritis? 222
ganglia
aspiration *vs.* steroid infiltration in,
238
simple aspiration or aspiration and
injection of corticosteroid and/or
hyaluronidase for, 232
median mononeuropathy at, effect of
body mass index and work activity
on, 107
mobilization, early, after Herbert screw
fixation and ligamentous repair of
transscaphoid perilunate
dislocations, 148
neuromas, painful, treatment by
relocation into pronator quadratus
muscle, 91
orthosis use during functional activities,
effect on surface electromyography
of wrist extensors, 20
pain, ulnar-sided, ulnocarpal stress test
in diagnosis of, 146

patients, postoperative, reliability of
isometric wrist extension torque
using LIDO WorkSET for late
follow-up of, 138
phylogeny of, 25
position, effect on testing light touch
sensation using Semmes-Weinstein
pressure aesthesiometer, 41
surgery, customized staple fixation in,
139
tissue cover, use of dorsal ulnar artery
flap in, 59
Writer's cramp
botulinum toxin does not reverse
cortical dysfunction associated
with, 251

Z

Z-plasty
radial, combined with ulnar excision for
radial dysplasia, 240

Author Index

A

Aaser P, 186
Abrahamsson SO, 115
Adolfsson L, 178, 217
Ahn JM, 34
Aiso S, 12
Akin S, 261
Albers JW, 107
Allieu Y, 62, 218
Allmann KH, 104
Alnot JY, 159
Al-Qattan MM, 5, 294
Al-Thunyan A, 294
Angermann P, 191
Antoniadis G, 126
Antonopoulos D, 59
Apredoaei C, 159
Armstrong AP, 114
Arner M, 179
Asfazadourian H, 199
Asnis-Ernberg L, 189

B

Backman C, 284
Bain GI, 28
Bakhach J, 67
Barrance PJ, 155
Barton NJ, 212
Beaton DE, 27
Becker GA, 43
Bednarkiewicz M, 2
Behrman MJ, 272
Bell MSG, 232
Belt EA, 222
Bhatia A, 199
Birklein F, 280
Bismuth J-P, 184
Bohannon RW, 36
Bolitho DG, 89
Bono C, 11
Bour C, 128
Bovenzi M, 257
Brady O, 212
Breitenseher MJ, 143
Brinker MR, 241
Brown RA, 291
Brzozowski D, 69
Buchanan TS, 13
Büchler U, 66, 183
Burke FD, 96
Butler TE, 163
Bynum DK, 80

C

Carey J, 151
Carlstedt T, 7
Catalano LW III, 177
Cayea D, 252
Ceballos-Baumann AO, 251
Chakrabarti AJ, 210
Chang J, 287
Chen C, 283
Chen H-C, 266
Chesney RB, 237
Chia J, 139
Chilvers CR, 38
Chipchase LS, 173
Cho BC, 270
Chung JI, 61
Cihantimur B, 261
Citron N, 233
Clement HG, 161
Clément P, 152
Cole RJ, 177
Conde A, 265
Coscoyuela MT, 193
Costa H, 265
Costi J, 219
Cox JA, 120
Cruchaga C A, 158
Culp RW, 208
Cunha C, 265

D

Dahlin LB, 204, 297
Davies DM, 114
Davis TRC, 212
Debono R, 59
Deeney VF, 284
De Gauzy JS, 187
De Groot PJM, 37
Delgado-Martínez AD, 100
Della Santa DR, 291
Delp SL, 13
del Pino JG, 113
del Valle EB, 193
Dijkstra PF, 243
Doi K, 200
Donoghue JO, 76
Dovelle S, 110
Drücke D, 299
Duthie RA, 237

E

Ebenbichler GR, 111
Eberhard D, 235
El-Gammal TA, 266
Elliot D, 68, 91
Endo T, 68
Engesμter LB, 182
Erhard L, 63
Escobedo EM, 205
Evanoff BA, 99
Ewashko T, 254

F

Fadili M, 174
Fairplay T, 160
Fehki S, 63
Fellinger M, 169
Fernández AD, 93
Ferry S, 108
Fikry T, 174
Finlay D, 49
Flinkkilä T, 168
Flodmark BT, 256
Flynn JR, 114
Fontes D, 194
Fossel AH, 118
Foucher G, 63, 207
Franzblau A, 106, 107
Freedman DM, 136
Frisén M, 217
Frot B, 159
Fryback DG, 101
Funk L, 40

G

Gabl M, 191
Gaebler C, 143
Gajisin S, 291
Galán V, 158
Gallagher P, 210
Garcia-Elias M, 136
Geary SP, 284
Gebhardt MC, 227
Geertzen JHB, 129
Gelberman RH, 177, 293
Genda E, 155
Germann G, 299
Gilbert SEA, 95
Gill DRJ, 162
Goldstein B, 205
Gonzalez MH, 209
Gonzalez RV, 13

González Della Valle A, 167
González del Pino J, 100
González González I, 100
Grechenig W, 161, 169
Green JS, 49
Griffin MJ, 257
Grossman JAI, 43, 275
Guggenheim PR, 213, 214
Guzzardella M, 50

H

Haddad FS, 109
Haerle M, 144
Hagberg L, 116, 179
Hage JJ, 37
Hallin RG, 7
Hämäläinen M, 168
Han S-K, 64
Hannah S, 138
Hansen PB, 46
Hansen TB, 46
Harburn KL, 247
Harfaoui A, 174
Hargens AR, 298
Hargreaves IC, 153
Hasson SM, 20
Heistand M, 123
Herbert TJ, 153
Hildreth DH, 241
Hirachi K, 94
Hjall A, 186
Hobby JL, 215
Hochwald NL, 11
Hodgetts K, 89
Hollstien SB, 99, 293
Hong C-Z, 125
Horch RE, 104
Horii E, 146
Hove LM, 182
Hovius SER, 243
Hudak P, 138
Hudson DA, 89
Hülsbergen-Krüger S, 242
Hunt J, 28

I

Ide J, 282
Illarramendi A, 167
Imaeda T, 31, 146, 148
Imanishi N, 12
Inoue G, 47, 148
Ireland DCR, 162
Irwin MS, 95
Ishii S, 89

Iwasaki N, 155
Izquierdo de la T J, 158

J

James CPA, 247
Jansen CWS, 20
Jeng O-J, 101, 103
Johansen S, 172
Jones DHA, 109
Jones SMG, 121
Jorgenson C, 296
Jörgsholm P, 178
Jupiter JB, 53

K

Kaarela K, 222
Kahan NJ, 298
Kanakamedala RV, 125
Kaneko K, 200
Kang HS, 34
Kang NV, 59
Kanje M, 297
Kany J, 187
Karlsson MK, 116
Karp N, 45
Kasabian A, 45
Kato H, 94
Katz JN, 118
Kaufman T, 127
Kautiainen HJ, 222
Kaye JJ, 284
Keir PJ, 249
Keith MW, 197
Keller RB, 118
Kelly P, 32
Kemmler J, 209
Kilgore KL, 197
Kim JS, 61
Kim W-K, 64
Kimata Y, 269
Kinahan A, 38
Kingma J, 171
Kish V, 16
Kitamura T, 282
Kitsis CK, 73
Klasen HJ, 171
Klose G, 279
Knapp M, 138
Ko DSC, 279
Kocher MS, 227
Komoto-Tufvesson Y, 204
Köppel M, 153
Kothari MJ, 123
Kour AK, 139
Kozuki K, 156

Kramer JF, 247
Kramer RC, 241
Krikler SJ, 73
Krishnan J, 173, 219
Kukla C, 143
Kulbaski M, 283
Kumta SM, 230

L

Lam WL, 239
Lamb DW, 239
Lamey D, 21
Laubenberger J, 104
Laulan J, 152, 184
Leandris M, 62
LeClercq C, 2
Lederman RJ, 203
Lee B-I, 64
Lee JH, 270
Lee M, 17
Lee WPA, 122
Leijnse JNAL, 201
Lerner R, 279
Leung PC, 230
Leupin P, 66
Li Z, 274
Lindau T, 116, 179
Lithell M, 284
Logan A, 78
Loh YC, 149
Long H-A, 125
Long Pretz P, 207
Looi KP, 139
Lovic A, 113
Low CK, 258
Low YP, 258
Loy S, 199
Luchetti R, 160
Ludlow KS, 120
Ludvigsen TC, 172
Lundborg G, 115, 256, 297
Lyall HA, 215

M

MacKenzie EJ, 254
Mähring M, 161
Manchester RA, 252
Mankin HJ, 227
Mariéthoz E, 2
Markolf KL, 21
Mathoulin C, 144
Matloub HS, 8
Mbubaegbu C, 83

McCarthy J, 45
McCarthy JA, 259
McCarthy ML, 254
McCormack TJ, 163
Meagher P, 291
Meggitt BF, 215
Mehdi S, 76
Mehta JA, 28
Merla JL, 120
Messina A, 74
Messina JC, 74, 233
Mielants H, 223
Mikkelsen S, 181
Millesi H, 235
Minami A, 94
Mink van der Molen AB, 8
Mizuo H, 269
Moiemen NS, 68
Moore JS, 103
Morgan WJ, 36
Moritomo H, 55
Moroni A, 50
Morsy AH, 283
Mosharrafa A, 17
Most D, 287
Mukouda M, 269
Munshi I, 83
Muradin MSM, 240
Murthy G, 298

N

Nagy L, 183
Nakajima H, 12
Nakamura R, 31, 47, 146
Nakayama Y, 68
Netscher D, 17
Neundörfer B, 280
Nicolakis P, 111
Noah EM, 296
Nyström Å, 284

O

Oberlin C, 128
Ochi T, 1
Okafor B, 83
Okutsu I, 3
Olea AG, 193
Olson SL, 20
Oskam J, 171
Oskarsson GV, 186
Osterman AL, 208
Özcan M, 261

P

Panchal J, 76
Park JJ, 61
Partecke B-D, 242
Parvizi J, 32
Passingham RE, 251
Pearcy M, 219
Peckham PH, 197
Peicha G, 169
Pilz SM, 240
Pollock DC, 274
Portilla Molina AE, 128
Potter HG, 189
Povlsen B, 119
Preisser P, 242
Pritchard T, 108
Propeck T, 151
Putz RV, 22

R

Raatikainen T, 168
Radwin RG, 101, 103
Ramos LE, 43
Razafimbahoaka F, 187
Reihsner R, 235
Rempel D, 249
Resch KL, 111
Revell M, 119
Richards RR, 27
Richter H-P, 126
Riedl B, 280
Ring D, 53
Robinson AHN, 210
Robinson PH, 129
Rock CL, 106
Rodgers JA, 259
Rollo G, 50
Romón MV, 113
Rosales RS, 93
Rosén B, 37, 115
Rosencrance E, 274
Ross DC, 69
Rothman ER, 110
Roux J-L, 62
Rozmaryn LM, 110
Rutkove SB, 123
Ryu J, 16

S

Sakuma M, 47
Sälgeback S, 204
Sandow MJ, 140
Sartoris DJ, 34
Schulz LA, 36

Scott H, 239
Segal E, 167
Seiler JG III, 288
Seki JT, 232
Sennwald GR, 133, 134, 213, 214
Seul J-H, 268
Shaieb MD, 289
Shakya IM, 156
Sheean G, 251
Shigetomi M, 200
Shionoya K, 31
Sicilia HF, 93
Sicre G, 152, 184
Silman AJ, 108
Singer DI, 289
Slater RR Jr, 80
Slavotinek J, 173
Smith SJM, 29
Smutz WP, 249
Soeda S, 68
Sood MK, 91, 96
Soragni O, 160
Sowa G, 22
Stahl S, 127
Stanec S, 87
Stanec Z, 87
Stanley JK, 149
Stark B, 7
Staunstrup H, 181
Steinau HU, 299
Stelnicki E, 287
Stothard J, 121
Strickland JW, 122
Stuart PR, 121
Sugamoto K, 1
Svenningsen S, 172
Sylaidis P, 78

T

Tada K, 55
Tanabe T, 3
Tanaka H, 156
Tang JB, 16
Taras JS, 272
Tarlton JF, 291
Tegnell I, 119
Terenghi G, 95
Tetro AM, 99
Tham S, 275
Tiedeman JJ, 259
Toby EB, 163
Tornetta P III, 11
Trail IA, 248
Turchin DC, 27

U

Usui M, 89

V

Vaghadia H, 38
Van Den Abbeele KLS, 149
Van den Bosch F, 223
van der Meulen JJNM, 240
Van de Wiele C, 223
Vang Hansen F, 181
Van Turnhout AAWM, 37
Vellodi A, 109
Vrieling C, 129

W

Wachtl SW, 213, 214
Wade PJF, 73
Wadhwani A, 151
Wayman J, 32
Wei F-C, 266
Weil J, 66
Weiland AJ, 189
Weinzweig J, 35
Weinzweig N, 35, 209, 270
Werner RA, 106, 107
Williams A, 296
Williams SC, 49
Winters SC, 288
Witthaut J, 2
Wong HP, 258
Woo S-H, 268
Woo SL-Y, 288

Y

Yamaga M, 282
Yamaguchi K, 293
Yamashita T, 89
Yan J-G, 8
Yang S, 21
Yip K, 230
Yoshida T, 55
Youatt M, 78
Young J, 205

Z

Zaza C, 253
Zbrodowski A, 2
Zdravkovic V, 133, 134
Zguricas J, 243
Zimmermann R, 191
Zuber Ch, 291